Neurodiverse Couple Therapy

This inclusive and comprehensive manual equips marriage and family therapists with the skills to identify, support, and provide Brain-Informed Care to neurodiverse couples.

Written from Murgado-Willard's unique perspective as a neurodivergent couple therapist, this book addresses a knowledge gap in the couple counseling field and helps therapists develop and maintain an ethical standard of care for neurodiverse couples. The text also introduces a new style of couple therapy for use in private practice settings: Brain-Informed Neurodiverse Couple Therapy (BINCT). Chapters begin by providing some historical context of neurodiversity before offering invaluable training on best practices, assessment, treatment planning, and using non-ableist, practical interventions for this population. Case studies that present a variety of sexual identities are featured throughout as well as a glossary of key terms and checklists that therapists can use immediately in their practice.

This book aims to implement a paradigm shift in the field and is essential reading for therapy students. It is invaluable reading for practicing therapists that did not receive training on working with neurodiverse clients.

Kelli Murgado-Willard is a licensed marriage and family therapist with over 12 years' experience. She writes from her first-hand experience of being neurodivergent and runs her own therapy practice, Love All the Brains, in Georgia, USA.

"Written with passion and intellectual rigor, this practical guide pulls readers into a unique approach that integrates the intersection of couple therapy and neurodiversity. With a foundation built on scientific evidence and theoretical rationale, Murgado-Willard offers a broad conceptual overview as well as specific techniques that can be implemented by therapists. Based on a decade of experience as a licensed marriage and family therapist, Murgado-Willard's innovative approach to neurodiverse couple therapy will appeal to graduate students expanding their base of knowledge as well as to seasoned clinicians seeking to continue their professional development."

    —**William F. Doverspike, PhD,** *Adjunct Professor, Emory University*

"Conversations with Kelli leave my head spinning with thoughts and possibilities. She approaches life with expertise, passion, and honesty. This book is no exception. My understanding of neurodiversity used to be limited in the past, but now I feel more confident and competent. I'm eager to apply these concepts and exercises in my work to best serve neurodiverse couples."

    —**Rachelle Colegrove, MA, CST,** *Co-Founder of*
The Fun Marriage Workshop

"Kelli adds an important, missing piece to the field of relationship therapy and mental health care in general. One size does not fit all in relationships, and this text provides a solid foundation for mental health professionals wanting to better serve our many neurodivergent clients."

    —**Dana Frederick, MA, LPC, LMFT**

Neurodiverse Couple Therapy

A Practical Guide to Brain-Informed Care

KELLI MURGADO-WILLARD

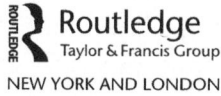

NEW YORK AND LONDON

Designed cover image: © Bruce Rolff/Stocktrek Images @ Getty Images

First published 2024
by Routledge
605 Third Avenue, New York, NY 10158

and by Routledge

4 Park Square, Milton Park, Abingdon, Oxon, OX14 4RN

Routledge is an imprint of the Taylor & Francis Group, an informa business

© 2024 Kelli Murgado-Willard

Library of Congress Cataloging-in-Publication Data
Names: Murgado-Willard, Kelli, author.
Title: Neurodiverse couple therapy : a practical guide to brain-informed
    care / Kelli Murgado-Willard.
Description: New York, NY : Routledge, 2024. | Includes bibliographical
    references and index.
Identifiers: LCCN 2023020806 (print) | LCCN 2023020807 (ebook) |
    ISBN 9781032397771 (hardback) | ISBN 9781032397764
    (paperback) | ISBN 9781003351337 (ebook)
Subjects: LCSH: Couples therapy. | Neurodiversity. | Neurodivergent
    people—Counseling of. | Neurodivergent people—Psychology. |
    Neurodivergent people—Mental health.
Classification: LCC RC488.5 .M874 2024 (print) | LCC RC488.5 (ebook) |
    DDC 616.89/1562—dc23/eng/20230814
LC record available at https://lccn.loc.gov/2023020806
LC ebook record available at https://lccn.loc.gov/2023020807

ISBN: 978-1-032-39777-1 (hbk)
ISBN: 978-1-032-39776-4 (pbk)
ISBN: 978-1-003-35133-7 (ebk)

DOI: 10.4324/9781003351337

Typeset in Dante and Avenir
by Apex CoVantage, LLC

To my children

Contents

Preface

Kelli Murgado-Willard, MA, LMFT

This book is the result of much contemplation, research, and discernment. It was not birthed entirely from a position of altruism, however, as I sincerely hope that my neurodivergent (ND) children and I also stand to benefit from the global paradigm shift the text encourages. My personal life experiences as a Gifted, late-diagnosed ADHDer and SPDer with some Autistic traits fueled the inception of this book. It is also informed by my clinical experiences as a practicing Licensed Marriage & Family Therapist (LMFT).

Going through the diagnostic process alongside my two children not only awakened me to my own neurodivergence, it also helped attune me to the client narratives being expressed within my private practice. ND client experiences so often mirrored aspects of my own life story, it wasn't long before certain trends and interpersonal patterns began to stand out. Specifically, the couple dynamics that differ between neurodiverse and neurotypical (NT) couplings started to become crystal clear. Why was no one talking about this? I felt an urgent calling to educate and empower my LMFT peers. With stereotypically neurodivergent vigor, my goal expanded to encompass bringing meaningful change to the mental health field at large. The need to increase availability of compassionate, competent therapeutic care for neurodiverse couples is very real: This book had to be written, and fast.

Neurodiverse couples, as a clinical population, are too often misunderstood and underserved. Yet, they are more common than many professionals realize and often desperate for help. Thankfully, professional interest in this topic does exist. My colleagues' ears never fail to perk up, in fact, when I speak about the reality of neurodiversity. Most offer encouragement as I talk about my desire to train up the first generation of unwaveringly neuroaffirmative therapists. Interestingly, therapists who are ND themselves never fail to express a mix of validation, uncertainty, and curiosity as we talk. They wonder not only how to best serve neurodiverse couples in a clinical setting and beyond, but also how this can involve utilizing their own atypical qualities.

To back up a bit, I've been fortunate enough to counsel hundreds of ND individuals and those in neurodiverse relationships over the years – but I didn't always know it. I humbly admit that I didn't properly recognize neurodivergence at the very start of my counseling career. Sadly, I had been ill-equipped by my therapy training programs to do so and I lacked a personal connection to the topic at the time. This is because I had not yet birthed ND children, nor had I recognized the complexity of my own brain! How might some of the earliest couples I served have benefitted from all that I've learned since then? While it's unrealistic to expect myself to have had a vast knowledge base in the early days of my career, it's not unrealistic to think that this professional narrative can change for others. It's thrilling to think of all the ways both current therapy students and established professionals can improve their treatment of neurodiverse populations, starting now!

This book is a love letter to myself, my family, the counseling field, and the world at large. It's written after over a decade of working in a private practice setting as a LMFT in the state of Georgia, over a decade of parenting ND children, nearly two decades in a neurodiverse marriage, and over 40 years as a multi-exceptional ND person myself. The text refines existing approaches to therapy by applying a new paradigm called Brain-Informed Care (BIC). Thank you to all past and present clients who have helped me develop and practice one specific application of this environment of care in particular, a method called Brain-Informed Neurodiverse Couple Therapy (BINCT). And, of course, I must thank the supportive colleagues who have pushed me to develop and teach these methods over the years.

I must also make two important acknowledgements. The first is that I am but a mere creator and author; I am not *The Creator* or *The Author*. All glory goes to Almighty God who originates and nurtures Earth's diversity in all its many forms. The opportunity to begin and complete this text in the midst of pandemic parenting, homeschooling, working, and experiencing significant personal loss is nothing short of a miracle. My second acknowledgement concerns privilege. I readily recognize and do not take for granted the fact that I've had access to education on this topic, as well as diagnostic resources. It's not lost on me that my own life, and that of my children, would have had a totally different trajectory were it not for the ability to seek out effective brain assessment and support. It's tragic that many around the world today simply do not have the same opportunities to learn, access fair diagnostic processes, receive ethical treatments, or benefit from social support. Misunderstanding, invalidation, stigma, and overt prejudice exists far too often. May this book be a small part of changing this.

We stand at the precipice of a new era in which ND therapy clients and their NT partners will be more seen and supported. Just as my own eyes were forever opened years ago, I pray a similar awakening happens for others around the world. The opportunity is at hand to elevate an understanding of neurodiversity principles and neurodivergent life experiences to the status of a core ethical competency. May clinicians, researchers, self-advocates, and allies work together across disciplines to promote inclusivity. And, may we each embrace our own brain features in the process.

Introduction

Couple therapists largely do good work. They know each client's brain characteristics and corresponding diagnostic labels (whether self-ascribed or formally diagnosed) have an enormous impact on relationship dynamics. Yet, many therapists are ill-equipped to properly assess and treat the neurodiverse couples they serve within private practice settings. For the purposes of this text, a *neurodiverse couple* is a partnership in which one person is neurodivergent (ND) and the other is neurotypical (NT). *Neurodivergence* implies deviation from socially determined norms in such neurological areas as cognition, sensory processing, communication, and more. *Neurotypicality* implies conformity to majority standards in these areas.

Neurodiversity discussions tend to revolve around first reporting emergent evidence of the biological reality of brain variations, and then framing them as differences rather than pathologies or deficits. Similarly, pro-neurodiversity professionals and self-advocates work toward the explicit acceptance of all neurotypes within an inclusive society. The Neurodiversity Paradigm provides the theoretical underpinnings for all this, and is also the foundation upon which the practical therapy guidelines in this book have been built. This book seeks to go beyond proving that no two people have the same neurological makeup, though. It also does not waste time justifying the fact that each person, regardless of neurotype, has inherent value. These principles are immediately accepted as a starting point for discussion, prompting a new knowledge base to build upon this firm foundation.

Of course, no single work can explain how best to apply Brain-Informed Care (BIC) across the numerous solo or group settings, organizations, or

DOI: 10.4324/9781003351337-1

agencies in which therapists and others provide services. There are many discoveries about the intersectionality of neurodiversity and related topics waiting to be made. The scope of this book is limited to current understanding of best practices for the treatment of neurodiverse couples within a private practice outpatient setting. It introduces a specific therapy method, Brain-Informed Neurodiverse Couple Therapy (BINCT), that is meant to support both the individual mental wellness of each partner and the relational health of ND persons and their NT partners. Readers are invited to thoughtfully implement and expand upon these concepts in their respective fields of study, whenever ethically and clinically appropriate to do so, and also to cite this text appropriately.

This book is divided into four sections: Foundational Concepts, Best Practices, Clinical Application, and Case Studies.

- **Foundational Concepts** includes a historical overview of the Neurodiversity Paradigm, definitions of key terms, explanations of biological mechanisms that underlie various neurotypes, and exploration of the types of issues most neurodiverse couples face. It also explains *Brain-Informed Care* (BIC).
- **Best Practices** encourages personal and professional development for neurodiverse couple counselors who work in private practice settings. It includes original exercises designed to promote self-insight and growth, which may be easily adapted for use with clients, as well as tips for the implementation of ethical marketing strategies.
- **Clinical Application** outlines hands-on approaches to the actual work of neurodiverse couple therapy, including the specifics of *Brain-Informed Neurodiverse Couple Therapy* (BINCT). It discusses how to conduct a thorough assessment and how to implement a wide variety of interventions that are central to the thoughtful application of BIC.
- Although clinical examples are featured throughout the text, the **Case Studies** section provides greater detail. Each fictional couple in this section receives Brain-Informed assessment and treatment, and their therapy experience across the four stages of BINCT is discussed.

Identity-First Language (IFL) is used intentionally throughout. Because linguistic preferences can change over time, the author humbly requests forgiveness should this or any other language used become outdated.

Each chapter includes a glossary of its **bolded** terms and a reference list.

Section I
Foundational Concepts

What's Neurodiversity?　1

Neurodiversity refers to the biological reality that neural variations between humans are organic, complex, and important. The fact that these differences are both coded by genetics and influenced by environmental factors has been proven time and time again via numerous discoveries. Neurodiversity is not just a theory or the product of postmodern social constructivism: Neurodiversity is science.

The structure and functionality of each person's own brain wiring is a fundamental aspect of how they experience life on Earth. Our planet, after all, is a **sensory multiverse** wherein each creature processes incoming stimuli according to their unique biological features. Every organism perceives things and formulates their corresponding thoughts, feelings, and reactions within the confines of their distinct capacities. For instance, a butterfly tastes through its feet while an ant communicates via pheromones. Thankfully, human feet never taste what they touch . . . and, we don't have to rely on chemical signals to communicate. (It's also a blessing that human noses smell far less than what dog noses smell.)

Given these different ways of "being" and "experiencing" from species to species, would you expect a butterfly, a dog, and a human to respond similarly when presented with identical stimuli? Of course not! Even if these different creatures were placed together inside the same room with the same environmental conditions, they would all experience this situation differently: To expect otherwise is illogical. Although it's equally illogical to expect two creatures of the same species to react similarly to identical stimuli, both

DOI: 10.4324/9781003351337-3

therapists and their clients make this assumption all the time! Neurotypicality is an expected, and often explicitly promoted, norm that glosses over the fact that neural nuances exist among humans and deserve attention.

The presumption that the response of two humans to identical stimuli should be more similar than different is problematic, especially for neurodiverse partners. Clients are bound to receive subpar care when couple therapy invalidates neurodiversity. This is particularly true when neurodivergence is labeled a defect worthy of elimination. **The Neurodiversity Paradigm**, on the other hand, promotes the recognition and acceptance of individual brain characteristics. It even goes so far as to pose the question, "Can neural diversions from society's usual expectations sometimes be a good thing?" While acknowledging the challenges inherent to some forms of neurodivergence, this paradigm paves the way for couple therapists and their clients to explore how neurology manifests on an interpersonal level. It reminds therapists that each client has their own neurological home base – and that they, themselves, have one as well. From this home base, each and every life experience is filtered.

Applying this paradigm can enhance a clinician's empathy and other counseling skills, perhaps especially if they consider how their own brain wiring impacts their personal and professional life. Commitment to ongoing discovery about one's own brain may actually represent a crucial, but overlooked, ethical competency within all of the helping professions. Unfortunately, relationship therapists have not always considered how the Neurodiversity Paradigm applies to their clients, let alone themselves. This is likely due to subconscious bias, overt prejudice, lack of knowledge, sociocultural factors, or any number of other reasons. Why is this detrimental? At best, ignoring neurodiversity misses out on providing neurodiverse couples a high standard of care. At worst, it may even cause harm.

There are many benefits to learning about neurodiversity and its historical context. First, the recognition of each client's neurological individuality informs customized intervention strategies. Next, exploring one's own brain wiring as a therapist may help to identify and process the specific types of countertransference experiences that tend to show up when working with neurodiverse couples. Finally, maintaining a neurodiversity-oriented mindset may lead to eliminating barriers to treatment for underserved populations desperate for support.

Popular opinion has always differed regarding whether or not certain forms of human diversity should be recognized, and brain variations are no exception. The Neurodiversity Paradigm is not universally accepted today, nor has it ever been in the past. In fact, societies around the world have shown a tendency to reject diversity ever since the earliest known human civilizations. Ancient Rome, for instance, had a law requiring fathers to drown or abandon to the elements any child born with an obvious physical deformity or mental challenge. This was deemed necessary in order to protect family assets, but also aligned with the Classical Greek philosopher Plato's concept of selective breeding. At the time, this was a state-sanctioned practice meant to maximize human potential. There's little doubt that **neurodivergent (ND)** persons suffered disproportionately during this era. Moving forward, it's also reasonable to assume the mass murders conducted during the Inquisition of medieval Europe included the deaths of many ND people. It was probably quite easy to be charged with heresy back then due to any display of atypical behavior. Being ND during the Salem Witch Trials was probably highly perilous, too, as ND traits may have led to accusations of being a witch or under the influence of witchcraft. Even in very recent history, equating neurodivergence with evil has certainly occurred in regions of Africa, South America, Asia, and other parts of the world.

Today, self-advocates, allies, and pro-neurodiversity professionals work towards greater acceptance and inclusion for all of society's **neurominorities** versus their manipulation or extinction.[1] They draw a clear line in the sand away from antiquated beliefs that deem brain differences (and their associated behaviors) as evidence of sin, magic, or genetic inferiority. In doing so, they frequently cite cutting-edge evidence from science inclusive of twin studies and other heritability research to explain that the biodiversity of human brain cells is natural.[2,3] They also note that geneticists have proved Autism is not a modern phenomenon. Rather, Autism genes have been located deep within the ancient human genome. Their preservation over all this time may indicate that they serve a positive purpose for society as a whole.[4] Why else would they have been passed on? A ND person's own anecdotes, self-descriptions, and family trends are generally considered valuable within these discussions. Accordingly, self-advocates are encouraged to openly share their lived experiences whenever safe to do so. NT persons are encouraged to amplify these minority voices and use their assorted privileges to make space for others to be heard. Collectively, the hands-on component of all these efforts forms the **Neurodiversity Movement**.

Much like the **Body Positivity Movement** states that a person can be healthy at any size, the Neurodiversity Movement asserts one can be mentally healthy with any **neurotype**. Just as thinness doesn't necessarily equate to physical wellness, neurotypicality doesn't always equate to mental wellness. Many liken this pursuit of social justice and thought reform with the efforts that took place during the era when homosexuality was once considered a disorder. Successful protests and advocacy work allowed its de-classification in the 1980 edition of *The Diagnostic and Statistical Manual of Mental Disorders* (DSM-III). Some envision a similar future for Autism, ADHD, and other "ways of being" which are currently categorized as mental disorders. They also assert that neurodiverse relationships can thrive, that neurodivergence affords society benefits that would otherwise not exist, and that bias and stigma against ND persons should be eliminated.

Regarding the Neurodiversity Movement in America, social precursors include both the 20th century Disability Rights Movements and previous Civil Rights Movements. It was not until the 1990s, however, that Autistic self-advocate Judy Singer first used the term *neurodiversity* during her formal sociology studies. Journalist Harvey Blume subsequently popularized this word in the media around 1998. Another primary influence during these years came from Jim Sinclair, an Autistic adult. His poignant 1993 essay, entitled "Don't Mourn for Us," asked parents around the world to embrace their child's neurological variations.[5] These linguistic and perspective shifts were incredibly meaningful at the time, galvanizing social groups of Autistic individuals and others who eventually began to meet online. Many began to refer to themselves as *different* versus *disabled*. (It's worth pausing here to note that the term Disabled has recently been reclaimed as a positive self-descriptor. Its users appreciate that this word acknowledges the challenges inherent to atypicality while proclaiming that it's not shameful to be Disabled. In the 1990s, however, using the term *disabled* had a very negative connotation. Rejection of this word in favor of the term *different* was considered radical. Ironically, today's reframe back to the word Disabled is also considered radical! Linguistics are constantly in flux.)

Fueled by new technologies that allowed unprecedented accessibility to social connection, ND cultures and Disabled identity narratives began to flourish from the 1990s on. The Internet united early neurodiversity advocates around a common goal: To educate and encourage society to put in the work necessary to impart Autistics, and all other ND persons, dignity, equality, and support. They made this request to friends and family, the public at large, specific professional communities, the American educational system, the medical field, specific fields of scientific study, and the government. Today's neurodiversity proponents around the world still advocate for respect, acceptance, and social justice. They assert neurodiversity is every bit as valuable as cultural diversity, racial diversity, and other human variations.

Historically, a lack of education and tolerance regarding brain atypicality has been a direct reflection of dominant social views and scientific beliefs.

This has contributed to terrible outcomes for ND persons in the past, such as when forced institutionalization was common. The systematic segregation of people with physical, behavioral, emotional, or neurocognitive differences can actually be traced as far back as the 17th century in some places. The mental asylum was a convenient manifestation of the world's disgust for differences, and its disinterest in inclusion.

In past eras, almost any behavioral or cognitive presentation that deviated from typical expectations could be deemed defective enough to warrant institutionalization. Women in the United Kingdom who talked too much or held opinions that were deemed too intense, for example, used to be sent away to asylums during the 19th century. When this was done by a husband, father, or brother, that male family member received all her assets. This occurred until the 1882 Married Women's Property Act changed this rule, yet the act of institutionalization still remained popular.

Forced psychiatric institutionalization became widespread across almost all Westernized countries between the 1800s and 1950s due to a profound lack of understanding of mental health, human brain anatomy, and physical disease processes. By 1900, almost every industrialized country in the world had developed its own formalized system to institutionalize any citizen that was deemed undesirable by majority standards. Alternatives to institutionalization were sometimes equally bleak. If a ND person was not institutionalized, they were likely to be hidden at home, sent away to a medical hospital for unethical and risky care, abandoned to the mercy of a nearby monastery or convent, or confined to a workhouse or prison.

The mental hospitals in Europe actually did resemble prisons at one time. For example, the Bicêtre Hospital in Paris, France forced its residents to wear chains. Some others used straightjackets as restraints and ice water baths as punishments. Conditions were abusive at both mental hospitals and asylums until French hospital superintendent Jean-Baptiste Pussin and physician Philippe Pinel started a movement in the late 1700s to encourage a more humane approach – according to the standards of their day, that is. By today's standards, their new methods cannot be called humane. Mental hospitals remained a place for physicians and others to explore new treatment methods aimed at molding almost any atypical human behavior toward a closer fit with social propriety. Obviously, these attempts to modify or "rehabilitate" patients usually failed. Tragically, horrific medical practices persisted long after advances led doctors to forgo such misguided treatments as bloodletting and purging. For instance, after the lobotomy was invented in 1935, about 60,000 Americans are believed to have undergone this procedure until its elimination in the 1970s.

Forced institutionalization and its associated injustices are a cruel stain on human history. Yet, as new fields of science emerged in the 19th century, things actually got even worse for ND people. After the study of genetics was introduced by Gregor Mendel, reproduction by a human with a mental or physical difference began to be seen as a distinct threat to the advancement of humanity which must be intentionally eliminated. Thus, discoveries regarding **genetic determinism**, heritability, and biodiversity within the plant and animal kingdoms did not nudge society towards the Neurodiversity Paradigm . . . they actually bolstered existing problematic beliefs. Almost all forms of human diversity at the time were devalued in **eugenics** discussions that promoted White, NT, non-disabled standards as superior.

Ten years after Charles Darwin wrote *On the Origin of Species* to declare evolution and **natural selection** the primary mechanisms behind biodiversity within the animal kingdom, his half-cousin Sir Francis Galton wrote a pivotal book in 1869. Galton's application of Darwin's concepts to mankind had far-reaching influence. He wanted to protect humanity from mediocrity, or worse, via selective breeding. This notion challenged the popular practice of simply sending away the weak to live in institutions. Instead, his argument promoted extinction of the genetically unfit. Because Galton asserted that civilized society should only cultivate strength, he proposed a British class structure in 1901 that emphasized limiting the reproductive capacity of anyone with low social or genetic value. He created a method to measure intelligence that was almost entirely based on a person's capacity to demonstrate a typical degree of sensory discrimination ability.

Eugenic beliefs and practices became widespread in Western culture from the late 19th century into the mid-20th century. As time went on, sometimes this stemmed from racism and sometimes from a desire to reduce human suffering. However, predominant social and scholarly ideologies were a complex combination of both. At the same time, new discoveries in medicine caused society to ponder the consequences of applying medical advancements to previously untreatable conditions. Whether to treat human defects or to prevent them from happening in the first place became a key question.

Eugenic beliefs were so widespread by 1915 that even Hellen Keller herself, a popular American Deafblind social activist, publicly defended the actions of a doctor who had refused to provide life-saving medical intervention to a baby born with significant impairments. She actually wanted there to be juries of expert doctors tasked with determining the value of each human life at birth. Keller wrote that this type of jury should have the power to refuse treatment to any baby born with severe mental or physical challenges, and that doing so would protect society from the likelihood of such a child growing up to be a criminal.[6] Although this view seems to sharply contrast with her humanitarian advocacy work to improve the quality of life for Deaf and working-class individuals, it is actually unsurprising given that she graduated from Harvard in 1904 and was a close associate with many eugenics-minded persons. Perhaps it mattered to Keller that she herself was not born Deaf or Blind, and thus her disability was not inborn: She had become disabled only after a childhood illness. Although she avoided institutionalization as a child due to privileged access to specialized educational opportunities and the loving care of lifelong tutor Anne Sullivan, she could not avoid dominant influences of her era: The emerging sciences, institutions of higher learning, and the media.

It was quite typical for educated people in the early 1900s, including politicians, to be influenced by Carnegie- and Rockefeller-funded propaganda produced from 1910 to 1935 at the Eugenics Records Office (ERO). There, American scientific eugenicists Charles and Gertrude Davenport and others conducted statistical analyses on hundreds of studies measuring desirable and undesirable human traits and human breeding patterns.

The committees within the ERO included prominent figures in their respective fields of study:

The Committee on Inheritance of Mental Traits (Robert M. Yerkes & Edward L. Thorndike; Comparative Psychology, Behavioral Psychology).

The Committee on Heredity of Deafmutism (Alexander Graham Bell; Physiology of Speech, Science, Engineering, and others).

The Committee on Sterilization (Harry H. Laughlin: Sociology, Government Policy).

The Committee on the Heredity of the Feeble Minded (Henry H. Goddard; Clinical Psychology, Education).

During this time period, textbooks like *Heredity in Relation to Eugenics*, written by Charles Davenport in 1911, were approved for use in medical schools. Terms like "idiot" and "imbecile" were widely circulated words to describe mental deficiency. Henry H. Goddard added the term "moron" to this list in 1908 after translating physician Théodore Simon and psychologist Alfred Binet's invention of the Intelligence Quotient (IQ) test from French into English. His popular 1912 work *The Kallikak Family: A Study in the Heredity of Feeble-Mindedness* spoke at length about the danger of allowing "morons" to breed. Goddard distributed the IQ test throughout America to identify and isolate those unfit for society, even regulating immigrants who entered through Ellis Island. Later, Lewis Terman published the *Stanford Revision of the Binet-Simon Scale* in 1916 and also applied this test far and wide. Events such as *The 1914 National Conference on Race Betterment* were well attended in America. Even magazines such as *Good Housekeeping* and *Popular Science* openly espoused racist, ableist, and eugenic beliefs.[7]

Interestingly, people like Hellen Keller are not, first and foremost, remembered as eugenicists. She is most known as a radical socialist who received the Presidential Medal of Freedom, helped found the American Civil Liberties Union (ACLU), and did many other remarkable things. Her close friend Alexander Graham Bell, to whom she dedicated her autobiography, is similarly remembered for his amazing inventions instead of his eugenic leanings. Other prominent historical figures whom history classes may overlook as eugenicists are: Sir Winston Churchill, Theodore Roosevelt, Woodrow Wilson, and George Bernard Shaw. To presume all eugenicists were simultaneously White supremacists, however, would be incorrect. Both the co-founder of the National Association for the Advancement of Colored People (NAACP), William Edward Burghardt Du Bois, and prominent sociologist Edward Franklin Frazier were Black Americans who advocated for selective breeding within the Black community.

Preventing what powerful, educated persons in Western society considered to be flawed genes from entering the human gene pool was the unfortunate target of political actions in the early 20th century around the world. The first sterilization laws actually originated in the United States, dating as far back as the 1907 *Indiana Eugenics Law*. This had enormous global influence, perhaps especially after 1927 when the Supreme Court ruled compulsory sterilization constitutional. Government-sanctioned, forced sterilization efforts for women were also enacted in the United Kingdom, Europe, Canada, and Australia. After Germany implemented its *Law for the Avoidance of Genetically Diseased Offspring* in 1934, approximately 400,000 individuals were sterilized by 1945. Puerto Rican governor Menendez Ramos also established sterilization laws in the 1930s.

Notably, the Catholic church has always openly opposed eugenics from its earliest discussions. Clergyman Thomas John Gerrar wrote about this in his 1912 text *The Church and Eugenics*, as did several other Catholic advocates during the 1920s and 1930s. Opposition on a larger scale, however, only emerged as the horrors of World War II began to unfold. Despite the Carnegies' removal of funding for the ERO in 1939, widespread negativity toward the Disabled, scientific bias, and forms of psychiatric abuse lingered. Their generational effects can still be felt today. And, we must not ignore that some of these abuses do still occur in certain places around the world!

The above discussion shows the overtness and recency of past efforts to eradicate human brain variability. Only a mere 100 years ago or so, a shocking absence of neurodiversity knowledge and acceptance contributed to a world climate so toxic that it was an enabling factor for the Holocaust itself. While it's impossible to know just how many people were killed during Adolf Hitler's evil regime, the American Holocaust Memorial Museum estimates approximately 6 million Jews lost their lives from the late 1930s to 1945.[8] Because Hitler also killed any child or adult deemed to carry undesirable racial, genetic, behavioral, or ideological traits, it's likely that thousands of ND persons were killed among those he deemed subhuman. Up to 250,000 institutionalized persons were murdered in a Nazi euthanasia program code-named *Aktion T4*.

Even though eugenics as a global movement is largely over, neurodivergence is still a death sentence in some isolated regions. The use of forced psychiatric institutionalization and/or unconsented sterilization practices remain vital humanitarian issues at the time of this text's publication. It's also important to recognize that certain selective breeding practices are far from a remnant of the past. One needs only to look at current abortion rates in Europe to argue that eugenics is alive and well. In Denmark, for instance, over 95% of pregnancies for which a universal, government-funded prenatal screening reveals a high likelihood of Down syndrome end in a decision (made by one or both parents) to terminate the pregnancy.[9] Neurotypicality, in modern times, is still highly favored.

Because of the high value modern society places on NT norms, or at least the outward appearance of NT behavior, specific behavior modification therapies emerged alongside advances in 20th-century brain research. The goal of these therapies was to shape ND individuals to more closely resemble NT individuals. Sometimes this was for safety purposes, i.e., to reduce self-harm. Sometimes, though, this was driven by questionable intentions and delivered in an unethical manner. In the not-so-distant past, for example, certain therapy modalities aimed at Autistic children and teens prioritized client compliance via the use of hitting, restraint, food deprivation, and even electric shock.[10,11,12] Although ethical standards have now increased drastically, behavior modification techniques continue to vary widely by geographic location. Neurodiversity proponents often heavily critique behavior-based therapies.

The use of behavior modification techniques often corresponds with application of the **Medical Model of Disability**. This represents the dominant mentality held by most doctors, psychiatrists, therapists, and other types of professionals from the 20th century until now. This perspective is deeply embedded within most scientific research, vocational systems, and educational programs of the modern era. It designates any brain characteristic that produces behavior that deviates from accepted norms as a defect to be cured. The Medical Model is problem-focused, and uses words such as *disorder* and *dysfunction*.

Critics state this model's focus on curing individuals – who may or may not actually wish to be cured – disrespects the wishes of many ND persons. They also say it promotes a hierarchy in society in which neurotypicality is judged superior. Its focus on aberrations within the individual, versus society itself, has been called too dismissive of context.[13] Some aspects of the modern Medical Model, however, are not necessarily incompatible with a **neurocosmopolitan** mindset. For example, there's a huge difference between a professional who diagnoses and treats a ND person to prove their inferiority versus one who does so to alleviate a ND person's own self-identified pain points.

The Medical Model has actually provided some amazing benefits to ND persons over the years. First, discovering certain medical conditions whose symptoms closely mimic neurodivergence has yielded vital information that can be used in differential diagnosis. Consider, for example, the similarities and differences between Autism and **Pediatric Acute-onset Neuropsychiatric Syndrome (PANS)** or **Pediatric Autoimmune Neuropsychiatric Disorders Associated with Streptococcal Infections (PANDAS)**. A debilitating illness, PANS/PANDAS involves a strong inflammatory brain response centered around the basal ganglia. This induces a variable presentation of intense and sometimes life-threatening obsessive-compulsive behaviors, anxiety, sensory sensitivities, restrictive eating, tics, extreme mood swings, cognitive inflexibility, and other distressing symptoms. To the untrained eye, some of this list may resemble Autistic characteristics. Yet, these symptoms have been found to result from poorly understood infectious responses, allergic reactions, and other somatic mechanisms waiting to be discovered. Some doctors have begun to refer to PANS/PANDAS as basal ganglia encephalitis, which is occasionally treatable but sometimes chronic.

Understanding what is going on with a client medically, versus what may be an inborn human characteristic, is crucial to discerning how to provide ethical treatment. Many ND self-advocates assert there are times it is most ethical to support a person versus cure a person – and vice versa. Using the example above, most are very quick to clarify that Autism is not a medical condition like PANS/PANDAS. They state that attempting to cure Autism is equally unethical to refusing to attempt to cure PANS/PANDAS.

An additional benefit from the Medical Model stems from its emphasis on formulating new pharmacological treatments. This has helped alleviate some of the suffering that stems from medical conditions that have been found to frequently co-occur with some neurotypes. Taking medication for such co-occuring conditions as anxiety, depression, gastrointestinal issues, sleep disturbances, and seizures can represent an important form of self-care for some ND persons. A number of Autistics, in particular, struggle with gastrointestinal issues, sleep disorders, or epilepsy.[14,15] Other assorted medical struggles have been found, with one survey showing 95% of the Autistic children studied had at least one co-occurring medical condition.[16,17] The ethical development and utilization of medication meant to improve a ND person's quality of life is generally viewed positively by self-advocates . . . provided that the use of medication is not forced, the medication does not eradicate neurological strengths, and the medication does not alter inextricable aspects of ND identity. Having the option to take certain medications has proved extremely beneficial for some ND persons, as well as having the option to attend supportive treatments like Occupational Therapy.[18]

Therapists must always view their clients' own self-care decisions regarding treatment options (either for co-occurring conditions or their neurotype itself) as deeply personal and often complex. Some ND persons may genuinely long to receive some yet-unknown treatment in order to minimize or eliminate their own personal neurodivergence, while others vocally speak out against the future development of any such option. These voices tend to loudly oppose the Medical Model in general, suggesting that its pervasive influence has unnecessarily pathologized neurodivergence and overemphasized "cure" language. They fear society's complicity with any belief or practice with actual or potential eugenic applications. As a result, most ND self-advocates tend to favor the **Social Models of Disability**. These models catapult each individual's particular context into focus. Arguably, they may even lend themselves to Disabled identity formation.

One example of a Social Model is the North American Social Model of Disability. This emerged alongside the U.S. Civil Rights Movement in the 1960s. Its perspective states that neurological and physical variations in humans must be seen from a much broader lens than the Medical Model allows. It encourages a strongly contextual approach that, upon first glance, is likely quite familiar to any Licensed Marriage and Family Therapist (LMFT) or other mental health professional who has been trained to operate from a systemic lens. In all the Social Models, society itself is the identified patient – not the ND client.

Proponents of the Social Models assert that ND clients do not need to be fixed because they are not broken. They seek to appropriately validate the challenging reality of being ND while working toward building a world in which more support exists. As such, they tend to fight for greater availability and access to accommodations in the workplace, vocational training opportunities, communication technology, and independent living supports. The Social Model asserts that those in power have a responsibility to reorganize oppressive systems in order to respect each individual's distinct neurological and physical needs.

Although not without some controversy, perhaps no community has made the leap away from the Medical Model toward the Social Models quite like the Autistic community. This is due in large part to the efforts of early Autistic self-advocates and those involved in today's **Autism Rights Movement**.[19,20] Perhaps this is because of the Social Models' emphasis on questioning norms and de-emphasizing conformity. Maybe the calls for practical support and justice for all neurotypes is particularly meaningful in light of oppressive experiences that may have personally affected them or their **neurokin**. Or, perhaps, it is their overall theme of acceptance that is appealing. The Social Models display much higher tolerance by avoiding negative linguistic terms in favor of defining impairment almost entirely via context, i.e., one is only "dysfunctional" to the degree society does not appropriately accommodate their specific support needs.[21] The models imply there is no shame in having support needs, but that it is certainly shameful that society does not accomodate these needs. Moreso than the Medical Model, the Social Models tend to leave room for neurodiverse couples to identify a ND partner's strengths and find flexible solutions for their relationship challenges together.

As this chapter comes to a close, it's important to note that many of the topics covered thus far can be quite polarizing among colleagues and clients. While some find pro-neurodiversity discussions incredibly validating, others find them overly optimistic. They feel they minimize the complexity and hardships inherent to being ND, living with a disability, or living with a ND and/or Disabled partner. Remember that not everyone rallies around the Social Models, or even the Neurodiversity Paradigm itself. Some fully embrace the Medical Model. Others disagree that there is such a thing as a typical brain versus an atypical brain in the first place.

A good therapist creates space within the therapy room for clients to safely explore all angles of the neurodiversity issues that may pertain to their life or are relevant to their neurodiverse relationship in some way. Providing unbiased psychoeducation, and perhaps a bit of historical context, is especially helpful when partners in a neurodiverse relationship disagree about the scientific facts regarding neurodiversity. Going one step further, a **neuroaffirming therapist** recognizes that one's access to financial resources, education, and other privileges matters when considering neurodiversity issues. Some clients may be in the process of learning about neurodiversity for the first time during therapy, while others may be longtime ND self-advocates or allies. Gender, race, power, and safety are all crucial considerations: It may not be feasible or safe for a client to learn about and express their own neurodivergence or advocate for others. It can be a luxury in some places of the world to apply some aspects of the Neurodiversity Paradigm, at least in public.

Neuroaffirming therapists address the concerns that neurodiverse couples bring into session while gently inviting each partner's brain features to take a central position within the counseling process – if the clients so desire. Respectfully, neuroaffirming therapists tend to question any treatment goal set by a client, psychologist, psychiatrist, researcher, or other service provider that prioritizes a ND client's attainment of NT norms.[22] This is because they recognize that each person's particular configuration of brain cells and biological features impacts every aspect of their life, particularly in regards to: Attention, learning, memory, and emotion regulation. Whether inborn or acquired, these features may be changeable via **neuroplasticity**, or unchangeable. Instead of attempting to change the unchangeable, they wonder, "What if neurodiverse couples were taught how to identify and understand the unique way each partner experiences the world? Can validating each partner's specific sensory and cognitive processes form a foundation for healthier relationship dynamics?"

To dispel a common myth, a truly neuroaffirming therapist is not biased in favor of the ND partner in a neurodiverse relationship. Nonetheless, NT partners tend to fear this type of therapist will enable their ND partner to use brain differences as an excuse to continue behaving in hurtful ways. Because neuroaffirming couple therapists believe all persons of any neurotype are inherently valuable, they seek to give each partner equal attention during the course of therapy and never enable either partner to skirt accountability. Each partner's relational boundary crossings and unhealthy coping strategies receive equal attention. Some other misconceptions about neuroaffirming therapists may be that they are always anti-medication or anti-diagnosis.

In summary, the breadth of issues in this chapter are relevant to the practice of neurodiverse couple therapy because of their complexity and polarizing nature. It's important to understand what neurodiversity is, as well as its historical context, in order to decide how this information will inform one's professional practices. Ultimately, the way each therapist conceptualizes neurodivergence, neurotypicality, disability, and neurodiversity issues impacts the type of services they provide. Rigid application of the Medical Model, for example, may lead to pathologizing ND traits. Application of the Social Models of Disability, on the other hand, may encourage a more systematic approach. Any therapist who chooses to incorporate aspects of the Neurodiversity Paradigm in their work may become more neuroaffirming in big or small ways. For instance, they may simply put more thought into tailoring clinical interventions to the brain-based needs of each client. Or, they may decide to pursue more specialized training. These efforts can potentially promote a paradigm shift toward greater inclusivity within the field of Marriage & Family Therapy and beyond.

Glossary of Bolded Terms

Autism Rights Movement Also known as the Autistic Acceptance Movement, the Autistic Self-Advocacy Movement, or the Autistic Liberation Movement. A social movement led by Autistic adults that promotes neurodiversity as natural versus something to be cured. Proponents fight for Autistic persons to have equal rights, genuine social inclusion, no stigma when they display Autistic traits and behaviors, and overall improved well-being.

Body Positivity Movement A social phenomenon begun in Victorian times by the rejection of corsets but rocketed lightyears ahead by the invention of social media in the 21st century. It embraces bodies of all shapes and sizes, rejecting dominant Western cultural standards for thinness and pointing to research that indicates thinness does not perfectly equate to physical health.

Eugenics The practice of (or belief in) the act of "selective breeding" to reduce so-called undesirable human features from the population and increase so-called desirable ones.

Genetic Determinism This view emphasizes that genetic factors are more important than contextual factors such as epigenetic, social, or environmental considerations.

Medical Model of Disability This view states disability is based solely on each individual's own physical, intellectual, and psychological capacities. As such, a person's own "pathology" is unrelated to society or other contextual considerations.

Natural Selection A natural process in which only those organisms best adapted to their immediate environment survive and reproduce.

Neuroaffirming Refers to therapy that demonstrates a pro-neurodiversity stance, stays up-to-date on research about the human brain, and validates the self-identifications and lived experiences of ND persons.

Neuroaffirming therapy provides intentional space for clients to explore their own neurodivergence or that of a loved one.

Neurocosmopolitan   Coined by Dr. Nick Walker, this term refers to one's ongoing willingness to learn about neurodiversity and its potential goodness.

Neurodivergent (ND)   A person with brain wiring that differs from the majority.

Neurodiversity   The biological fact that variations in the way each human brain thinks, feels, interprets social cues, processes incoming stimuli, etc. are naturally-occurring and akin to other forms of human diversity.

Neurodiversity Movement   A social movement that promotes neurodiversity as a scientific reality, highlights aspects of actual ND lived experience, amplifies ND voices, and fights for systemic changes in order to eliminate barriers to inclusivity.

Neurodiversity Paradigm   The reframe that asserts human neurological variations are not inherently pathological, but rather organic and valuable. Note that it does not seek to deny the challenges associated with neurodivergence.

Neurokin   Other people who share one's own neurotype.

Neurominorities   Groups of persons who differ from the neurotypical majority in terms of their brain wiring.

Neuroplasticity   The human brain's ability to modify its connectivity on a cellular level to allow development across the lifespan, healing after trauma, and recovery from injuries. It also allows people to create new ideas and learn new skills.

Neurotype   The moniker used to identify a specific set of brain-based features while still allowing individual variance, e.g., NT, ND, ADHD, etc.

Neurotypical (NT)   A person with brain wiring that matches the majority.

Pediatric Acute-onset Neuropsychiatric Syndrome (PANS)/Pediatric Autoimmune Neuropsychiatric Disorders Associated with Streptococcal Infections (PANDAS)   Potentially devastating autoimmune disorders that affect the basal ganglia. Triggered by infection or other unknown causes, they induce multiple neuropsychiatric symptoms that both laypersons and professionals may erroneously confuse with Autism. Note that Autism and PANS/PANDAS can co-occur. Differential diagnosis is important to determine what type of treatment or support may be available.

Sensory Multiverse   The concept that all life is divided into distinct planes of sensory perception. Sensory perception is relative due to the biological reality that every organism processes stimuli according to neurology, physical attributes, and context. Even in the presence of identical stimuli, each partner in a neurodiverse couple can only directly experience their own sensory plane.

Social Models of Disability   These views state that one's own experience of Disability depends on their own physical, intellectual, and emotional capacities <u>plus</u> significant contextual factors dictated by mainstream society.

Notes

1 Rosqvist, H. B., Chown, N., & Stenning, A. (Eds.). (2020). *Neurodiversity studies: A new critical paradigm*. Routledge.

2 Chaste, P., & Leboyer, M. (2022). Autism risk factors: genes, environment, and gene-environment interactions. *Dialogues in clinical neuroscience*.

3 Sandin, S., Lichtenstein, P., Kuja-Halkola, R., Hultman, C., Larsson, H., & Reichenberg, A. (2017). The heritability of autism spectrum disorder. *JAMA, 318*(12), 1182–1184.

4 Casanova, E. L., Switala, A. E., Dandamudi, S., Hickman, A. R., Vandenbrink, J., Sharp, J. L., . . . & Casanova, M. F. (2019). Autism risk genes are evolutionarily ancient and maintain a unique feature landscape that echoes their function. *Autism Research, 12*(6), 860–869.

5 Sinclair, J. (1993). Don't mourn for us. Our voice. *Autism Network International, 1*(3).

6 Nielsen, K. E. (2009). *The radical lives of Helen Keller* (Vol. 1). NYU press.

7 Pernick, M. S. (1997). Eugenics and public health in American history. *American Journal of Public Health, 87*(11), 1767–1772.

8 The American Holocaust Memorial Museum. (2020, December 8). *Documenting Numbers of Victims of the Holocaust and Nazi Persecution*. Holocaust Encyclopedia. Retrieved January 6, 2023, from https://encyclopedia.ushmm.org.

9 Lou, S., Carstensen, K., Petersen, O. B., Nielsen, C. P., Hvidman, L., Lanther, M. R., & Vogel, I. (2018). Termination of pregnancy following a prenatal diagnosis of Down syndrome: A qualitative study of the decision-making process of pregnant couples. *Acta obstetricia et gynecologica Scandinavica, 97*(10), 1228–1236.

10 Lovaas, O. I., Schaeffer, B., & Simmons, J. Q. (1965). Building social behavior in autistic children by use of electric shock. *Journal of Experimental Research in Personality*.

11 Morton-Bentley, D. W. (2010). On punishments: The continuing debate over aversive therapy on punishment: New York State, the Judge Rotenberg Center and the continuing debate over aversive therapy. *Holy Cross JL & Pub. Pol'y, 14*, 113.

12 Chance, P. (1974). After you hit a child, you can't just get up and leave him; you are hooked to that kid. *O. Ivar Lovaas Interview. Psychology Today, 7*(8), 76–84.

13 Pellicano, E., & den Houting, J. (2022). Annual Research Review: Shifting from 'normal science' to neurodiversity in autism science. *Journal of Child Psychology and Psychiatry, 63*(4), 381–396.

14 Madra, M., Ringel, R., & Margolis, K. G. (2020). Gastrointestinal issues and autism spectrum disorder. *Child and adolescent psychiatric clinics of North America, 29*(3), 501–513.

15 Al-Beltagi, M. (2021). Autism medical comorbidities. *World journal of clinical pediatrics*, *10*(3), 15.

16 Soke, G. N., Maenner, M. J., Christensen, D., Kurzius-Spencer, M., & Schieve, L. (2018). Prevalence of co-occurring medical and behavioral conditions/symptoms among 4- and 8-year-old children with autism spectrum disorder in selected areas of the United States in 2010. *Journal of autism and developmental disorders*, *48*(8), 2663–2676.

17 Neumeyer, A. M., Anixt, J., Chan, J., Perrin, J. M., Murray, D., Coury, D. L., . . . & Parker, R. A. (2019). Identifying associations among co-occurring medical conditions in children with autism spectrum disorders. *Academic Pediatrics*, *19*(3), 300–306.

18 Sterman, J., Gustafson, E., Eisenmenger, L., Hamm, L., & Edwards, J. (2022). Autistic Adult Perspectives on Occupational Therapy for Autistic Children and Youth. *OTJR: Occupation, Participation and Health*.

19 Kapp, S. K. (2020). *Autistic community and the neurodiversity movement: Stories from the frontline* (p. 330). Springer Nature.

20 Leadbitter, K., Buckle, K. L., Ellis, C., & Dekker, M. (2021). Autistic self-advocacy and the neurodiversity movement: Implications for autism early intervention research and practice. *Frontiers in Psychology*, 782.

21 Oliver, M. (2013). The social model of disability: Thirty years on. *Disability & Society*, *28*(7), 1024–1026.

22 Armstrong, T. (2015). The myth of the normal brain: Embracing neurodiversity. *AMA journal of ethics*, *17*(4), 348–352.

What's Brain-Informed Care (BIC)? 2

Respect for individual differences is a core competency for any mental health profession. Because of this, clients can reasonably assume their therapist will be willing and able to validate multiple aspects of personhood. As clinicians practice joining early in the therapy process, they have many opportunities to demonstrate genuine curiosity and offer unbiased support. This establishes good rapport and a firm foundation upon which the therapeutic alliance can blossom. Each client should feel deeply cared for, valuable, safe, and seen throughout their entire therapy experience.

Rightfully, couple therapists around the world are trained to recognize and respect a number of aspects of human diversity. The most current *Code of Ethics* at the time of this publication was issued by the American Association for Marriage & Family Therapy (AAMFT) on January 1, 2005. It clearly indicates:

> 1.1 Non-Discrimination. Marriage and family therapists provide professional assistance to persons without discrimination on the basis of race, age, ethnicity, socioeconomic status, disability, gender, health status, religion, national origin, sexual orientation, gender identity or relationship status.[1]

Even the most eloquently written statements do not ensure the application of perfect ethics each time a therapist interacts with clients, but these aspirational expectations serve as an essential guideline nonetheless. Individual practitioners are charged with ensuring their own compliance,

DOI: 10.4324/9781003351337-4

while professional licensing boards and other regulatory bodies assign consequences for their noncompliance. These combined efforts establish a standard of care that reassures the public. Yet, where is the explicit mention of neurodiversity? To assume the inclusion of neurodivergence in the above list of human diversities seems insufficient to fully recognize its significance. Intrapersonal brain differences are worth much more explicit attention than they currently receive in most private practice therapy settings.

Neurodiversity, after all, is an indisputable and meaningful aspect of being human. The reality that each person's neural pathways are as unique as the lines in their fingerprints has been demonstrated time and time again, such as in 2017 when researchers were able to identify individual study participants by brain anatomy alone.[2] Every client's personal configuration of brain cells and structures represents just one example within an endless number of combinations.

The average human brain has approximately 86 billion neurons and approximately 85 billion non-neuronal cells, i.e., Glial and endothelial cells.[3] If the largest brain map ever created by scientists to date is a connectome of a fruit fly (which only has about 25,000 neurons and approximately 20 million synaptic pathways), how much more immeasurably complex is each human brain?[4]

To properly recognize neurodiversity in the couple therapy process, therapists are invited to take a cue from a recent paradigm shift in the field of mental health. Increased interest in the psychological and physical impacts of trauma after the 1970s has inspired numerous studies and practical changes that have benefited the public. Some of the most notable trauma research of the late 1990s includes both the *2-year Adverse Child Experiences Survey (ACE)* by Dr. Robert Anda and Dr. Vincent Felitti and the *5-year Women, Co-Occurring Disorders and Violence Study sponsored by the Substance Abuse and Mental Health Administration (SAMHSA)*. Learning more about the individual and relational effects of trauma created an imperative for modern counselors to create new therapy guidelines. **Trauma Informed Care** (TIC) developed to promote optimal care for all clients, but especially those with a traumatic background. Its founding concepts and best practices seek to avoid unintentional retraumatization of clients en route to their healing.

The Five Guiding Principles of TIC were originally explained as: Safety, choice, collaboration, trustworthiness, and empowerment. However, the model has recently been expanded to emphasize certain individual factors and contextual considerations.[5,6] Since 2014, updated TIC guidelines have been covered in great detail in such publications as *SAMHSA's Concept of Trauma and Guidance for a Trauma-Informed Approach* and others.[7,8]

The Six Principles of a Trauma-Informed Approach[9]

1. Safety.
2. Trustworthiness and transparency.
3. Peer support.
4. Collaboration and mutuality.
5. Empowerment, voice, and choice.
6. Cultural, historical, and gender issues.

TIC has proved invaluable to clients, therapists, and organized care systems worldwide. First, opening up intentional dialogue about trauma has allowed widespread de-stigmatization. Second, increasing the educational opportunities available for mental health professionals regarding trauma has afforded the public greater access to competent care. Even therapists who do not specifically specialize in serving traumatized populations tend to have an expanded knowledge base these days based on the integration of TIC within continuing education programs. For new therapists in training, the mental health field before TIC seems unimaginable. What if a similar paradigm shift occurred regarding neurodivergence?

The intentional recognition and de-stigmatization of neurodiversity seems the next logical step to continue the momentum begun by TIC. Learning how to support neurodiverse populations is, in fact, an incredibly important responsibility within the field of Marriage & Family Therapy and other helping professions. Sadly, there is currently a lack of scholarly research and training opportunities available pertaining to the care of neurodiverse couples. Presenting a comprehensive model for **Brain-Informed Care (BIC)** could inspire change.

BIC promotes effective clinical support for neurodiverse populations in private practice and outpatient settings through the therapist's appropriate recognition and valuation of neural complexity. (This includes careful consideration of the therapist's own brain qualities, as well.) BIC therapists are encouraged to avoid unhelpful professional practices as they help each client safely explore their interoceptive and interpersonal experiences over the course of treatment.

There are six foundational tenets of BIC. Each one focuses on either the therapist's own mindset or a characteristic of their professional behavior. The overall framework of BIC lends itself to integration with almost all of the existing therapy approaches currently in use. BIC is not a therapy modality in and of itself: Much like TIC, BIC simply provides an environment of care.

The Six Tenets of Brain-Informed Care

1. Commitment to non-ableist practices.
2. Promotion of sensory security.
3. Presumption of competence and strengths.
4. Acceptance of atypicality without manipulation or toxic positivity.
5. Validation of neurodivergent lived experience.
6. Therapist authenticity.

Commitment to Non-Ableist Practices

In a therapy context, **ableism** can be defined as any belief, action, or inaction by a therapist that promotes neurotypicality as a superior way of being. Ableism can be either explicit or implicit, intentional or unintentional. But, it is always a form of discrimination. Most ableism involves one's view of others, but a special type of ableism involves one's own self-concept. An example of **internalized ableism** is when a ND therapist views their own brain variations as shameful defects they try to hide in order to appear NT.

Explicit Ableism

Example 1. Emphasizing eye contact and/or close physical proximity between relationship partners during couple therapy.
NT social norms in American culture tend to emphasize eye contact and closeness during in-person communication. Actually, these behaviors receive strong and continual emphasis within the field of Marriage & Family Therapy. Language about eye contact even exists in the DSM-V-TR, and it is used in some empirically validated screening questionnaires for Autism. This is because these behaviors are widely regarded as the "best" way to convey respect, focus, and concern. It's important to note, though, that not everyone thinks this way. Not every person can provide eye contact to begin with! It's a good thing that conversations with our visually-impaired friends remind us this is not a mandatory component of communication. Similarly,

our Deaf friends remind us that the ability to hear spoken words is not a requirement of a good conversation.

Some ND clients find the expectation to give and receive eye contact overwhelming. Some consider making eye contact physically uncomfortable, emotionally draining, or physiologically agitating. (Others may have zero issues with eye contact whatsoever.) A therapist's commitment to inclusivity means understanding that each client has a different physiological and psychological experience regarding eye contact. One's communication preferences and expectations are highly influenced by their biological capacities, cultural factors, gender, and other social factors like power, rank, or age.

What if a NT client expresses a deep need for eye contact from their ND partner in order to feel heard, respected, and connected? In this case, it's acceptable to encourage the ND partner to consider the potential relational benefits to learning ways to use intentional eye contact from time to time . . . but only to the degree the client has the biological capacity and genuine desire to do so. A therapist should never push either client in a neurodiverse relationship to exceed their personal limits in the name of pleasing their partner: This is a recipe for resentment and burnout.

Sometimes, creative solutions to the above scenario are possible. The therapist may ask the ND partner to consider the potential relationship benefits to the following: Physically turning their body toward their NT partner as they speak while looking above their forehead, at their mouth, or at their nose. This provides an effective illusion of eye contact that could be a win-win for both. This is potentially a less taxing, more sustainable way for a ND partner to meet their NT partner's communication needs. When this type of compromise is combined with a commitment from the NT partner to not demand eye contact or pathologize the lack of it, more effective interpersonal connection may result.

Regarding physical closeness during in-person communication, each client's preferred distance from their conversational partner may remain constant or vary. Allowing each client the autonomy to choose whatever proximity feels best at any given time conveys respect.

BIC therapists . . .

Encourage each client to direct their own gaze wherever they find most comfortable when communicating: Eye contact is never mandated or touted as an essential life skill.

> Provide multiple seating options so that each client may communicate at their preferred proximity to others during therapy sessions.

Example 2. Encouraging a client to maintain a "calm body" during sessions and/or promoting stillness as a superior method of self-regulation.
Most NT clients will not use repetitive body movements and/or vocalizations during therapy to self-regulate, whereas many ND clients might. One reason for this could be that NT persons tend to prefer to self-regulate in public settings in ways that are not likely to draw attention to themselves.

ND clients tend to prefer a pathway to physiological soothing that involves movement rather than stillness, which can certainly sometimes persist regardless of their social context. The use of repetitive movements with or without accompanying vocalizations is affectionately called **stimming** by Autistic self-advocates and others. Common ND stims include: Rocking back and forth, clenching and unclenching fists, spinning, hand flapping, making big or small dance moves, humming, rubbing something that has a pleasant texture, looking at visually interesting objects, tightly hugging an object, or any number of other behaviors. Stims are as unique as the person who uses them.

NT people stim, too, of course, but usually in more socially "acceptable" ways such as nail biting or foot tapping. Research shows that Autistics and ADHDers tend to stim the most, and that this really can help with self-regulation.[10] Also, a detailed interview of 32 Autistic adults in 2019 highlighted the importance of stimming as a way for ND people to express strong feelings, e.g., happiness, fear, or anxiety. These researchers emphasized the importance of de-stigmatizing the act of stimming in public settings.[11]

There may be times when a ND client's stims become exceptionally distracting to the therapy process or their NT partner expresses frustration with them. For example, consider the stim of lightly rubbing one's own lips with their fingertip or a pencil eraser. If this action makes it difficult to understand the client's spoken words, or is frustrating to their partner for any other reason, the therapist can simply invite collaboration towards replacing this stim with an alternative. Conversing about the meaning, purpose, and physiological effects of the original stim is important. This informs the search for something that still provides personal benefit, but is less interpersonally problematic. The ND client should always be allowed to choose their new stim: Stims should not be dictated by the therapist.

Rarely, a client may use a stim in the therapist's presence that is either unsafe or blatantly inappropriate. A BIC therapist can use the following steps to respond to any adult client who uses an injurious stim (e.g., hitting one's own face) or a stim with genital involvement (e.g., stroking one's own penis over their clothes) during a counseling session.

Addressing an Injurious Stim or a Stim with Genital Involvement

1. Pair a brief process comment with a clear request to stop:
   "That action makes me uncomfortable. Please stop."
2. Review ethical expectations regarding safety, boundaries, and consent in therapy:
   "Self-harm is never ok, even if you meant this for self-regulation or self-expression instead of injury. If this continues, a higher level of care than I can provide you in a private practice setting may be required."
   "Even if you meant this for self-regulation or self-expression instead of erotic stimulation, touching your own genitalia is never appropriate during therapy. I did not give consent to witness this. I do not consent to witness this in the future, either, so I cannot engage in therapy with you if this continues."
3. Collaborate:
   "Can we work together to understand what this stim does for you? Perhaps there is something else you can choose to do."

If an unacceptable stim persists despite intervention, it may be necessary to end the therapeutic relationship. This should only be done after thoughtful discussion about the purpose of the stim and potential reasons why the client has not found an alternative stim. A comprehensive referral should be given in order to best support the client's underlying dysregulation, compulsivity, impulsivity, cognitive capacity, trauma, etc.

BIC therapists . . .

Invite clients to stim freely during therapy sessions as needed.
  Do not attempt to redirect any stims that are not of an excessively distracting, self-harming, or blatantly inappropriate nature

Example 3. Refusing to use a client's preferred language to describe themselves or their loved ones and/or correcting a client's linguistic choices regarding neurodivergence. Consider the difference between the phrases "I have Autism"/"I'm a person with Autism" (Person-First Language; PFL) and "I'm Autistic"/"I'm an Autistic person" (Identity-First Language; IFL). The use of PFL or IFL is a crucial distinction for many ND people, although some assert these two phrases mean exactly the same thing. No group is ever homogenous!

Psychologist Beatrice Wright first proposed PFL in America around 1960, but it did not become popular until 20 years later when the AIDS crisis unfolded.[12] In an attempt to counteract negative stigma, advocacy groups intentionally chose to use PFL to assert that persons with HIV and AIDS were, first and foremost, human beings. PFL soon began to appear in U.S. government documents to describe "persons with disabilities" in a favorable light. After *The Americans with Disabilities Act* used PFL in 1990, this language became widespread across many professions. Despite feedback from ND and/or Disabled communities who argue for the discontinuation of PFL, some training facilities around the world still teach it. It is also still in use by certain influential organizations.

The majority of today's self-advocates point out that using PFL implies what makes someone different deserves to be distanced from their identity, and also warrants clarification of their innate personhood. IFL users assert that no one's humanity should ever need clarification. They appreciate that IFL emphasizes neurodivergence and/or Disability is inextricable from identity. For example, Autism is not something a person <u>has</u> . . . it's part of who they <u>are</u>.

IFL is currently promoted as proper etiquette for mental health professionals due to its popular use within ND communities and the fact that scholars have documented this shift away from PFL quite well.[13,14] Obviously, some ND persons still prefer to use PFL. Each client has the right to use whatever language they choose.[15]

BIC therapists . . .

Acknowledge the distinction between Person-First Language (PFL) and Identity-First Language (IFL) along with its historical context.[16]
   Accept each client's choice to use PFL, IFL, or both.
   Follow updated guidelines regarding the use of either PFL or IFL when conducting therapy, writing, or speaking.[17]

Example 4. Using "cure language" or promoting cure-directed efforts.
BIC never aims to cure a client's neurodivergence. Rather, it validates clients' personal and interpersonal challenges while offering empathetic therapy support.

Because curing neurodivergence implies the elimination of ND people, it's understandable that most ND persons find "cure language" and the practice of cure-directed efforts highly offensive. It's also important to recognize discussions on these topics may trigger traumatic memories. Some misguided caregivers – usually led astray by persons posing as quasi-medical professionals – have attempted to rid their children of Autism or other brain differences through bleach enemas, pharmaceutical chelation agents, or eccentric diets.[18,19,20] This and other forms of abuse may have even resulted from interventions by doctors, religious authorities, or mental health professionals.

Recently, ND self-advocates and researchers alike have raised important concerns about the unethical clinical interventions historically tied to Applied Behavior Analysis (ABA) around the mid-20th century.[21] Undoubtedly, ABA in its original form was both cure-directed and abusive. Some fear that the updated versions of ABA currently in use with Autistic youth and others are no better, while others disagree.[22,23] Enthusiastic support for today's ABA generally comes from NT parents of ND children, whereas ND adults generally stand in strong opposition. Therapists who work with neurodiverse populations should recognize this controversy and follow it closely for new developments. For example, both personal anecdotes from adult Autistics and emerging scholarly data suggest exposure to ABA may indeed induce symptoms of Post-Traumatic Stress Disorder (PTSD).[24,25]

BIC therapists . . .

Recognize that pathologization of a ND client's atypical features may have resulted in physical harm and/or psychological trauma – sometimes even at the hands of caregivers, doctors, or mental health professionals.

Avoid any therapy modality that seeks to cure, eliminate, conceal, or devalue aspects of ND culture.

Example 5. Refusing to make reasonable accommodations for a client's executive functioning challenges and/or sensory needs.
ND persons process everyday sensory input differently than NT persons, sometimes even responding with extended Fight, Flight, Freeze, or Fawn

states.[26] This is especially true for those with concurrent PTSD.[27] Some ND individuals report that certain sensory sensations can be physically painful, confusing, or overwhelming, while others require a high level of input to even recognize some kinds of stimuli at all.[28,29]

Knowledge of the eight key **executive functioning skills**, as directed by the prefrontal cortex, is essential for any therapist. These essential skills relate to: Working memory, task initiation, planning, organization, cognitive flexibility, self-monitoring, impulse control, and emotional control.[30] Similarly, every therapist should understand how the eight human sensory systems and their corresponding body parts function. They should be willing and able to provide this information to clients via psychoeducation in order to collaborate toward greater recognition of the brain processes that likely underlie their presenting issues. As the therapist customizes the therapy experience accordingly, reasonable accommodations should be made as needed.

Some of the somatic mechanisms that account for ND and NT sensory processing differences have been demonstrated using neuroimaging technology.[31] These differences are generally referred to as forms of either **hypersensitivity** or **hyposensitivity**. Hypersensitivity can result in sensory-avoiding behavior due to the body's over-responsiveness to stimuli, while hyposensitivity may result in sensory-seeking behavior due to the body's under-responsiveness. These categories are not mutually exclusive, though. It's possible for the same person to over-respond to some sensations, yet under-respond to others. (Furthermore, one's degree of sensory sensitivity can vary from day to day! An example of this occurs when a person who usually requires heavily spiced food in order to taste it at all happens to one day notice the slightest hint of a particular seasoning.) Each client's sensory processing characteristics usually follow a consistent rhythm across their lifespan, but some people experience less predictability.

BIC therapists . . .

Understand the body's eight sensory systems and the brain's key executive functions.

Recognize each client's sensory needs and executive functioning challenges differ, fluctuate, and deserve reasonable accommodation.

Table 2.1 Sensory chart

Sensory System	Function	Body Parts Involved	Hyposensitive Examples	Hypersensitive Examples
Auditory	Hearing	Outer ear, middle ear, and hair fibers of the cochlea (located in the inner ear). Processed by the thalamus, primary auditory cortex (located in the temporal lobe), nonprimary auditory pathways (located in the brain stem), and cerebral cortex.[32]	Listens to music at high volumes; Unaware of their own high volume at times; Frequently misses someone speaking directly to them or calling to them across a room.	Uses ear defenders to block out sounds in noisy or crowded environments; Overwhelmed in situations where many types or layers of sounds occur at once.
Gustatory	Tasting	Taste buds on the tongue. Processed by the thalamus, brainstem, and gustatory cortex (located within the insular lobe and frontal lobe). Works closely with the olfactory system.[33]	Prefers highly seasoned food; Likes very sour candy; Enjoys trying new menu items at restaurants.	Prefers bland foods; Eats a small and consistent set of foods; May taste each and every nuance in a recipe before anyone else.

(Continued)

Table 2.1 (Continued)

Sensory System	Function	Body Parts Involved	Hyposensitive Examples	Hypersensitive Examples
Olfactory	Smelling	Nose Odors bypass the thalamus to be first processed by the olfactory bulbs and olfactory cortex (a component of the limbic system located in the temporal lobe). Only after the amygdala, hippocampus, and hypothalamus connect smells to our memories and emotions do signals reach the thalamus and frontal cortex. Works closely with the gustatory system.[34]	Does not notice the unpleasant smells that others do; May not notice that the trash needs to be taken out or that a baby's diaper needs to be changed; Accidentally wears much more perfume or cologne than what is typical; Not bothered by indoor pet odors; Holds their nose close to something and breathes in deeply in order to register its smell; Uses heavily scented laundry detergent and household cleaners; Enjoys essential oil diffusers, scented candles, and room sprays.	Nauseated by the slightest foul odor; Is the first to notice a scent in the air; Gets a headache when someone nearby smokes or wears a fragrance; Avoids scented deodorants, perfume, cologne, and household cleaning products; Avoids shopping at stores known for heavy scents; May not be able to be in the same room as an aversive smell; Pumps gas quickly to escape the scents of gasoline and car exhaust; Avoids the meat and fish counter of the grocery store; Avoids nail salons, barber shops, or beauty salons due to their strong smells.

Sense	Function	Processing	Seeking behaviors	Avoiding behaviors
Visual	Seeing	Eyes	Enjoys looking at spinning wheels, bright lights, neon colors, and complex images; Finds it difficult to focus on one page of a book at a time or a static image on a screen; Decorates their room with numerous items.	Avoids bright lights/wears sunglasses; Prefers darkness or dim lighting; Finds it difficult to take in all parts of a complex image at once; Anxious or uncomfortable in cluttered rooms; Closes eyes when overwhelmed.
		Processed by the thalamus, brainstem, and occipital lobe; They work closely with the hippocampus, parietal lobe, and frontal lobe to interpret what we see.[35]		
Tactile	Sensing textures, pain, vibrations, temperature, pleasure, etc.	Dermis and epidermis, mouth, esophagus, digestive system, hairs in the inner ear canal.	Does not notice when food crumbs remain on their face after eating; Gives very firm hugs and handshakes; Touches things in order to fully experience them; Seeks out pleasing clothing textures; Needs high sexual stimulation to register erotic sensation.	Avoids touching wet or messy textures; Does not like to be touched, especially without warning; Ticklish; Bothered by heat or cold; Dislikes wearing jewelry; Avoids certain fabrics altogether; Avoids tight clothing and garments with noticeable seams; May find sexual contact overwhelming or unpleasant.
		Processed by the thalamus, somatosensory cortex (located in the parietal lobe), and prefrontal cortex.[36]		
Vestibular	Sensing balance and movement.	Inner ear.	Likes bouncing; Appears to move constantly by fidgeting, pacing, or using fast movements; Spins without getting dizzy; Doesn't mind long car rides; Enjoys amusement park rides, jumping, and dancing.	Gets motion sickness easily in a plane or car; Gets dizzy easily; Dislikes roller coasters, merry-go-rounds, and swings; Afraid of falling; Does not like to be off the ground; Prefers sedentary activity.
		Processed in the cerebellum, brainstem, and somatosensory cortex.		
		Works closely with the proprioceptive system.[37]		

(Continued)

Table 2.1 (Continued)

Sensory System	Function	Body Parts Involved	Hyposensitive Examples	Hypersensitive Examples
Proprioception[38]	Sensing the location of where one's own body is within a given space.	Skin, muscles, tendons, ligaments, and joints. Processed in the cerebellum, brainstem, and somatosensory cortex. Works closely with the vestibular system, the visual system, and the nervous system.[39]	Inadvertently stands a little too close or too far from others; Bumps into things or people; Likes running and jumping activities; Prefers tight clothing and firm hugs; Bites nails or chews pencils.	Seems uncoordinated or perhaps lethargic; Has difficulty catching a ball; Ladders and stairs are hard to climb; Slumped posture; Uses a mobility aid; Avoids exercise or sports.
Interoception[40]	Sensing the body's internal states: Emotions, hunger or fullness, thirst, bathroom needs, heart rate, muscle tension, cramps, etc.	Muscle tissue, joints, organs, and bones. Processed in the insular cortex.[41]	Unaware of their need to urinate until the sensation is intense; Has a high pain tolerance; Unaware of their hunger or thirst cues until starving or parched; May struggle to articulate how they feel emotionally.	Experiences every itch, scrape, and bump on their body quite intensely; Easily flooded by their own emotions; Very "in touch" with themselves; May be prone to panic attacks; Struggles to focus elsewhere when preoccupied by internal body states.

Implicit Ableism

Example 1. Promoting face-to-face verbal communication as the gold standard for couple communication and/or ranking interactions from "Most Intimate" (i.e., speaking face-to-face) to "Least Intimate" (i.e., communicating electronically).

This practice elevates NT expectations while devaluing the very modalities some ND persons find most accessible, and perhaps even most conducive to emotional connection. Additionally, it ignores that both partners in a neurodiverse relationship may stand to benefit from the use of various forms of electronic communication. For example, typing out one's own thoughts in an email or text may allow more time alone to think through a response. Removing the pressure or anxiety involved with being together in-person to discuss certain hot topics may also help both partners remain actively engaged in effective back-and-forth conversation for a longer duration . . . instead of becoming overwhelmed, defensive, critical, controlling, or irrational.

Each client's capacity for interpersonal communication, as well as their preferred method of engaging, is usually consistent over time. But it can also change depending on personal, interpersonal, or environmental factors. For example, an Autistic person who generally prefers to speak aloud may sometimes choose to utilize *Augmented and Alternative Communication (AAC)* instead during times when they have much to say, when they are experiencing sensory overload or executive functioning difficulties, when the act of speaking feels draining, or when they simply prefer to do so.

BIC therapists . . .

Recognize texting, e-mailing, and utilizing AAC devices as valid forms of communication between partners.

   Accept that communication needs may be fluid. They encourage clients to use whatever communication style they wish.

Example 2. Giving backhanded compliments such as, "I would have never guessed you were Autistic!"

The above phrase, and those like it, are often said as a therapist innocently offers encouragement. However, this can actually be invalidating. Misguided attempts at praise usually rely on stereotypes to highlight ways clients behave that seem to defy the therapist's assumptions about ND people. Since many ND persons already experience an incredible amount of invalidation and misunderstanding from society, they certainly should not have to experience this from their therapist as well.

Additionally, backhanded compliments about a client's neurodivergence are usually based on the premise that every ND person views their brain wiring as something they wish to conceal from others, eliminate, or overcome. IFL users generally do not feel this way.

BIC therapists . . .

Understand there is no uniform "look" to persons of the same neurotype.
   Use discernment when giving compliments.

Example 3. Taking on the role of an infallable expert within the therapy room.
Skilled therapists draw upon their own specialized education and experiences to offer clients competent psychoeducation and psychotherapy services without inflating themselves to a position of undue authority.

BIC therapists . . .

Recognize each client as the expert of their own life.
   Serve as educated, collaboration-minded professionals in the therapy room.

Example 4. Presuming that each client has NT executive functioning skills.
It's ableist to presume all brains function the same way, period. Regarding executive functioning, almost all ND clients struggle more than NT persons. Each client's strengths and challenges in this area must be assessed with accuracy.

BIC therapists . . .

Understand that NT and ND brains generally differ regarding executive functioning.

Promotion of Sensory Security

It's well-known that quality couple therapy environments strive to offer each partner a consistent degree of emotional and physical security. Accordingly, therapists are well-versed in ways to meet clients' needs in these areas. They are generally less attuned to sensory concerns, however, because these are simply not on their radar . . . unless a clinician happens to be ND, that is.

It's easy for NT professionals to take for granted the way their own brain detects, organizes, interprets, and responds to sensory input in the environment. These are, after all, generally automatic processes that occur with little conscious thought or energy expenditure. For many ND individuals, however, sensory processing challenges are obvious and quite draining. Repeated aversive sensations over time can sometimes feel like shaking a can of soda. Eventually, the can explodes. Chronic understimulation can sometimes feel equally unsettling. Certain acute, intense sensations may even induce significant physiological distress.

How frequently do brain-based sensory challenges occur in society? Studies estimate 30% of Disabled children and 5–10% of Non-Disabled children have obvious sensory challenges that interfere with everyday life.[42,43] Regardless of age or neurotype, those who have experienced trauma can also have these difficulties. Research on PTSD has long proven that acute or chronic trauma can impact a person's sensory experience. (A clear demonstration of this occurs when a sudden loud noise triggers the sympathetic mode and/or dorsal vagal response in some veterans.[44]) Those born prematurely sometimes experience sensory processing challenges, too.[45,46] Statistically, though, those who are Autistic and/or have ADHD are the most likely to experience sensory challenges due to physical differences in their brains' white matter areas.[47,48]

It should be an explicit ethical standard for every private practice environment to foster each client's experience of **sensory security** during couple therapy. Sensory security occurs when the brain does not perceive any aversive sensory stimuli, and thus retains free access to the parasympathetic mode of the autonomic nervous system. Sensory security is not optional; it is a vital prerequisite to the receipt of support. **Sensory insecurity**, on the other hand, occurs when defensive brain tactics are activated in response to negative sensory stimuli. It's impossible to learn, heal, and grow optimally while in this state. If a client feels they are not able to cope with the sensory threats involved with attending therapy, or that they cannot trust their therapist to make reasonable accommodations, the therapeutic alliance will be negatively affected.

Obviously, total environmental perfection during neurodiverse couple therapy is not a realistic goal – nor should it be. The sensory stimuli within the therapy room at any given time contribute, but do not <u>solely</u> determine, clients' immediate experiences of sensory security or insecurity. There are actually a few dimensions involved:

1. *External factors*, e.g., the sensory stimuli in the therapy room and surrounding area.
2. *Internal factors*, e.g., the client's unique brain features related to sensory processing capacity, level of interoceptive awareness of their own internal body sensations and emotions, trauma history, stress level, degree of accumulated stimulation up to this point, coping skills, level of fatigue, etc.
3. *Interpersonal factors*, e.g., the client's communication skills regarding reaching out for help, level of trust in their partner's ability to appropriately respond to them, level of trust in the therapist's ability to provide them support, etc.

This list explains why a client with sensory processing challenges may suddenly have a huge, negative reaction to a relatively small sensation that otherwise would not have been bothersome. At that moment, the sensation likely became the proverbial straw that broke the camel's back and triggered overload. It also explains why a client who normally expresses distaste for bright light may suddenly request brighter lighting during a session. They may be understimulated or physically tired, in need of a neurological pick-me-up. Finally, it reveals a new perspective on why some clients continually struggle to cope and/or communicate.

Neurodiverse couple therapists are tasked with remaining curious and accommodating regarding the sensory needs of two clients who experience the same environment . . . but from very different neurological home bases. There are times when the sensory needs of a ND partner and a NT partner are diametrically opposed. It can be difficult for a therapist to juggle multiple brain-based needs at once, including their own! Nonetheless, these efforts are necessary and worthwhile.

Note that most ND clients in a private practice environment are able self-regulate in response to mild instances of sensory insecurity via stimming or other coping skills. This may be visible or invisible to the therapist. When self-regulation is not possible, however, some clients will be quite comfortable asking the therapist to make changes to the environment while others will be far too uncomfortable to ask. Gender and cultural considerations may or may not be a factor in this.

At first a therapist should not rely on clients to initiate communication about their sensory needs. Expecting a new ND therapy client to speak up for themselves, unprompted, may enable their needs to remain unmet. This is because assertive communication skills, and self-advocacy in general, can be extremely difficult for some ND people. This is especially true in scenarios that involve a perceived authority figure. Poignantly, too, some ND clients come to therapy with no understanding of their own sensory needs. Or, perhaps they do know their needs but have zero reason to believe that bringing them up will result in their validation. Perhaps a lifetime of negative data gleaned from invalidating experiences with close family members, schools, jobs, peers, and social systems has taught them that these needs either don't exist or don't matter.

It is a best practice for neurodiverse couple therapists to periodically initiate conversation about the seen and unseen ways a ND client may be attempting to regulate their sensory system during sessions. They should also, of course, discuss anything that triggers dysregulation. It is simple, but meaningful, to briefly check-in with each client at the start of each session regarding their level of sensory security. It is also simple to learn how to quietly observe the visible aspects of a client's physiology that indicate sensory insecurity, wondering aloud if an alteration to the room's lighting, seating, scents, or sounds may be helpful. All of this demonstrates care and respect for individual neurology to a degree many clients have never experienced before, providing a corrective emotional experience to the ND client and valuable behavioral modeling to the NT partner.

For some neurodiverse relationships, telehealth options provide the most sensory secure environment. This allows clients free access to their preferred sensory regulation supports, which are very frequently pets. They may also feel more freedom to make body movements or vocalizations in ways that are judged socially awkward in public settings, and less anxiety in general. For these reasons and more, ND persons and their NT partners may be especially motivated to seek telehealth. It allows a level of control over their sensory experience to a degree that traditional therapy can never replicate.

Sensory Insecure Example and Discussion

During an Intake session with a neurodiverse couple, a therapist warmly greets her clients by inviting them to sit down together on a large sofa within her vanilla-scented office. Sunlight floods the room, providing what she considers to be a cheery atmosphere conducive to conversation. Although both clients appear at ease at first, the ND husband soon begins to rub his head while shifting back and forth in his seat. He apologizes for this, explaining that he is currently experiencing a bit of brain fog. The therapist makes a mental note that this behavior began as his NT partner described details of their most recent argument. She surmises he has high anxiety regarding interpersonal conflict, heightened by reduced social skills related to his neurodivergence. "What this couple really needs," the therapist thinks to herself, "are some good conflict resolution strategies." She proceeds to provide psychoeducation regarding ND versus NT social skills.

After a few weeks pass without hearing from these clients, the therapist wonders why this couple has not booked a second visit.

How is the therapist above practicing casual ableism?
When a professional presumes that each client's brain detects and reacts to sensory stimuli similarly, they lose sight of their responsibility to inclusiveness. The interior design in this example strongly favors NT preferences and assumptions regarding sensory processing. Remember that the very environmental conditions that read as "welcoming" to most NT clients may be extremely off-putting to some ND clients.

The ND client in this example may have been both cognitively and physiologically distracted by the bright lights and smells in the therapy room. He may have had no other way to describe his experience of sensory insecurity other than as "brain fog." Fidgeting may have been a form of stimming in order to cope, especially because the room provided only one seating option.

An environment inclusive of potentially aversive sensory stimuli, along with a therapist who does not take the initiative to inquire about their clients' sensory experiences, reflects insensitivity. In this example, this actually even led to a premature conclusion that the ND husband is "conflict-avoidant" with "reduced social skills."

What could have been different if the therapist had cultivated a sensory-friendly environment from the start, or inquired about each client's sensory experience?
The therapeutic alliance may have been strengthened instead of severed.

Can sensory insecurity occur even when a therapist consistently cultivates a sensory-friendly environment?
Yes! Sometimes a ND client will come to therapy already overwhelmed due to circumstances that have nothing to do with the therapy environment. They may have been in heavy traffic on the way to the office, or perhaps they've had to stop at the shopping mall to run an errand that day. Using

process comments can be very helpful, e.g., "I noticed you are squinting a bit to the lighting in the room today. Have you had a taxing sensory day or week so far?" Suggesting an accommodation in this scenario shows flexibility and care, e.g., "If the lights are too bright for you today for any reason, I'm happy to dim them a bit."

Sensory Secure Example

During an Intake session with a neurodiverse couple, a therapist warmly greets her clients by inviting them to sit in one of several seating options within her neutrally-scented office. As they begin talking, the clients appear at ease. However, the ND husband soon begins rubbing his head and shifting back and forth in his seat. He attributes this behavior to "brain fog" and apologizes. The therapist makes a gentle process comment, wondering aloud if anything in the therapy environment may be a contributing factor. She briefly explains the concept of sensory security and her commitment to foster this. "It's not just one of the ways I'd like to demonstrate support for you both as people," she says "it's also something all brains need on a neurological level to be able to heal, learn, and grow."

The therapist first invites the ND husband to share his physiological experience of the room's design: Lighting, seating, smells, sounds, etc. He pauses to think before stateing that the room's lighting may be too bright for him right now. "Sometimes light bothers me on days that have already been stressful at work," he says. The therapist thanks him for sharing his internal experience, offering to alter the window shades in a way that lets less light into the room – after checking that this would be ok with the NT partner. Next, she invites the NT partner to share their unique sensory experience of the room. They state they are perfectly comfortable, and that no further accommodations are needed. A rich discussion follows about the clients' presenting relationship issues as therapy continues. The clients schedule another session right away.

How does the therapist in this example differ from the first?

This therapist displays sensitivity to each client's sensory experience and flexibility regarding accommodations to the therapy environment. She also provides psychoeducation regarding sensory processing and gives explicit permission for sensory security or insecurity to be discussed at any time.

The ND client in this example is able to quickly pinpoint the aversive stimulus and communicate his sensory needs. What if this was not the case? How can a therapist support a client who is unable to identify their sensory needs and/or communicate about them?

The therapist can provide psychoeducation regarding interoception and collaborate with the client to assess what may be changeable or unchangeable in this area for them. The therapist can encourage assertiveness, learn about the client's communication style, and provide opportunities to practice identifying sensory needs and talking about them together during sessions.

BIC therapists . . .

Recognize the importance of sensory security.

Challenge their own assumptions about clients' responses to stimuli.

Validate clients' sensory experiences, regularly initiating dialogue about them.

Presumption of Competence and Strengths

It's unethical to presume a lack of competence in any client. This undervalues their strengths and stunts autonomy and growth. Yet, therapists can easily fall into this trap when working with neurodiverse couples. For example, a well-meaning therapist may inadvertently provide too much scaffolding as they teach strategies to improve executive functioning. To avoid this, a client's capacities should always first be assessed without bias and then the least amount of scaffolding should be provided. Unnecessary scaffolding should be removed over time as the client demonstrates improvement.

Of course, identifying a client's brain-based strengths and challenges will always be an imperfect process. Not only does this rely on the clinician's mindset and clinical skills, it also depends on the client's desired level of authenticity in the therapy room. Some clients have learned to camouflage, or outright deny, their challenges. Others have learned to minimize their talents and strengths in order to fit in. While accurate assessment is sometimes difficult, it's important to presume competence and strengths without over- or underinflating a client's actual abilities.

Example of Not Upholding this Tenet

Over the phone, a therapist schedules an initial couple counseling session with a neurodiverse couple in which the wife is an AuDHDer. He then emails all the necessary Intake paperwork <u>only</u> to the NT husband, requesting they each complete a copy and bring it to their first visit.

Why is the above action problematic?
The therapist in this example has, either consciously or subconsciously, presumed that the ND partner is incompetent. Perhaps this is due to the therapist's own negative assumptions about AuDHDers' capacities. Or, perhaps their past experiences have proven that bypassing the ND partner in a neurodiverse relationship with regards to Intake paperwork tends to result in more timely completion of the forms. This is not ok.

Although the therapist in this example may justify their strategy by saying it is driven by a sense of efficiency versus ableism this practice is unprofessional and disrespectful nonetheless. Neither client requested for the NT partner to be in charge of paperwork: The therapist simply presumed it should be that way. This can reinforce a common stereotype about neurodiverse partnerships: That the NT person must "manage" the ND partner and/or handle all important relationship tasks for them to get done. It's unfair to make this global assumption of ND persons, and also unfair to assign NT partners this role. It's most ethical for a neurodiverse couple therapist to provide Intake paperwork to both the ND partner and the NT partner equally and simultaneously, offering the option of other accommodations as desired.

BIC therapists . . .

Presume clients' competence, accurately assess their strengths and challenges, and avoid enabling unhealthy stereotypes.

Acceptance of Atypicality Without Manipulation or Toxic Positivity

A therapist's overt respect for a ND client's atypicality allows the therapy environment to be a sacred space where corrective emotional experiences are possible. This can potentially help counteract a lifetime of negativity from media sources, doctors, mental health professionals, teachers, family members, peers, and more. It may be especially impactful if protective factors have been absent in a client's history, such as the lack of a neuroaffirming caregiver.

It's important for therapists to refrain from pathologizing harmless aspects of a ND client's physical appearance, style of dress, hobbies, mannerisms, hairstyle, etc. What may be perceived by the dominant culture as "odd," "quirky," or "abnormal" across many professional disciplines may simply represent a different way of being human. ND self-expression can vary from dominant culture. Additionally, whenever practical, a client's own preferred stim toys or nontraditional emotional support animal (e.g., a reptile) should be allowed in the therapy room. Intense interests should be incorporated into sessions. If needed, extra time should be given for ND clients to process questions before expecting an answer. Focusing on a client's tone of voice to the degree their message is ignored, called **tone policing**, should always be avoided.

These efforts to promote individuality represent a commitment to support each neurodiverse couple toward therapy success on their own terms . . . not manipulate them to conform. Sadly, the helping professions have historically focused on neurodivergence as an undesirable deficiency to be molded into something more palatable. The achievement of neurotypical relationship norms has been emphasized, although humanistic and positive psychology represent notable exceptions to this rule. It is encouraging that most helping professions seem to have begun to take a less manipulative approach to treatment these days as human diversity is becoming more recognized.

While manipulation of ND clients represents one behavioral extreme, exaggerated glorification of ND client features is another. Of course, celebrating one's own neurodivergence or that of others is certainly acceptable. Doing so affirms the inherent value of ND persons and promotes social inclusion. To imply that neurodivergence is nothing but a gift, though, represents **toxic positivity**. This view glosses over very real challenges. Often promoted by parent-led advocacy groups, toxic positivity can also feel infantilizing and condescending.

A recent example of this tension occurred after *Time Magazine* selected Greta Thunberg, an Autistic teenager, as their Person of the Year in 2019. (Interestingly, *Time Magazine* selected an Autistic individual for this title again in 2021 when Elon Musk earned the honor.) ND representation is an amazing thing, so having Thunberg's face on the cover of such a prominent magazine proved meaningful for many around the world. However, controversy arose after Thunberg was widely quoted in the media stating she views Autism as her "superpower."[49] Obviously, one can certainly choose to label their own neurodivergence this way: Everyone is allowed to self-identify however they wish. Problems with this language only began after the general public took her words as permission to refer to <u>every</u> ND person's neurotype as their personal superpower. Some enjoy this reframe, but many find it an off-putting example of toxic positivity.

Interpretation of one's own neurodivergence is extremely personal and varies from person to person. A therapist should not refer to a ND client's neurotype as their superpower unless the client themselves uses this language.

BIC therapists . . .

Accept clients' atypicality.
  Avoid manipulation, tone policing, and toxic positivity.

Validation of Neurodivergent Lived Experience

Willingness to listen to real life stories is essential to ensure that a therapist's interventions actually align with clients' needs. Yet, existing scholarly literature lacks research centered around the actual lived experiences and opinions of ND persons. Even fewer studies exist that consider neurodiverse couples. Many studies focus on identifying and improving social deficits.

It's encouraging that a recent study that reviewed 315 articles published by the *Washington Post* between 2007 and 2017 noted a shift in favor of neurodiversity topics and strength-based considerations.[50] As researchers become more aware of the potential for NT bias in research, and the actual desires of neurodiverse populations, hopefully this trend will expand.

Certain themes tend to emerge when ND voices are amplified. First, they express concern about society's lack of inclusivity. They are thankful technology provides accessible options for support in the form of websites, podcasts, hashtags, chat features, and other ND community-building tools, but wish this could expand to encompass more in-person opportunities. Another theme is a lack of access to neuroaffirming diagnosis and treatment experiences. Stories about negative experiences with mental health professionals are common. Regarding diagnosis itself, there are also concerns that NT bias and stereotypes may be embedded within diagnostic criteria and assessment tools. ND culture tends to view self-diagnosis as equally valid – or even more valid – than professional diagnosis as a result. Finally, themes of invalidation emerge as clients lament the ways others tend to emphasize either their shortcomings or their talents versus their holistic selves.

Each ND client has a unique life story. However, research does show some alarming trends:

- ND persons tend to struggle in areas such as employment, sexual relationships, and mental health. A recent survey of 7,491 people by Autistic advocate Chris Bonnello revealed 69% of Autistic respondents reported anxiety, 59% reported depression, 36% reported PTSD, 22% reported an eating disorder, and 17% reported Obsessive-Compulsive Disorder (OCD).[51]
- Statistics for suicide within ND populations reveal an urgent need to provide targeted support. Sadly, a 2019 study of over 21,000 Autistic adults enrolled in Medicare found that 4% had experienced suicidal ideation or attempted suicide.[52] A Danish population-based study of over 6.5 million people over a 10-year period observed that Autistics had a threefold incidence of suicidal attempts or deaths over those who were not Autistic.[53] Among Autistics, researchers found a higher rate of suicidality for females. Researchers in a statewide study in Utah noticed this as well, which is possibly due to higher rates of depression in females regardless of neurotype.[54] Possible contributing factors include various forms of abuse, bullying, discrimination, co-occurring anxiety, and other considerations.
- ND people disproportionately experience sexual trauma.[55,56,57] Shockingly, a recent French study found nine out of ten Autistic females reported a sexual trauma history.[58]
- It's a horrible reality that Disabled children and adults still die from caregiver abuse in our modern era. Zoe Gross, former director of advocacy at the *Autistic Self Advocacy Network (ASAN)*, has designated March 1st of each year since 2012 as an International Day of Mourning to memorialize Disabled persons who have been murdered by the very adults who were supposed to provide them loving care.[59]

Obviously, not all ND lived experience is negative. A ND person's experiences, especially pertaining to interoceptive sensations, may actually sometimes differ from that of a NT person in an amazing way. ND persons often describe feeling extremely pleasant sensations while listening to music, dancing, observing patterns in nature, running, reading, or doing any number of other activities. Explained as an intense, energetic, full-body feeling, **Autistic joy** may include happy stimming (either alone or alongside a friend with the same neurotype, an **allistic** friend, or a validating NT partner). This is usually in response to a positive somatic, emotional, or cognitive experience involving a special interest. But, it can also result from solving a complex problem, connecting previously unrelated ideas, repeating something enjoyable, or lots of other circumstances. Autistic joy is almost never appropriately recognized by society, nor is it usually explored in couple therapy.

BIC therapists . . .

Listen to clients' actual life experiences and needs.

Recognize ND persons are at a higher risk for psychological, physical, and sexual harm than NT persons.

Invite clients to explore any aspect of their neurology they experience positively.

Therapist Authenticity

The notion of therapist authenticity is closely related to Irvin Yalom's concept of genuineness, an existential psychotherapy practice.[60] A therapist's genuineness establishes good rapport and offers clients the opportunity to work with a professional who is sincere.[61]

In the context of BIC, being an authentic therapist may or may not include personal disclosure of their neurotype. A therapist should never feel forced to reveal this or anything else about themselves, of course, as they can certainly uphold professional standards for both genuineness and authenticity without doing so.[62] Yet, it is interesting to consider how the appropriate disclosure of a therapist's own neurodivergence may potentially strengthen the therapeutic alliance or contribute to positive neurodiverse couple therapy outcomes.[63]

Therapist disclosure of their own gender, race, sexual orientation, and religious self-identifications is starting to become a common topic debated within counselor training programs. Why not add a therapist's own brain wiring to this list of personal characteristics? When safe, wise, and clinically relevant to do so, a therapist's ethical disclosure of their neurotype may powerfully model self-acceptance.

As a final note, regardless of disclosure, this tenet also reminds therapists who are ND that authenticity involves attending to their own physiological needs during each session. Even though therapists should seek to prioritize the client's sensory security over their own, it's crucial that a ND therapist does not deny themselves access to self-regulation strategies when needed. These coping skills may be clearly visible to a client (e.g., when a therapist squeezes a stress ball in one hand during a session), or they may be invisible mental processes. A therapist's visible stims may inspire discussion that normalizes stimming in front of others, as well as valuable behavioral modeling. Making a sensory accommodation for oneself during a session (e.g., altering the temperature of the room to be more comfortable) shows clients it is ok to have needs, and to advocate for them. These actions should occur in a professional manner so as not to divert attention away from the client's intended focus for the session or detract from their overall experience of care.

BIC therapists . . .

Acknowledge that every person (including themselves) has the right to determine whether or not to disclose any kind of personal information.

Follow applicable ethical guidelines when choosing to appropriately disclose their own neurotype and/or associated characteristics.

Attend to their own sensory needs as they manifest in the therapy room, discussing their personal coping strategies whenever clinically relevant to clients' goals.

Glossary of Bolded Terms

Ableism   Refers to a biased set of beliefs and/or behaviors that promote NT, Non-Disabled existence as superior.

Allistic   A descriptor for someone who is ND, but not Autistic. For example, many ADHDers are not simultaneously Autistic. An ADHDer who is not also Autistic is referred to as Allistic. (An ADHDer who is simultaneously Autistic is described as an AuDHDer).

Autistic Joy   An extremely pleasant response to positive stimuli, interpersonal interactions, one's special interests, or other good circumstances. It usually involves happily stimming.

Autistic Meltdown   Also known as a neurological emergency. This brain-based response and associated behavior occurs as a defense mechanism when an Autistic person experiences distress that exceeds their ability to cope. It can result from a single aversive stimulus, the accumulation of aversive stimuli over time, interpersonal dynamics, or chronic sensory understimulation.

Brain-Informed Care (BIC)   A therapeutic environment that promotes holistic treatment via application of the Neurodiversity Paradigm and commitment to non-ableist practices.

Executive Functioning Skills   Behaviors largely dictated by the prefrontal cortex, e.g., paying attention, staying organized, making and following through with plans, self-monitoring, controlling impulsiveness, and regulating emotions.

Hypersensitivity   In the context of human sensory perception, this refers to a person responding very highly to an incoming sensation.

Hyposensitivity   In the context of human sensory perception, this refers to a person responding minimally (or not at all) to an incoming sensation.

Internalized Ableism   This occurs when a ND and/or Disabled individual sets personal goals based on NT and/or Non-Disabled standards. It can sometimes result in burnout.

Sensory Insecurity   A person's experience of physiological and psychological discomfort based on the sum of any aversive internal and external stimuli in their immediate presence.

Sensory Security   A person's experience of physiological and psychological comfort based on the sum of any neutral to positive internal and external stimuli in their immediate presence.

Stimming   The conscious or subconscious act of using repetitive motions and/or vocalizations to self-stimulate towards greater physiological balance or express strong emotion. Both ND and NT persons stim.

Tone Policing   In the context of a neurodiverse couple relationship, this occurs when one partner dismisses what the other has to say due to their misperception that the message itself was delivered in a negative manner.

Toxic Positivity   Unrelenting optimism that lacks appropriate empathy and may block healthier forms of insight and coping.

Trauma Informed Care (TIC)   An atmosphere of care that recognizes the reality and effects of various forms of trauma while attending to the specific needs of traumatized individuals.

Notes

1 American Association for Marriage & Family Therapy. (2005, January 1). *Code of Ethics*. AAMFT. Retrieved January 6, 2023, from https://www.aamft.org/Legal_Ethics/Code_of_Ethics.aspx

2 Valizadeh, S., Liem, F., Mérillat, S. *et al.* (2018). Identification of individual subjects on the basis of their brain anatomical features. *Sci Rep 8*, 5611.

3 Herculano-Houzel, S. (2016). *The human advantage: A new understanding of how our brain became remarkable.* Cambridge, MA: The MIT Press.

4 Xu, C. S., Januszewski, M., Lu, Z., Takemura, S. Y., Hayworth, K. J., Huang, G., . . . & Plaza, S. M. (2020). A connectome of the adult drosophila central brain. *BioRxiv.*

5 Harris, M. & Fallot, R. D. (Eds.) (2001). *Using trauma theory to design service systems. New directions for mental health services.* San Francisco: Jossey-Bass.

6 Butler, L. D., Critelli, F. M., & Rinfrette, E. S. (2011). Trauma-informed care and mental health. *Directions in Psychiatry, 31*(3), 197–212.

7 Huang, L. N., Flatow, R., Biggs, T., Afayee, S., Smith, K., Clark, T., & Blake, M. (2014). *SAMHSA's concept of trauma and guidance for a trauma-informed approach.*

8 Center for Substance Abuse Treatment. (2014). Trauma-informed care in behavioral health services.

9 Huang, L. N., Flatow, R., Biggs, T., Afayee, S., Smith, K., Clark, T., & Blake, M. (2014). *SAMHSA's concept of trauma and guidance for a trauma-informed approach.*

10 Charlton, R. A., Entecott, T., Belova, E., & Nwaordu, G. (2021). "It feels like holding back something you need to say": Autistic and Non-Autistic adults accounts of sensory experiences and stimming. *Research in Autism Spectrum Disorders, 89.*

11 Kapp, S. K., Steward, R., Crane, L., Elliott, D., Elphick, C., Pellicano, E., & Russell, G. (2019). "People should be allowed to do what they like": Autistic adults' views and experiences of stimming. *Autism, 23*(7), 1782–1792.

12 Wright, B. A. (1960). *Physical disability: A psychological approach.* Harper & Row.

13 Dunn, D. S., & Andrews, E. E. (2015). Person-first and identity-first language: Developing psychologists' cultural competence using disability language. *American Psychologist, 70*(3), 255.

14 Ferrigon, P., & Tucker, K. (2019). Person-First Language vs. Identity-First Language: An examination of the gains and drawbacks of Disability Language in society. *Journal of Teaching Disability Studies.*

15 Best, K. L., Mortenson, W. B., Lauzière-Fitzgerald, Z., & Smith, E. M. (2022). Language matters! The long-standing debate between identity-first language and person first language. *Assistive Technology, 34*(2), 127–128.

16 Bulluss, E. (2019, October 1). *Talking About Autism.* Psychology Today. Retrieved January 6, 2023, from https://www.psychologytoday.com.

17 Bottema-Beutel, K., Kapp, S. K., Lester, J. N., Sasson, N. J., & Hand, B. N. (2021). Avoiding ableist language: Suggestions for autism researchers. *Autism in Adulthood, 3*(1), 18–29.

18 Zadrozny, B. (2019, May 21). *Parents are poisoning their children with bleach to "cure" autism. These moms are trying to stop it.* NBC News. Retrieved January 6, 2023, from https://www.nbcnews.com.

19 Lardieri, A., Cheng, C., Jones, S. C., & McCulley, L. (2021). Harmful effects of chlorine dioxide exposure. *Clinical Toxicology (Philadelphia, Pa.), 59*(5), 448.

20 James, S., Stevenson, S. W., Silove, N., & Williams, K. (2015). Chelation for autism spectrum disorder (ASD). *Cochrane Database of Systematic Reviews,* (5).

21 Wilkenfeld, D. A., & McCarthy, A. M. (2020). Ethical concerns with applied behavior analysis for autism spectrum "disorder". *Kennedy Institute of Ethics Journal, 30*(1), 31–69.

22 Gorycki, K. A., Ruppel, P. R., & Zane, T. (2020). Is long-term ABA therapy abusive: A response to Sandoval-Norton and Shkedy. *Cogent Psychology, 7*(1).

23 Sandoval-Norton, A. H., & Shkedy, G. (2019). How much compliance is too much compliance: Is long-term ABA therapy abuse? *Cogent Psychology, 6*(1).

24 Kupferstein, H. (2018). Evidence of increased PTSD symptoms in autistics exposed to applied behavior analysis. *Advances in Autism.*

25 Anderson, L. K. (2022). Autistic experiences of applied behavior analysis. *Autism.*

26 Schaaf, R. C., Benevides, T. W., Blanche, E., Brett-Green, B. A., Burke, J., Cohn, E., . . . & Schoen, S. A. (2010). Parasympathetic functions in children with sensory processing disorder. *Frontiers in Integrative Neuroscience, 4,* 4.

27 Harricharan, S., McKinnon, M. C., & Lanius, R. A. (2021). How processing of sensory information from the internal and external worlds shape the perception and engagement with the world in the aftermath of trauma: Implications for PTSD. *Frontiers in Neuroscience, 15.*

28 Miller, L. J. (2006). *Sensational kids: Hope and help for children with sensory processing disorders.* New York, Putnam Press.

29 Robertson, A. E., & Simmons, D. R. (2015). The sensory experiences of adults with autism spectrum disorder: A qualitative analysis. *Perception, 44*(5), 569–586.

30 Goldstein, S., & Naglieri, J. A. (2014). *Handbook of executive functioning.* Goldstein, S & Nagliere, J. A. (eds), Springer, Cham.

31 Marco, E. J., Hinkley, L. B., Hill, S. S., & Nagarajan, S. S. (2011). Sensory processing in autism: A review of neurophysiologic findings. *Pediatric Research, 69*(8), 48–54.

32 Moerel, M., De Martino, F., & Formisano, E. (2014). An anatomical and functional topography of human auditory cortical areas. *Frontiers in Neuroscience, 8,* 225.

33 Jaime-Lara, R. B., To, L., & Joseph, P. V. (2021). Anatomy, physiology, and neurobiology of olfaction, gustation, and chemesthesis. In *Sensory Science and Chronic Diseases* (pp. 3–20). Springer, Cham.

34 Jaime-Lara, R. B., To, L., & Joseph, P. V. (2021). Anatomy, physiology, and neurobiology of olfaction, gustation, and chemesthesis. In *Sensory science and chronic diseases* (pp. 3–20). Springer, Cham.

35 De Moraes, C. G. (2013). Anatomy of the visual pathways. *Journal of Glaucoma, 22,* S2–S7.

36 Rullmann, M., Preusser, S., & Pleger, B. (2019). Prefrontal and posterior parietal contributions to the perceptual awareness of touch. *Scientific Reports, 9*(1), 1–8.

37 Baloh, R. W., Honrubia, V., & Kerber, K. A. (2010). *Baloh and Honrubia's clinical neurophysiology of the vestibular system.* Oxford Academic.

38 Blanche, E. I., Reinoso, G., Chang, M. C., & Bodison, S. (2012). Proprioceptive processing difficulties among children with autism spectrum disorders and developmental disabilities. *The American Journal of Occupational Therapy, 66*(5), 621–624.

39 Taylor, J. L. (2009). Proprioception. *Encyclopedia of Neuroscience,* 1143–1149.

40 Trevisan, D. A., Parker, T., & McPartland, J. C. (2021). First-hand accounts of interoceptive difficulties in autistic adults. *Journal of Autism and Developmental Disorders, 51*(10), 3483–3491.

41 Suksasilp, C., & Garfinkel, S. N. (2022). Towards a comprehensive assessment of interoception in a multi-dimensional framework. *Biological Psychology, 168,* 108262.

42 Baranek, G. T. (1998). Sensory processing in persons with autism and developmental disabilities: Considerations for research and clinical practice. *Sens. Integr. Spec. Interest Sect. Q, 21*, 1–3.

43 Ahn, R. R., Miller, L. J., Milberger, S., & McIntosh, D. N. (2004). Prevalence of parents' perceptions of sensory processing disorders among kindergarten children. *The American Journal of Occupational Therapy, 58*(3), 287–293.

44 Van der Kolk, B. A. (2006). Clinical implications of neuroscience research in PTSD. *Annals of the New York Academy of Sciences, 1071*(1), 277–293.

45 Niutanen, U., Harra, T., Lano, A., & Metsäranta, M. (2020). Systematic review of sensory processing in preterm children reveals abnormal sensory modulation, somatosensory processing and sensory-based motor processing. *Acta Paediatrica, 109*(1), 45–55.

46 Wickremasinghe, A. C., Rogers, E. E., Johnson, B. C., Shen, A., Barkovich, A. J., & Marco, E. J. (2013). Children born prematurely have atypical sensory profiles. *Journal of Perinatology, 33*(8), 631–635.

47 Miller, L. J. (2014). *Sensational kids: Hope and help for children with sensory processing disorder (SPD)*. Penguin.

48 Mulligan, S., Douglas, S., & Armstrong, C. (2021). Characteristics of idiopathic sensory processing disorder in young children. *Frontiers in Integrative Neuroscience, 15*, 9.

49 Ryalls, E. D., & Mazzarella, S. R. (2021). "Famous, beloved, reviled, respected, feared, celebrated:" Media construction of Greta Thunberg. *Communication, Culture and Critique, 14*(3), 438–453.

50 Lewin, N., & Akhtar, N. (2021). Neurodiversity and deficit perspectives in *The Washington Post*'s coverage of autism. *Disability & Society, 36*(5), 812–833.

51 Bonnello, C. (2022, March 23). *Results and Analysis of the Autistic Not Weird 2022 Autism Survey*. Autistic Not Weird. Retrieved January 8, 2023, from https://autisticnotweird. com/autismsurvey/

52 Hand, B. N., Benevides, T. W., & Carretta, H. J. (2019). Suicidal ideation and self-inflicted injury in Medicare enrolled autistic adults with and without co-occurring intellectual disability. *Journal of Autism and Developmental Disorders*.

53 South, M., Costa, A. P., & McMorris, C. (2021). Death by suicide among people with autism: Beyond zebrafish. *JAMA Network Open, 4*(1).

54 Kirby, A. V., Bakian, A. V., Zhang, Y., Bilder, D. A., Keeshin, B. R., & Coon, H. (2019). A 20-year study of suicide death in a statewide autism population. *Autism Research, 12*(4), 658–666.

55 Brown, K. R., Peña, E. V., & Rankin, S. (2017). Unwanted sexual contact: Students with autism and other disabilities at greater risk. *Journal of College Student Development, 58*(5), 771–776.

56 Ridout, S., & Murphy, S. (2021). Neurodiversity, autism and sexual violence. *Good Autism Practice (GAP), 22*(1), 97–98.

57 Dike, J. E., DeLucia, E. A., Semones, O., Andrzejewski, T., & McDonnell, C. G. (2022). A systematic review of sexual violence among autistic individuals. *Review Journal of Autism and Developmental Disorders*, 1–19.

58 Cazalis, F., Reyes, E., Leduc, S., & Gourion, D. (2022). Evidence that nine autistic women out of ten have been victims of sexual violence. *Frontiers in Behavioral Neuroscience, 136*.

59 (n.d.). Disability Day of Mourning – Remembering the Disabled Murdered by Caregivers. Retrieved January 6, 2023, from https://disability-memorial.org.

60 May, R., & Yalom, I. (1989). Existential psychotherapy. *Current psychotherapies*, 363–402.

61 Schnellbacher, J., & Leijssen, M. (2009). The significance of therapist genuineness from the client's perspective. *Journal of Humanistic Psychology, 49*(2), 207–228.

62 Henretty, J. R., & Levitt, H. M. (2010). The role of therapist self-disclosure in psychotherapy: A qualitative review. *Clinical Psychology Review, 30*(1), 63–77.

63 Barrett, M. S., & Berman, J. S. (2001). Is psychotherapy more effective when therapists disclose information about themselves? *Journal of Consulting and Clinical Psychology, 69*(4), 597.

What's a Neurotype?   3

The new discoveries about the human brain that occur every day allow a neurodiverse couple therapist's knowledge base to expand at the rate of scientific advancement. Sadly, though, myths and misinformation confound this potential.

The brain's incredible complexity affords humanity a wide variety of cognitive, behavioral, physiological, emotional, and psychological attributes that deserve recognition. To do so, without devaluing individual differences, it's practical to group together neurologically-based features which frequently co-occur. A **neurotype** is the name given to a recognized cluster of brain characteristics. These are usually inborn, but also may be acquired. Therapists have an important ethical imperative to pursue lifelong learning about the science behind neurotypes. They also must consider their own personal embodiment of their neurotype and listen to each client's lived experience of theirs.

Most professionals and clients consider the terms *neurotype* and *diagnosis* equal nomenclature, using them interchangeably. However, those who reject the concept of diagnosis all together do not. This is because of their perspective that brain wiring should always be viewed from a completely non-pathological lens. They believe the act of giving a diagnostic label imparts unnecessary negativity. This controversy aside, most people agree with a popular analogy: A neurotype is to a brain as an operating system is to a computer.

Are neurotypes rooted in genetics?
Yes. Scientists have found biological evidence behind some of the mechanics involved with each known neurotype. Neurodivergence can sometimes

DOI: 10.4324/9781003351337-5

even be detected in the womb! For example, researchers recently used *magnetic resonance imaging (MRI)* to observe neurobiological differences in developing fetuses. These features were later linked to either neurotypicality or Autism.[1]

Other research shows certain involuntary and voluntary behaviors associated with some forms of neurodivergence are observable during early infancy. Regarding automatic behavior, a 2022 study showed that larger pupil dilation in response to nonsocial sounds (an indicator of an alertness) occurred in infants thought to be genetically predisposed to having the Autistic neurotype.[2] Regarding voluntary behavior, other researchers noticed male infants thought to have a higher probability of later being identified as ADHDers behaved differently than the infants thought to have a higher probability of neurotypicality.[3] Another study, too, found that one year old children genetically predisposed to being ADHDers displayed more behavioral and temperament-related challenges than others.[4] None of this is surprising. Numerous genetic studies and observational studies of children before the age of two show that neurodivergence tends to run in families.[5]

Despite strong evidence for heritability, though, no neurotype has been found to be 100% inheritable. The way each person's unique interactions within their environment affect their gene expression is an important topic called **epigenetics**. Concepts from the **Diathesis-Stress Model** are vital to consider, as they may explain how genes switch on or off according to experiences and biologically-based vulnerabilities.

The age-old *nature versus nurture* debate is alive and well in the discussion of neurotypes. On the environmental front, researchers today consider both the positive and negative conditions that may be involved in the development of one's brain operating system. In particular, study topics tend to revolve around the question of whether or not exposure to toxins creates the Autistic and/or ADHD neurotype.[6,7,8]

To date, no single genetic or environmental pathway has been found to directly explain the way any neurotype comes about. We do, however, know a few things that are <u>not</u> causally related. For example, science has repeatedly proven that vaccines do not cause Autism.[9,10]

How does a neurotype compare with certain psychological terms and/or constructs? The term neurotype refers to one's actual, unique neural configuration. It is not a theoretical concept. Furthermore, neurotypes are permanent –although neuroplasticity does allow some degree of growth through the improvement of one's pre-existing strengths, as well as the acquisition of new skills.

Even though a neurotype is strongly related to temperament, personality, and identity, it is not synonymous with any of these.

- **Identity** is a psychological construct that consists of many personal components. Generally, though, it refers to one's holistic view of themselves. This is subjective and often quite flexible. Self-identifications are ultimately determined within one's own mind.
- **Personality** refers to the sum of one's salient attributes, traits, beliefs, attitudes, actions, and the way these manifest. Some parts of personality may be genetically determined, while others may be learned. Still others may be intentionally selected and integrated. Thus, personality is partially fixed and partially flexible.
- **Temperament** refers to one's general, inborn predisposition. This is thought to be genetic, permanent, and unchangeable. One's temperament sets both the pace that a person thinks, feels, and behaves and intensity with which they do so.

To compare and contrast the above terms, let's consider two main ideas: Permanence versus choice. One's neurotype, temperament, and personality will always have some degree of permanency because they directly relate to genetics; No one can <u>choose</u> their neurotype, temperament, or certain aspects of their personality. (Temperament and personality have actually been linked to inflammatory molecules and hormones released in the gut microbiome.[11] There is presently a lot of scientific interest in how the gut relates to neurotypes, as well.) At the same time, however, most people usually have at least some level of choice regarding how they outwardly present themselves and behave. For most people, it is possible to choose what parts of their own neurotype, temperament, and personality to display or suppress within different social environments.

Far from permanent, one's holistic identity framework has the potential for a high degree of flexibility and choice. As such it may or may not include aspects of neurotype, temperament, and personality at any given time. This is because each person's own self-identifications are subjective and can shift over the course of their lifespan; Identity in the postmodern era is fluid. The components of one's identity rely almost entirely on their own mental interpretations. Most Americans today feel free to amplify, minimize, alter, or ignore any of their personal attributes at whim . . . at least in private. This includes genetic and/or biological characteristics. Every person with the cognitive capacity to do so can formulate whatever personal self-identifications they wish. Whether or not they choose to embody these identifications in public is another matter entirely. One's own preferences, religious beliefs, level of self-esteem, media influences, social sphere, safety concerns, cultural factors, vocation, and economic status often mediate that choice.

Neurodiverse couples may benefit from an invitation by the therapist to learn more about each partner's temperament, personality, neurotype, and identity. It can be invaluable for clients to explore what may be *changeable* versus *unchangeable* about themselves and their relationship. Therapists are encouraged to support clients' process of discovery while showing the utmost respect for their preferences, beliefs, safety concerns, self-identifications, and sociocultural context. Clients deserve to receive unbiased psychoeducation and compassionate support as they sort through these sensitive aspects of personhood.

Is a person's neurotype always visible to others?
Not always. One's neurotype may or may not be associated with anything observable. Sometimes, of course, one's atypicality is on permanent display. Much like a wheelchair user cannot hide their wheelchair, for example, a non-speaking Autistic person who utilizes *Augmented and Alternative Communication (AAC)* cannot usually hide their device. (This is not to suggest these supports should be hidden. Rather, it's simply an acknowledgment that invisibility is not always an option.) Of course, visibility also depends on the eye of the beholder: Society sees what it wants to see. Autism, ADHD, Dyslexia, and other neurotypes are sometimes referred to as **invisible disabilities** because of their potential to go unnoticed.

It's each client's undeniable right to choose how, when, and why to express or conceal any personal aspect of themselves – including their neurotype. A poignant example of this occurs when a ND person engages in **masking** their atypical features, which is sometimes referred to as *camouflaging* in professional literature.[12] Masking is a survival strategy used to avoid negative social consequences. These consequences may be particularly dire for ND persons of color, who experience a disproportionate amount of discrimination.

Many ND persons rely on masking behaviors to help them stay safe and "belong" within majority NT spaces. The defensive coping mechanisms involved are often ingrained, lifelong, automatic reflexes – some clients may not even feel free to express certain ND qualities in the presence of their own partner. Many ND persons learned how to mask all on their own through attempts to meet the demands of NT parents, society at large, and to avoid harm. However, occasionally, an older ND mentor or well-meaning NT caregiver sometimes teaches masking as an intentional life strategy. Whether or not a ND client is consciously aware of their masking habits varies from client to client. Frequently, clients do not realize their specific masking behaviors or how they developed until they stumble upon neuroaffirming resources on the internet that explain this concept.

Therapists should never push any client towards unwanted public expression of any part of themselves in the therapy room or anywhere else. Despite the fact that studies have shown chronic masking/camouflaging behavior has been associated with suicidality, client autonomy remains a supreme ethic.[13] It's never a therapist's job to out their clients, as doing so may cause significant harm. Only certain pockets of society currently provide truly inclusive spaces where ND persons may safely practice **unmasking**. Generally, these are majority ND spaces.

If a client wishes to practice intentional unmasking in the therapy room, the therapist should provide a safe space to experiment. Nothing about the therapist or the therapy environment itself should hinder this effort. Additionally, those clients who are very aware of their own masking behaviors may appreciate the opportunity to process any emotional fatigue stemming from **code-switching** back and forth between majority ND and NT spaces.

Can a ND person have more than one neurotype at once?
Absolutely. Science confirms that some neurotypes co-occur quite frequently. ADHDers are sometimes simultaneously Dyslexic, for example. According to research, ADHD and Dyslexia each have unique biomarkers, yet co-occur as much as 40–50% of the time.[14,15] It's also fairly common for an ADHDer to simultaneously be Autistic. A 2022 study found this was true for 23.3% of its adult ADHD participants.[16] Researchers estimate between 20–50% of kids diagnosed as ADHDers may also be Autistic, and between 30–83% of Autistic children may actually be AuDHDers.[17,18] In light of this data, it's unfortunate that the DSM-IV used to forbid dual diagnosis of ADHD and Autism! The fact that this ban persisted all the way up until its 2013 revision has, undoubtedly, led to the invalidation of many ND persons. Thankfully, neuroimaging studies corrected the myth that ADHD and Autism are always mutually exclusive.[19] (A few researchers have now even gone so far as to propose ADHD and Autism may actually share a single genetic pathway.[20,21,22] They believe ADHD is just one of many **neurosubtypes** of Autism.[23] However, to date, no shared pathway has been found.)

Any person with more than one neurotype may refer to themselves as **Twice-Exceptional** or **2e**. This term is most commonly used by those who are Gifted and simultaneously either Autistic, ADHD, or Dyslexic. It's also possible for a person to be 3e or 4e. This is referred to as being **Multiexceptional**. Self-advocates have devised creative self-descriptors to combine their neurotypes into terms like *AuDHD* (i.e., Autism + ADHD) and others. They also encourage researchers and clinicians to acknowledge that a person can meet full diagnostic criteria for one neurotype while also having traits of another neurotype that fall short of full diagnostic standards. It's perhaps especially common for an ADHDer to have a few meaningful Autistic qualities but not meet full diagnostic criteria for Autism or vice versa.[24]

Should a therapist view a neurotype as synonymous with physical and/or mental illness?
Self-advocates, researchers, and different kinds of helping professionals often hold varying opinions on this topic. Their thoughts may be consistent or vary on a case-by-case basis. Some consider subjective variables as the highest indicator of whether or not a neurotype represents an illness, (e.g., quality of life). Others consider whether or not the ND person was born with their brain qualities, or if they were acquired via a specific medical condition or injury.

It's important to recognize that most self-advocates and pro-neurodiversity professionals make an emphatic distinction between the term *neurotype* and *illness*. Brain features associated with recognized neurotypes such as Autism, ADHD, etc. are never referred to as illnesses in the Neurodiversity Paradigm. Any neural configuration which represents a person's way of "being" is generally referred to as their neurotype. (This may also be the person's *disability*, yet not all ND persons consider themselves Disabled. Professionals should be aware that self-identifying as Disabled is a personal choice.)

Whenever there's an obvious, significant level of neural deterioration from a recognized disease process or injury which interferes with a person's way of "being" (e.g., epilepsy), it's generally acceptable to refer to this as stemming from *physical illness*. That which causes obvious, significant deterioration away from a person's mental wellness baseline (e.g., depression or anxiety) is generally referred to as *mental illness*.[25]

Gray areas do exist, of course. There is ongoing controversy about whether or not some forms of neurodivergence (e.g., Schizophrenia, Bipolar) represent neurotypes, physical illnesses, or mental illnesses.

Should a neurodiverse couple therapist view the ND partner as having a disorder?[26]
Neuroaffirming professionals generally dislike the term *disorder* and often advocate for its disuse. Within the counseling room, however, each client's personal preferences about using this terminology should receive priority.

Remember, too, that this linguistic choice may also revolve around complex factors that may or may not align with one's actual preferences. For example, specific language is often required when seeking insurance reimbursement or requesting accommodations in the workplace. In the absence of these limitations, a therapist's use of the word *disorder* in their professional endeavors comes down to a personal decision. This choice typically reflects their own brain-based life experiences, self-identifications, sociocultural context, educational background, and clinical experiences with neurodiverse populations.

Know that using *neurotype* versus *disorder* in publications, marketing materials, presentations, and other career-related activities does matter to some potential clients and colleagues. To them, this choice reveals whether or not the clinician is well-attuned to the needs and trends within the ND community at large. It also reveals how the person may interpret, and apply, information in the *Diagnostic and Statistical Manual of Mental Disorders (DSM-V-TR)*.

The fact that the *DSM-V-TR* unequivocally uses the term *disorder* in its title is an important consideration within this discussion. Consider, too, the connotation of the title of the *International Statistical Classification of Diseases and Related Health Problems (ICD-11)*. Both of these extremely influential resources clearly follow the Medical Model of Disability, and their use is often mandated. Insurance companies, of course, rely on formal diagnostic codes set by these sources to justify covered services. A client's qualification for certain government or private sector services also depends on using the diagnostic criteria and terminology within these sources.

Is the term neurotype listed in the DSM-V-TR?
No, the term *neurotype* has never been listed in this or any other version of the *DSM*. Like past editions, it stands accused of NT bias on both a conceptual and criterion level.[27]

Why do self-advocates and neuroaffirming therapists discourage the use of functioning labels when discussing neurotypes?
In reality, people do not arrange themselves on continuum from "severe" to "mild" like brands of salsa on a grocery store shelf. (Some Autistic self-advocates have a sense of humor in response to this common discussion point. They like to joke that their own personal form of neurodivergence is *Spicy Autism*.) This is because everyone, regardless of brain wiring, experiences fluctuations in their own personal capacities and support needs. To illustrate this variability, a popular drawing by the artist Rebecca Burgess eloquently suggests that ND traits related to language, movement, perception, executive functioning, etc. should be viewed as dynamic points on a color wheel. . .not a rigid continuum.[28] This type of visual model accounts for both neural individuality and environmental variability.

Rather than clarifying a person's capacities, the use of functioning labels can actually have the opposite effect. For example, if an Autistic person is nonspeaking and/or intellectually Disabled, they're often labeled *severely Autistic* or *low-functioning*. When an Autistic person speaks and/or lives independently, on the other hand, they're usually labeled *mildly Autistic* or *high-functioning*. Yet, each person's lived experiences day-to-day are far more nuanced than this dichotomy allows. So-called mildly Autistic persons are still likely to need intense support on occasion, but their assigned labels may minimize access to services. Meanwhile, those labeled severely Autistic may be misunderstood and passed over for growth opportunities because of others' view that they are permanently incapable.

Helping professionals are encouraged to say things like, "This client uses *AAC* to communicate" instead of using functioning labels. If, however, a ND client does self-ascribe themselves a functioning label then their therapist should respect this choice.

Neurotype Summaries

It's essential for neurodiverse couple therapists to learn as much as they can about each known neurotype in order to provide their clients up-to-date psychoeducation. This can help clients develop a clearer picture of their own brain attributes, as well as those of a partner or child. While avoiding overgeneralization, a series of summaries follows. Only Autism, ADHD, Dyslexia, Giftedness, and Sensory Processing Disorder (SPD), are explored below – but this does not imply that other neurotypes are unimportant.

Remember that no two people of the same neurotype are ever the same; There can be vast differences between people who share the same neurotype. Causal factors are deliberately excluded from this chapter, as there's currently no agreement about the exact role prenatal exposure, environmental toxins, specific genes, or other factors play. Finally, detailed information about medication and therapy modalities is not included because it exceeds the scope of this text.

Autism

History[29,30,31,32]

For an insightful deep dive, please see *Neurotribes* by Steve Silberman.[33]

- Case studies exploring the characteristics we now associate with the Autistic neurotype date back to the 18th century.

- Replacing the names *Dementia Infantilis* and *Childhood Schizophrenia* given in the early 1900s, the term *Autism* was first used in 1911 by German psychiatrist Eugen Bleuler. However, this did not change its strong association with Schizophrenia. Observations of children with Autistic traits during this era resulted in very different opinions. Most reflected the psychological theories of the day – namely, those of Sigmund Freud.
- Notable papers by American psychiatrist Leo Kanner and Austrian psychiatrist Hans Asperger emerged in 1943 and 1944, respectively. (Asperger had already, actually, described a group of children as *Autistic Psychopaths* in 1938.[34]) Kanner and Bruno Bettelheim went on to attribute *Infantile Autism* to frigid mothering. This was a problematic perspective in America that continued all the way through the 1960s. Meanwhile, Asperger wondered about a possible genetic link as he observed "high functioning" males and their fathers.
- Autism remained associated with Schizophrenia through the 1950s until the Psychology field shifted to behaviorism in the 1960s. The acquisition of spoken language and other forms of overt communication were strong areas of focus during this time due to their observable nature. Representing an outlier perspective for the year 1964, psychologist Bernard Rimland was perhaps the first to publish a theory that Autism might result from neurobiology.
- Widespread consideration of Autism as a developmental issue did not occur until the 1970s when heritability began to receive more attention. The 1980 edition of the *DSM-III* finally removed *Childhood Schizophrenia*, replacing it with a category called Pervasive Developmental Disorders. There were four diagnoses at the time: *Infantile Autism, Childhood Onset Pervasive Developmental Disorder, Residual Autism*, and *Atypical Autism*.
- In the 1980s, British psychiatrist Lorna Wing described Autism in terms of cognitive deficits. She asserted these challenges varied from person to person along a spectrum of abilities. Referencing the work of Hans Asperger, she coined the term *Asperger's Syndrome* to describe "high-functioning" Autism. This diagnosis was not yet listed in the *DSM*, however.
- The 1980s and 1990s saw a gradual explosion of research devoted to neural, genetic, and environmental considerations for Autistic traits. Autism began to be regarded as a mostly brain-based phenomenon. The *DSM-III-R* (1987) consolidated previous diagnostic distinctions into one diagnosis, *Autistic Disorder*. This disorder had three distinct domains of dysfunction: Reciprocal Social Interaction, Communication Impairments, and Restricted Interests/Resistance to Change Plus

Repetitive Movements. Additionally, *Pervasive Developmental Disorder Not Otherwise Specified (PDD-NOS)* became a new, separate diagnosis.

- Next, both the *DSM-IV* (1994) and the *DSM-IV-TR* (2000) began to formally embrace Wing's earlier conceptualization of an Autism spectrum. This spectrum expanded to include five distinct diagnoses: *Autism, PDD-NOS, Asperger's Syndrome, Childhood Disintegrative Disorder (CDD)*, and *Rett Syndrome*.

- 2013 brought a significant change to the *DSM-V* in the form of a major revision to Autism terminology. The terms *Asperger's Syndrome, PDD-NOS*, and *Autism* were removed altogether.[35] Instead, it introduced just one diagnosis: *Autism Spectrum Disorder (ASD)*. It also established two domains of dysfunction: Social Interaction/Communication and Restricted and Repetitive Interests/Behaviors. Lastly, it introduced a severity continuum: *Level 1 – "Requiring Support"; Level 2 – "Requiring Substantial Support"; and Level 3 – "Requiring Very Substantial Support."* A totally separate disorder, *Social (Pragmatic) Communication Disorder*, was also named in 2013 within the Communication Disorders section.

- The *DSM-V-TR* (2022) made only one minor change to the *ASD* diagnostic criteria in order to clarify some of the wording used within the Social Interaction/Communication domain.[36]

- Rather than using the term *ASD*, today American self-advocates tend to simply say *Autism*. Some people around the world, though, still identify with the old term *Asperger's* by referring to themselves *Aspies* – particularly in England and Australia. A few researchers argue for the reinstatement of *Asperger's Syndrome* to the DSM as an Autism subtype.[37] Usually, though, current literature tends to denounce this term based on Hans Asperger's association with Naziism and other beliefs of his day.

Strength-Based Description

No single stereotype regarding Autism is ever fully accurate. Autistics can be any ethnicity, religion, or gender. There are Autistic extroverts and Autistic introverts. Some enjoy eye contact, hugs, and loud rock concerts. Others need solitude, quiet, and sameness. Some have advanced degrees, a marriage, children, etc. Others struggle to work, to live independently, etc. Autistic people have any combination of these qualities, and so much more.

Many Autistics work without significant daily support, often as experts in their field. Others require assistance, either periodically or on an ongoing basis, to obtain and maintain employment; Autistic persons have a higher rate of unemployment than the general population.[38] Despite legislation in America to improve workplace inclusivity, it can sometimes be a struggle to obtain proper workplace accommodations.

About two thirds of Autistics have average to high intelligence as measured by standardized cognitive tests, whereas about one third have below average scores.[39] Autistic persons with a co-occurring intellectual disability frequently have high support needs, which may also involve health and safety concerns.

Some Autistics are nonspeaking or minimally speaking, while others consistently utilize verbal communication. Any Autistic person may choose to utilize *AAC*. One's preferred method of communication may be consistent across settings or vary. For example, a speaking person may not speak (either by choice or as a result of physiological processes) during times of extreme stress.

An Autistic person's particular deviations from NT standards in areas like language acquisition, socialization, self-regulation, sensory processing, learning, eating, and sleeping may or may not be noticeable to caregivers during childhood. Discovering one's own Autistic qualities sometimes happens for the first time as a teenager or adult.

Autistic persons may or may not find the following aspects of social interactions challenging. This is not an exhaustive list. Importantly, also, the degree to which a person struggles in these areas is both unique to their brain wiring and dependent on their sociocultural and environmental context. Some of a person's challenges can certainly remain consistent amidst all their circumstances. However, it's likely that some struggles are lessened (or eliminated) within wholly supportive conditions.

An Autistic Person's Potential Social Concerns

1. Interpreting nonverbal communication such as physical gestures and facial expressions.
2. Giving and receiving eye contact.
3. Maintaining the back-and-forth flow of conversation.
4. Knowing how to start up a conversation or begin a behavioral interaction.
5. Self-regulating in response to internal and external stimuli in order to remain interpersonally engaged.
6. Participating in small talk.
7. Identifying each partner's needs in an intimate relationship and communicating about them.

8. Interpreting "hidden meanings" behind certain idioms, metaphors, and abstract language.
9. Knowing when to end a conversation or behavioral interaction.
10. Setting and maintaining interpersonal boundaries.
11. Recognizing personal overwhelm from socializing, taking a break, and re-engaging.
12. Regulating the tone, inflection, or volume of their own voice and interpreting these qualities in others.

For those with the Autistic neurotype, knowing the "right" thing to say or do in social situations may not be intuitive. This is because they tend to not automatically grasp the structure or purpose of unspoken social hierarchies and their associated expectations. Instead, they may gravitate towards their strong interests, no matter what they may be, with little regard for what others may think of them for doing so. An Autistic extrovert may seek out interactions with others that relate to these interests, while an Autistic introvert may not.

NT persons tend to prematurely label Autistic people as awkward, rude, weird, aloof, single-minded/rigid, immature, or quirky – especially if they eschew NT social norms in visible ways. For example, some Autistic people have a strong dislike for small talk and avoid it at all costs. These persons find expending energy to identify and interpret the underlying subtext of conversation exhausting. Their preference for having direct, efficient conversations may be misunderstood.

Autistic persons often appreciate extra support to decipher the logistics, demands, and dynamics of their relationships with NT persons, as well as the social complexities of their school or work environments. Establishing and maintaining healthy interpersonal boundaries may be a particularly challenging area. Skill-building opportunities may be needed to help reduce an Autistic person's vulnerability to mistreatment in society.

Sometimes the repetition of phrases, vocalizations, motor movements, or patterns of interaction with people or objects can serve a meaningful purpose to Autistic persons. This may be due to their tendency to pay close attention to details, aptitude for pattern recognition, and style of sensory processing. Stimming may help an Autistic person express their own strong feelings, or aid in physiological and emotional self-regulation.

Autistics frequently show a strong preference for sameness in their food choices, clothing textures and styles, personal schedule, environmental conditions, etc. They may become visibly distressed when the need to transition from one activity to another arises, or when they're interrupted. Even small changes to an established, meaningful routine may be incredibly difficult to cope with. Many times this relates to sensory insecurity on a physiological level. However, this may also relate to executive functioning strain. Sleeping, eating, and personal hygiene may be affected.

Autistic brains process sensory input differently than NT brains. This can result in either <u>more</u> or <u>less</u> enjoyment of certain life experiences. For instance, some Autistic persons can experience physical pain or intense emotional distress when overwhelmed by one or more kinds of sensory input. Others can experience intense physical and emotional joy in response to one or more kinds of sensory input. (Most Autistic persons will experience a combination of both!) Sensory regulation can be an ongoing challenge that requires curiosity, empathy, and accommodation from loved ones and society.

Seeing things from another person's point of view may or may not be challenging for an Autistic person. Some Autistic persons have a huge amount of empathy and are able to express this in ways that NT society can recognize. Others may appear to "lack empathy" due to the fact they struggle to intuitively see things from another person's perspective and/or display this ability a bit differently than what may be expected.

Some Autistic people easily demonstrate reciprocal connectivity within their social relationships in ways that NT society can recognize, while others find this type of interpersonal engagement extremely difficult. Additionally, Autistics tend to attempt interpersonal connection in ways NT persons may not intuitively recognize.

Areas of the Brain Involved

- For Autistics, an enlarged amygdala can emerge in the first year of life. This may contribute to an increased fight or flight response.[40] There are also differences in brain regions that work very closely with the amygdala.[41] Amygdala differences have actually been noted in the womb, along with enlargement of the hippocampal commissure and insula.[42]
- Gray and white matter differences, plus reduced glial cells and other factors, may lead to excessive connectivity and/or underconnectivity within and across the various brain regions of Autistic persons.[43,44]
- There may be differences in the cerebellum's structure and function for Autistics, which can affect interpersonal interaction and cognition.[45]

- Autism may involve a different thickness of the brain's cortex.[46]
- Autistics may have excessive cerebrospinal fluid when compared to others.[47]
- There are neurotransmitter differences in Autistic brains, particularly regarding GABA, which may involve the gut-brain axis or other factors.[48]
- There is currently particular interest (i.e., Connectivome Theory) in how an Autistic person's immune system, sensory-motor system, and gut-brain axis interacts with connective tissues.[49]

Prevalence

The steady rise in Autism prevalence over the last few decades is most likely due to increased knowledge, the changes made to diagnostic assessments and criteria, and more frequent reporting.[50]

To estimate how many Autistic children currently live in America, *The Centers for Disease Control and Prevention (CDC)* relies on data collected by the *Autism and Developmental Disabilities Monitoring (ADDM) Network* regarding eight year olds located in eleven states. As of 2020, this showed about 1 in 36 American children may be Autistic.[51] In 2022, a report that averaged 99 different Autism prevalence calculations contained within 71 studies that had been conducted across the globe estimated 1 in 100 children may be Autistic.[52] The difference between these prevalence rates could be due to socioeconomic factors, racial bias, cultural norms, lack of accessibility to healthcare, lack of knowledge, and many other considerations.[53]

Another consideration is the complexity of differential diagnosis between ADHD and Autism, as they can be easily confused for one another. When a child has both neurotypes, ADHD characteristics tend to be identified first. An average of .7 to 1.8 years passes before concurrent Autistic characteristics are properly identified.[54]

DSM-V-TR Considerations

Autism is characterized in the *DSM-V-TR* as a **Neurodevelopmental Disorder**. A recent review of studies published globally between 2012 and 2019 reports the average age study participants received their Autism diagnosis was around three to ten years old. The same report estimates the current global average age of diagnosis for Autism, however, is closer to five years old or younger.[55]

In America, the CDC presently estimates the average age to receive an initial Autism diagnosis is around 4 years old.[56]

Nonetheless, not receiving an Autism diagnosis until Middle School, or well past this, still frequently occurs. Some researchers found that over half of the female participants in their study received their Autism diagnosis at age 18 or later, with a mean age of 25 years old.[57]

Options for Diagnosis

The *American Academy of Pediatrics (AAP)* recommends pediatricians screen all children for Autistic qualities at their 18 and 24 month well visits.[58] Most screenings rely heavily on parent questionnaires to assess whether or not a child is reaching typical developmental milestones. A few screenings, however, encourage behavioral observation by a clinician with specialized training.

Certain professionals can provide a formal Autism diagnosis to children as young as two or a little younger. To do so, a comprehensive battery of standardized assessments is usually given by a developmental pediatrician, neuropsychologist, pediatric neurologist, child psychiatrist, or child psychologist. This may include some of the following tests: *The Autism Diagnostic Observation Schedule™ (ADOS™-2), The Autism Diagnostic Interview™ Revised (ADI™-R), The Autism Behavior Checklist (ABC), The Childhood Autism Rating Scale (CARS), The Monteiro Interview Guidelines for Diagnosing the Autism Spectrum – 2nd Edition (MIGDAS-2),* and *The Pre-Linguistic Autism Diagnostic Observation Schedule (PL-ADOS).*

Most, but not all, of the above tests focus on the child's observable behavior. Caregiver and teacher observations are considered. Additional tests to assess hearing, vision, intelligence, speech and language, adaptive functioning, motor skills, sensory sensitivities, executive functioning, and neurological processes may also be used to aid in differential diagnosis. Some examples are: *The Wechsler Intelligence Scale for Children – Fifth Edition (WISC-V), The Autism Spectrum Rating Scale (ASRS), The Developmental Test of Visual-Motor Integration – 6th Edition (VMI),* and *The Social-Responsiveness Scale – 2nd Edition (SRS-2).*

If not identified earlier, many Autistic children may receive their diagnosis through the American public school system. Autistic features may be noticed by an educator or a caregiver, either of whom may request that the school system conduct an evaluation. *The Individuals with Disabilities Education Act (IDEA)* mandates this evaluation be comprehensive and conducted by a professional, multidisciplinary team. These results, as well as information from any private sector evaluations, form the basis for an Autistic child's *Individualized Education Plan (IEP)*.

For adults, a comprehensive battery of standardized assessments is usually given by a psychiatrist, psychologist, or neuropsychologist. This likely includes the following tests, many of which tend to focus on observable behavior: *The Social Communication Questionnaire (SCQ)*, *The Autism Spectrum Quotient (AQ)*, *The Adaptive Behavior Questionnaire*, *The Autism Diagnostic Observation Schedule™ (ADOS™-2)*, and *The Autism Diagnostic Interview™, Revised (ADI™-R)*. Additional tests to assess hearing, vision, intelligence, speech and language, adaptive functioning, motor skills, sensory sensitivities, executive functioning, and neurological processes may also be used.

Controversially, whether or not a Licensed Professional Counselor (LPC), Licensed Marriage & Family Therapist (LMFT), Licensed Clinical Social Worker (LCSW), or equivalent can officially diagnose Autism varies in America from state to state. An important consideration is the practicality of providing a client a diagnosis at the Master of Arts (M.A.) or Master of Science (M.S.) level. An Autistic person's receipt of workplace accommodations, Social Security payments, Medicaid reimbursement, commercial insurance reimbursement, and other services usually depends on formal diagnosis and documentation provided by a higher-level professional (e.g., Ph.D. or M.D.).

A variety of free online self-screening tools are available to promote insight, such as: *The Autism Quotient (AQ)*, *The Empathy Quotient (EQ)*, *The Systemizing Quotient-Revised (SQ-R)*, *The Ritvo Autism Asperger Diagnostic Scale-Revised (RAADS-R)*, *The Aspie Quiz*, *The Camouflaging Autistic Traits Questionnaire (CAT-Q)*, and *The Repetitive Behavior Questionnaire (RBQ-2A)*.

A non-invasive diagnostic technique for Autism that utilizes structural *magnetic resonance imaging (MRI)* information is currently under review, with encouraging results.[59] However, it is not yet a standard practice to diagnose Autism.

Options for Support

The kind of support available to Autistics varies widely. There tend to be far more options for children than adults. Any or all of the following aspects of the Autistic neurotype may benefit from specific, ethical intervention: Cognition, emotion regulation, communication, sensory integration, mobility, independent living skills, vocational skills, learning strategies, interpersonal skills, and more. Any co-occurring medical or mental health conditions also deserve attention. The following professionals may be helpful to Autistic people, depending on their specific needs:

- Occupational Therapist (OT).
- Speech-Language Pathologist (SLP).
- Neurologist.
- Gastroenterologist.
- LPC, LMFT, LCSW, or equivalent clinician.
- Vocational counselor.
- Life coach / Executive functioning skills coach.
- Music therapist.
- Animal assisted therapist.[60]
- Yoga instructor and / or personal trainer.[61]

Other Considerations

A recognized minority profile of Autism is **Pathological Demand Avoidance (PDA)**. First identified in the 1980s by Elizabeth Newson, this term did not appear in professional literature until 2003.[62] It's also sometimes called *Extreme Demand Avoidance, Rational Demand Avoidance,* or *The Demand Avoidance Phenomena.*[63] There's currently no uniform definition for PDA, and no consensus about how often it occurs. A free online screening test for PDA is *The Extreme Demand Avoidance Questionnaire (EDA-QA)*.

PDA may either be noticed in childhood or not until later. It's characterized by mood swings and intense resistance to actual (or perceived) interpersonal demands.[64] Individuals with PDA may appear chronically defiant and controlling. Their tendency to make excuses, deny responsibility, blame others, become aggressive, or utilize passive-aggressive communication is likely a brain-based defensive response. PDA could someday be found to either be a spontaneous trait, or perhaps that it stems from sensory insecurity exacerbated by trauma.[65] Far more research is needed to support individuals with this set of characteristics.[66]

Alexithymia involves significant difficulty identifying one's own emotions and body sensations due to interoceptive challenges.[67] The brain wiring of Alexithymic people is believed to differ from that of NT persons in regions that impart the ability to sense, label, and discuss internal experiences. Once thought to be a core feature shared by all Autistics, research shows that actually only about half of Autistic individuals experience this.[68] Free online screening tests include *The Online Alexithymia Questionnaire (OAQ)* and *The Toronto Alexithymia Scale (TAS)*. Alexithymia can also be experienced by non-Autistic people, particularly those with a trauma background.

Hyperlexia involves an intense interest in letters and exceptionally advanced reading skills from a very young age. Hyperlexic toddlers are not specifically taught how to read – they just do! However, their reading comprehension may lag behind. First labeled in 1967 by Norman and Margaret Silberberg, current research estimates that between 6% and 20% of Autistics are also Hyperlexic.[69] You do not have to be Autistic to be Hyperlexic.

Hypernumeracy involves an intense interest in numbers and the ability to both conceptualize math and work with numbers in highly advanced ways from a very young age. Hypernumeric children and adults tend to think in numbers, attempt to quantify everything numerically, and enjoy working with numerical data sets. You do not have to be Autistic to be Hypernumeric.

Attention Deficit/Hyperactivity Disorder (ADHD)

History[70,71,72]

- Descriptions of people who may have been ADHDers can be found in art, literature, and historical records that date back to the era of Hippocrates (493 BC). The ancient Greeks believed distractibility, overactivity, and emotional frustration resulted from an imbalance of a person's internal humors, i.e., too much "fire" versus "water" in the body.
- Child physicians and psychiatrists from Germany, France, Great Britain, and Scotland described certain ADHD features as early as 1775. These characteristics were attributed to poor parenting, a child's lack of internal discipline or motivation, or perhaps "dysregulation of cerebral fibers." These ideas persisted until the 19th century. If medical causes were considered at all in this era, the following terms were used: *Attention Deficit, Disease of Attention, Nervous Child, Mental Instability/Derangement, Unstable Nervous System*, and *Simple Hyperexcitability*.
- In 1902, influential British physician Sir George Frederic Still suggested that ADHD characteristics represented a "defect in moral character" due to brain damage, environmental conditions, and genetics. German physicians Franz Kramer and Hans Pollnow later coined the term *Hyperkinetic Disease* in 1932.

- American medical director and neurological researcher Charles Bradley first medicated children with the stimulant Benzedrine in 1937. His accidental discovery that this improved behavior paved the way for Ritalin and Adderall to be prescribed during the 1950s and 1960s. Terms like *Minimal Brain Dysfunction Syndrome, Hyperkinetic Impulse Disorder,* and *Hyperactive Child Syndrome* were used at the time.
- The *DSM-I* did not list any disorder based solely on a person's inattentiveness, impulsivity, or hyperactivity upon its release in 1952. In 1968, however, the *DSM-II* included the diagnosis *Hyperkinetic Reaction of Childhood* to account for these qualities. The *DSM-III* (1980) later renamed this to *Attention-Deficit Disorder (ADD)* and described two subtypes: *With Hyperactivity* or *Without Hyperactivity.* The 1987 text revision later consolidated these subtypes into one diagnosis, *Attention Deficit/Hyperactivity Disorder (ADHD).*
- In 1994, The *DSM-IV* formally acknowledged that *ADHD* can extend into adulthood. It expanded to include three subtypes: *Inattentive, Hyperactive/Impulsive,* and *Combined.* The *DSM-V* retained this terminology in its 2013 edition, and again in the 2022 revision. These subtypes are now called "presentations," however, and are acknowledged to sometimes shift across the lifespan. Other specifiers currently include severity levels (i.e., *Mild, Moderate, Severe*) and whether or not symptoms are *In Partial Remission.*

Strength-Based Description

The popular global stereotype for an ADHDer is an American boy who can't pay attention in class because he's too busy bouncing off the walls. In reality, though, ADHDers represent people of all ages, all ethnicities, and all genders. They embody a wide variety of visible and invisible characteristics. Usually, however, almost all ADHDers can be described as having an interest-based neurology plus a here-and-now focus. That is, they tend to be most motivated by that which they find interesting, new, urgent, critical, exciting, and right in front of them.

ADHD is often, but not always, first noted in childhood by caregivers or teachers who observe hyperactive, impulsive, or inattentive behavior. The child may also experience clear academic, emotional, or social difficulties. These may be heightened if the child's home environment includes negative parenting dynamics, socioeconomic concerns, or critical life events.[73] Regarding adult

ADHDers, a person's struggles may go largely undetected – until, at some point, they become impossible to cope with. ADHD adults can experience significant challenges at work and in their relationships due to executive functioning differences and emotion regulation concerns.[74,75]

Any or all of the activities listed below tend to come more naturally to NT persons than ADHDers. The degree to which these challenges affect one's daily life varies.

An ADHDer's Potential Concerns

1. Staying focused when a topic is uninteresting.
2. Maintaining an organized home, car, and/or workspace.
3. Prioritizing multiple high-priority interpersonal demands, e.g., a deadline at work and partner's request.
4. Remembering and implementing multi-step directions.
5. Getting started on a task/Avoiding procrastination.
6. Remembering important dates, times, and details.
7. Forming helpful routines and sticking to them.
8. Coping with stress without totally numbing out.
9. Managing intense emotions and/or impulsivity.
10. Juggling everyday responsibilities such as: Preparing meals, working, cooking, maintaining personal hygiene, caring for children and pets, attending to a partner's needs, paying bills, etc.
11. Following through with commitments.
12. Avoid risky behaviors.
13. Coping with boredom from understimulation.
14. Time management.

The ADHD brain tends to notice incoming environmental and interpersonal stimuli all at once instead of sequentially.[76] Furthermore, each stimulus tends to be received with the same degree of intensity. The fact that ADHDers appear easily distractible to others has earned them the reputation of being inattentive. Yet, ADHDers do not lack attention – they have it in excess! For example, consider the scenario of a dog barking outside a classroom. To an ADHDer, the barking may register to the same auditory degree as the teacher giving her geography lesson. It's difficult to filter out the barking because the sensory receptors and executive functioning parts of the ADHD brain struggle to organize incoming information into a priority-based hierarchy. Autistic brains can struggle with this, as well. However, most NT brains do this easily and automatically.

ADHDers tend to experience sleep disturbances and nutritional challenges that vary from person to person. Research suggests up to 20% of ADHD children may experience a co-occurring eating disorder.[77] Access to supportive people and resources mediate an ADHDer's acquisition of the kinds of coping skills that can lead to healthy routines for sleeping and eating.

Many successful ADHDers have learned to be skilled multitaskers who think and learn best when their body is in motion. Note that the type of motion and speed must be set by the ADHD individual themself. Being forced to learn or work at a pace that is too slow, too rigid, too chaotic, or too understimulating may be exceptionally difficult. It's not uncommon for an ADHDer to have learned how to overcompensate for the challenges they don't want others to notice by intentionally building up their skills and creating support systems. In fact, some use highly creative mental strategies plus social support to achieve their desired outcomes. This can be a huge energy expenditure, though, that is sometimes fueled by poor self-esteem.

ADHDers who are unable to cope with life's demands may find themselves chronically overwhelmed and underperforming. A pervasive sense of failure tends to enable further underperformance, leading to feeling stuck, and the cycle continues. The inability to manage personal responsibilities and/or thrive in intimate relationships may be a factor that leads some ADHDers to self-medicate with substances like alcohol, nicotine, marijuana, or others.[78] A recent metastudy found that 21% of those with a *Substance Use Disorder (SUD)* had ADHD, which translates to roughly 1 in 5 persons.[79]

Some ADHDers may pursue risky or compulsive behaviors as a way to escape, as a way to feel good, or a way to simply feel normal. This is because the ADHD brain differs in terms of its reward pathways and processes, which are areas related to dopamine.[80] In simple terms, ADHDers are chronically low in dopamine. So, they tend to pursue dopamine-rich activities in order to self-regulate. Food, sex, gambling, video games, internet use, substance use, and other areas may be especially problematic for ADHDers because they represent fast sources of dopamine.[81,82,83,84]

Many ADHDers feel restless in their mind and body. This may manifest in childhood as physical activity, impatience, or perhaps talkativeness. In adulthood this may manifest similarly, or perhaps also as rapid mental processing, drivenness, or always being "on the go." Exercise can be a helpful channel for this energy, as it has been shown to improve cognitive performance in children with ADHD.[85]

When an ADHDer's energy is channeled in pursuit of a strong interest, it may be so strong that they may not attend to their basic needs such as eating, sleeping, going to the toilet, or drinking water. This is called **hyperfocus**. It is perceived as either positive or negative depending on circumstances. When combined with an ADHDer's tendency to procrastinate, for example, hyperfocus can be an invaluable way to meet an important deadline. If hyperfocus occurs at an inopportune time, however, there may be negative social affects.

ADHDers frequently describe alternating between periods of hyperproductivity and hypoactivity. The latter is generally a response to overwhelming emotions, physical sensations, deadlines, or interpersonal demands. It can also result when something is perceived as "looming" on one's schedule. **ADHD paralysis** does not involve physical paralysis, but rather intense brain fog that makes task initiation impossible. It is the brain's attempt to cope by shutting down executive functioning ability. This may involve sleeping, engaging in low-demand activities, or mild dissociation, e.g., scrolling on social media or playing video games.

ADHDers are frequently considered fun people and are often well-liked, perhaps in part due to their tendency to have good conversational skills. Even though ADHDers may appear to be not listening at times, they are usually tracking quite well. It's true that sometimes their attention may be divided in response to environmental conditions, stress, and emotional dysregulation. On these occasions, engaging in effective problem-solving may be a challenge.

Areas of the Brain Involved

- Research using resting-state *functional magnetic resonance imaging (fMRI)* scans reveals that ADHD likely involves variations in connectivity between multiple brain networks, as well as differences in the neurotransmitters dopamine and norepinephrine. ADHD brains are chronically understimulated, which explains why ADHDers tend to chase dopamine in impulsive ways. It also explains why they've earned the reputation of having a short attention span, as ADHDers usually move away from things associated with low dopamine and move towards things associated with high dopamine.[86]
- ADHDers may have reduced availability of the neurotransmitters GABA and serotonin.[87]
- The most important brain structures involved with ADHD are thought to be the prefrontal cortex, the corpus striatum, and the cerebellum.[88,89]

- Studies using *MRI* scans reveal the nucleus accumbens (which plays a crucial role in emotions, motivation, rewards, learning, and motor skills) is reduced in ADHD. Additionally, these studies also show ADHDers have hippocampus and amygdala differences.[90]
- *Single photon emission computed tomography (SPECT)* imagery notes ADHDers have lowered cortical activity in the prefrontal cortex and parietal lobes.[91] This may relate to executive functioning challenges and the processing of somatosensory information. Dr. Daniel Amen reports using SPECT imagery in part to identify seven clinical subtypes of ADHD: *Classic, Inattentive, Over-focused, Temporal Lobe, Limbic, Ring of Fire,* and *Anxious.*[92]
- As with Autism, the relationship of the gut-brain axis to ADHD is starting to receive more attention. This is due to the fact gut microbiota helps produce neurotransmitters.[93]

Prevalence

A 2022 study that reported data from *The National Survey of Children's Health,* a survey which included over 100,000 children ages three to seventeen, estimated that between 6.1% to 16.3% of American children are ADHDers.[94] Global estimates indicate about 5% of children and 6.76% of adults have a diagnosis of ADHD.[95] As previously mentioned, the overlap between ADHD traits and Autistic traits makes differential diagnosis somewhat complicated.[96] Note that prevalence numbers may also vary due to other factors, including: Sociocultural expectations for learning, focus, and behavior; Diagnostic criteria and practices; and racial bias.[97]

Researchers and the general public tend to question whether or not ADHD is currently overdiagnosed in America.[98] Interestingly, though, self-advocates and neuroaffirming therapists assert the ADHD neurotype may actually be underrecognized – especially in females.

DSM-V-TR Considerations

ADHD narrowly escaped being placed in the Disruptive, Impulse-Control, and Conduct Disorders chapter of the *DSM-V-TR.* Instead, it's considered a Neurodevelopmental Disorder. A recent literature review reports the average age to receive an ADHD diagnosis around the world is between 4.9 years old and 9.8 years old.[99] Data from *The National Survey of Children's*

Health regarding children ages four to seventeen indicates the median age of ADHD diagnosis in America is between four and seven years old.[100] It's not uncommon, though, for ADHD traits to remain misunderstood and misidentified until a much later age.

Options for Diagnosis

Evidence supports that ADHD does not always begin in childhood, as the onset of ADHD characteristics can seemingly also occur in adulthood.[101,102] What may appear to be adult-onset ADHD, however, may actually represent an ever-present neurotype that was masked (or simply missed) prior to adulthood. As with some other neurotypes, ADHD may only become clear when a person's environmental and interpersonal demands exceed their capacity to cope.[103,104] Similar to female Autistics, female ADHDers are particularly prone to slipping through the cracks until adulthood – perhaps even as late as the onset of menopause! Researchers suspect that certain hormonal changes may play a role in amplifying inattention, hyperactivity, and impulsivity.[105] Pubescent and postpartum periods are also areas of interest regarding the onset of ADHD challenges.

The *AAP* recommends pediatricians screen patients for ADHD if they are between the ages of four to eighteen years old and have difficulty at school, behavior challenges, inattention, hyperactivity, or impulsivity. However, not all pediatricians provide standardized assessment. A 2014 study discovered the pediatricians it surveyed diagnosed ADHD solely on the basis of their own clinical examination process and experience about 50% of the time.[106]

Pediatricians, and perhaps nurse practitioners, that do utilize standardized measurements may rely on some of the following: *The Attention and Executive Function Rating Inventory (ATTEX), The Childhood Executive Functioning Inventory (CHEXI), The Vanderbilt ADHD Rating Scales, The Child Attention Profile (CAP), The Behavior Assessment System for Children (BASC), The Brown ADD Scales for Children, The Child Behavior Checklist/Teacher Report Form (CBCL),* and *The Conners Rating Scale (CBRS).*[107,108] These all tend to focus on a child's observable behavior as reported by parents and teachers. Additional tests to assess hearing, vision, intelligence, and neurological processes may be used to aid diagnosis.

A developmental pediatrician, neuropsychologist, child psychiatrist, or child psychologist may or may not offer a more comprehensive assessment than a pediatrician. They will likely rely on some of the same tests listed above, which tend to focus on observable behavior. Sometimes, electronic *Continuous Performance Tests (CPTs)* may also be offered to quantify sustained attention.

A neurologist may use *The Neuropsychiatric EEG-Based Assessment Aid System (NEBA)*, a scan that measures brain waves in children ages six through seventeen, or perhaps utilize certain *electroencephalogram (EEG)* microstates to help identify ADHD.[109] These tests do not stand alone as a diagnostic tool, however. Neither do other brain scans such as *SPECT, MRI*, and *Quantitative Electroencephalography (qEEG)*. Nonetheless, they may yield helpful data. Currently, results of any of the above tests are always used as only one part of a comprehensive ADHD assessment.

If not identified sooner, many children receive an initial ADHD diagnosis through the American public school system. When ADHD traits are noticed by an educator or a parent, either party can request that the school system conduct a formal evaluation. IDEA mandates this evaluation is comprehensive and conducted by a multidisciplinary team. These results, as well as information from any private evaluations, are the basis for writing an ADHD child's IEP.

For adults in America, a primary care doctor may diagnose ADHD. A more official battery of standardized assessments, however, is generally only offered by a psychiatrist, psychologist, neurologist, or neuropsychologist. This process may include some of the following tests, which tend to focus on behavior: *The Adult ADHD Clinical Diagnostic Scale (ACDS), The Brown Executive Function/Attention Scales, The World Health Organization ADHD Self-Report Scale (ADHD-ASRS v1.1)*, and *The ADHD Lifespan Functioning Interview (ALFI)*.

Whether or not a LPC, LMFT, LCSW, or their equivalent can provide an official diagnosis of ADHD is a matter of debate. This ability varies by state. Additionally, the usefulness of a diagnosis given by a professional at this level of education varies. Requirements related to the receipt of workplace accommodations, Social Security payments, Medicaid reimbursement, commercial insurance reimbursement, and other benefits tend to mandate diagnosis from a higher source.

A variety of free online self-screening tools for adults are available to promote insight, such as: *The World Health Organization ADHD Self-Report Scale (ADHD-ASRS v1.1), The ADHD Self-Report Scale for DSM-5 (ASRS-5)*, and *The Executive Skills Questionnaire (ESQ)*.

Options for Support

An ADHDer who is struggling in any or all of the following areas may benefit from ethical intervention: Learning, attention, executive functioning skills, emotion regulation, sensory integration, vocational skills, interpersonal skills, and more. Co-occurring medical conditions may also need attention. The following professionals may be especially helpful:

- Neurologist.
- LPC, LMFT, LCSW, or equivalent therapy professional.
- Vocational counselor.
- ADHD coach / Executive functioning coach.
- Professional organizer.
- Registered dietician.
- Sleep specialist.

Other Considerations

Rejection Sensitive Dysphoria (RSD) is a risk factor for depression.[110] It involves frequent, brief bursts of extreme difficulty coping with actual or perceived criticism to the extent that mood and self-esteem are affected. Anyone can experience RSD. However, it is very often associated with ADHD.[111] Persons with RSD have heightened emotional sensitivity and intrusive thoughts related to social rejection. They tend to misinterpret the thoughts, feelings, and actions of others. Negative interpretation bias reinforces their negative core beliefs about themselves, leaving them feeling chronically insecure. To defend against intense shame, people with RSD tend to display tendencies towards perfectionism, conflict avoidance, and people-pleasing.

Deficient Emotional Self-Regulation (DESR) is a term coined in 2015 by Dr. Russell Barkley to describe emotional impulsivity plus self-regulation challenges. It's not currently included within the diagnostic criteria for ADHD, however, despite its increased recognition as a core feature.[112] ADHDers tend to find self-soothing to be extremely challenging at times. Improving frustration tolerance, learning delayed gratification strategies, and reducing impulsivity are usually important goals for any therapist who supports individuals with DESR. Note that DESR may also occur with other neurotypes, such as Autism and Dyslexia.[113,114]

Time Blindness is a common experience for many ADHDers that likely has a neurological explanation.[115] Autistic individuals may struggle with this as well.[116] Time blindness means a person struggles with time management to an extreme degree – particularly in regards to estimating the amount of time it will take to complete an activity. This can also explain some ND persons' lack of specificity when discussing the timing or other details of past events; Things either happen "right now" or "not right now." The insula and hippocampus may be involved in these cognitive processes.

Body-Focused Repetitive Behavior (BFRB) such as skin-picking, check or lip biting, and nail biting may occur more frequently among ADHDers.[117]

Dyslexia

History[118]

- Dyslexia used to be called *Word Blindness* in the late 19th century. Its nearly exclusive association with brain functionality (versus a disease process, mental disorder, or social problem) occurred relatively early in comparison to some other neurotypes. In 1877, German neurologist Adolf Kussmaul noted extreme reading impairment in some persons persisted despite adequate reading instruction and lack of visual impairment. German physician Rudolf Berlin first used the term *Dyslexia* in 1887 to describe these challenges.

- Case studies and investigations into the relationship between Dyslexia and sight occurred in the early 20th century by James Hinshelwood, Samuel Torrey Orton, Clement Launay, and others. The theory that Dyslexics may have a "lack of cerebral dominance" was proposed and refuted during this time.

- In 1952, the *DSM-I* categorized Dyslexia as a *Learning Disorder* within the Special Symptom subcategory of Personality Disorders. Interest in the cognitive development of persons with Dyslexia peaked in the 1960s. In this period, neurologist Macdonald Critchley and psychologist Tim Miles opened a London facility called *The Word Blindness Centre*.

- Dyslexia's official definition was set by *The World Federation of Neurology's Research Group on Developmental Dyslexia and World Illiteracy* in 1968. Dyslexic children were agreed to experience an innate cognitive disability independent of both their intelligence and opportunities to receive reading instruction. That year, the *DSM-II* removed Dyslexia from the Personality Disorders section and called it a *Specific Learning Disruption* instead.

- Pivotal research about the causes of Dyslexia and how best to educate Dyslexic children flourished in the 1970s. Two seminal works, Critchley's *The Dyslexic Child* and Sandhya Naidoo's *Specific Dyslexia*, are still referenced today. However, Dyslexia was frequently considered an excuse made by middle- and upper-class parents to justify their children's inability to perform in school. This myth persists in geographic locations without accurate information and supportive resources.

- *The Education for All Handicapped Children Act of 1975* defined the term *Learning Disability* in America, inclusive of Dyslexic characteristics. It would not be until 2008, though, that *The Americans with Disabilities Act Amendments Act (ADAAA)* added this to the list of things an employer cannot discriminate against within the workplace.

- In 1980, the *DSM-III* designated the diagnosis *Developmental Reading Disorder* within the Primary Disorders in Childhood and Adolescence section. At this time, this was to be diagnosed by a professional based on a person's slow reading, reduced reading comprehension, and word distortions as compared to the expected norms for their age and IQ.

- Neuroimaging advancements in the 1980s and 1990s provided insight into the brain-based features of Dyslexia, as it became known to involve distinct differences in the phonological, auditory, and magnocellular areas of the brain. These differences cause the brain's "reading circuit" to be altered. The *DSM-IV* (1994) added the term *Reading Disorder* to a Learning Disorders category and recognized this could continue into adulthood.

- In 2000, the *DSM-IV-TR* noted that *Reading Disorder* is sometimes not diagnosed until adulthood. It also acknowledged there may be accompanying social or employment difficulties. Diagnosis at this time required a discrepancy of over two standard deviations between a person's measured reading achievements and their IQ score.

- In 2013, the *DSM-V* listed a Specific Learning Disorders category in which it designated a *Specific Learning Disability with Reading Deficit* that existed along a continuum of mild to severe. Dyslexia was formally stated to be a neurodevelopmental disorder rooted in one's biology, yet impacted by epigenetics and socio-environmental factors. The IQ score and achievement discrepancy criterion was eliminated at this time. Instead, four new criteria were introduced: At least one of six listed symptoms of learning difficulty persists despite customized education for at least six months, academic skills have been proven impaired as compared to age norms, symptom onset occurred during childhood or early adulthood, and certain intellectual and physical disorders plus adverse social conditions have been ruled out.

- Currently, Dyslexia is thought to run in families due to its link to specific genes which determine the brain's ability to process language.[119] The *DSM-V-TR* categorizes it as a Specific Learning Disorder that is neurodevelopmental in nature.

Strength-Based Description[120,121]

Dyslexic children have marked difficulty learning letters and connecting them to the sounds they make. Because decoding words does not come automatically, learning to read through conventional methods of education is not effective. This also makes it extremely difficult to learn how to write, spell, and form fluent sentences.[122] Children who are provided access to customized instruction and social support often greatly improve these areas. Nonetheless, some reading, writing, and spelling challenges can still persist across their lifespan.

It's a myth that Dyslexics lack intelligence; Dyslexic persons, by definition, have typical to high intelligence. They do, though, experience varying degrees of cognitive challenges related to short-term recall and sequencing. Some may also have brain-based difficulty maintaining their physical balance or coordinating their body movements.[123] This may make them appear clumsy to others.

Research shows that Dyslexic brains work far harder than NT brains to complete language-based tasks.[124] Grammar and vocabulary, in particular, may be especially draining. Yet, society rarely recognizes how much effort is involved with doing the kinds of tasks NT brains do easily and automatically. This can lead Dyslexic persons to feel misunderstood and wrongfully criticized. For example, despite their best efforts, poor spelling in emails or texts may be mislabeled as "sloppy" by others.

Understandably, Dyslexic persons can experience anxiety and low self-esteem within learning environments that lack specialized instruction or social environments that lack understanding. They may suffer when incorrectly presumed to be uneducated or unintelligent, or when accused of making errors due to "carelessly rushing through" language-based tasks. Support from parents, teachers, and peers is essential to both a Dyslexic child's academic success and their overall mental health.[125]

Some Dyslexic persons may find participating in verbal conversations challenging. This is due to not being able to easily recall the kinds of words they'd like to use to express themselves. Most others, however, excel conversationally. Similarly, some Dyslexics may have difficulty processing the spoken words of others, while others do not experience this challenge.

At school, home, and the workplace, simple accommodations can make a big difference for Dyslexic persons. For example, a teacher allowing the use of a computer to create an interactive presentation instead of requiring a lengthy written report can allow a Dyslexic person's talents to shine. Indeed, the development of specific kinds of assisted technology has allowed many Dyslexic persons to thrive.

Many, but not all, Dyslexics tend to be highly creative and artistically inclined. Studies confirm high rates of Dyslexia among art school students.[126,127]

Areas of the Brain Involved

- Structurally, Dyslexic brains differ from others with regard to the cerebral cortex, thalamus, and other regions. The left hemisphere has been found to be underactive, while both the primary motor cortex and anterior insula have been found to be overactive.[128]
- *MRI* scans reveal gray matter differences in Dyslexic persons, while *positron emission tomography (PET)* scans show abnormal Broca's area activation.[129]
- In Dyslexics, the volume of the right anterior lobe of the cerebellum is usually noted to differ from other people.[130]
- The brain stems of Dyslexic people tend to show more variability in auditory response to speech.[131]

Prevalence

Dyslexia is common, with most estimates placing between 5% and 10% of the American population as Dyslexic.[132] However, some researchers think up to 20% of people may actually be Dyslexic.[133] Researchers emphasize the importance of screening persons across all levels of reading ability and achievement, not just those who outwardly struggle.[134]

DSM-V-TR Considerations

The *DSM-V-TR* considers Dyslexia both a Specific Learning Disorder and a Neurodevelopmental Disorder.

Options for Diagnosis

A review of 11 studies conducted in English-speaking countries between 2013 and 2021 revealed the need for universal guidelines for psychologists in order to more accurately diagnose Dyslexia around the world.[135] Not only does a lack of diagnostic precision cause Dyslexia to be underidentified and undersupported in impoverished areas, it also explains why Dyslexia can be missed until High School or later – even in relatively affluent areas.[136,137]

The diagnostic process varies worldwide. For example, there is no single test used to diagnose Dyslexia in America. Diagnosis is a process that generally involves coordination between the public school system, parents, and other professionals. Shockingly, though, at least one Western country (Denmark) relies on a single electronically-administered test to identify Dyslexia.[138] This approach is generally considered insufficient.

Because Dyslexia is the most common learning disability, American public schools are legally required to identify children who may be showing early signs. Some or all of the following may be noted by teachers between Kindergarten and First Grade: Difficulty learning whole words or parts of words, matching words with their meanings, speaking certain letter sounds or blends, reading out loud, rhyming, or learning to write.

Screening tests such as *The Predictive Assessment of Reading (PAR)*, *Dynamic Indicators of Basic Early Literacy Skills (DIBELS)*, *The Texas Primary Reading Inventory (TPRI)*, *The Shaywitz DyslexiaScreen (SDS)*, and *The AIMSweb Screening Assessments* may be used by the public school system to help identify students who may be Dyslexic as early as possible. Those considered at risk will not be given a diagnosis at this point, but will instead receive specialized support during school hours. Data is collected to determine if this support results in academic improvement. If not, the diagnostic process may begin alongside a formal IEP process.

The International Dyslexia Association recommends that any official evaluation for Dyslexia be comprehensive, such as what is offered by a licensed educational psychologist. Their report should consider information collected from parents, teachers, a speech language pathologist, a school psychologist, and other professionals (such as a neurologist) as needed. A vision and hearing screening is necessary, too, along with standardized measurements of attention and performance on language-based tasks.

One-on-one specialized education for Dyslexic students in most public-school classrooms within most U.S. states is provided by either a special education teacher, school psychologist, or SLP.

New tests, such as *The Dyslexia Marker Test for Children (Dysmate-C)*, are being developed all the time.[139] In the near future, research indicates neuroimaging techniques such as *fMRI* and *EEG* may be helpful in diagnosing Dyslexia.[140] Eye movement trackers may also prove helpful.[141]

Options for Support

- School psychologist.
- SLP.
- Special education teacher.
- Certified Structured Literacy Dyslexia Specialist (C-SLDS).
- Orton-Gillingham certified educator or tutor.
- Accredited multisensory structured language educator or tutor.
- Neurologist.
- Licensed educational psychologist.
- Neuropsychologist.
- OT.
- Other learning specialist or reading specialist.

Other Considerations

Stealth Dyslexia, also known as *Hidden Dyslexia*, is a term first used in 2005 by Brock and Fernette Eide to refer to challenges otherwise masked by intellectual Giftedness. A person with Stealth Dyslexia usually expresses themselves far better when talking than in writing. This is because they have some of the same brain-wiring configurations associated with classic Dyslexia. They, too, struggle with word decoding, handwriting, spelling, and may even have issues with visual/auditory processing and motor skills. Yet, their reading ability and academic achievements can still sometimes appear typical. Why? Advanced problem-solving skills and creativity from their Giftedness allows them to overcompensate. This coping strategy may be successful only until a person experiences elevated stress or is faced with very difficult language-based tasks . . . making Stealth Dyslexia more visible.

Dyslexia may or may not co-occur with **Dysgraphia**, a specific learning disorder involving spatial awareness difficulties and impaired handwriting.[142]

Dyslexia may or may not co-occur with **Dyscalculia**, a specific learning disability involving impaired mathematical comprehension.[143]

Sensory Processing Disorder (SPD)

History

- Dr. Jean Ayres first coined the term *Sensory Integration Dysfunction* in the 1960s and 1970s in her work as an OT, psychologist, and neuroscientist.

She developed Sensory Integration Theory, assessments, and treatment interventions. She noted children with Sensory Integration Dysfunction had poor motor planning, difficulty using both sides of their body at the same time, tactile defensiveness, visual processing differences, and auditory-language problems.

- Three broad categories of *Sensory Processing Disorder (SPD)* were introduced by Dr. Lucy Jane Miller and colleagues during the early 2000s: *Sensory Modulation Disorder*, *Sensory Discrimination Disorder*, and *Sensory-Based Motor Disorder*.[144] The modulation category included three subtypes: *Sensory Over-Responsive*, *Sensory Under-Responsive*, and *Sensory Seeking/Craving*. The motor disorder category included two subtypes: *Postural Disorder* and *Dyspraxia*. Miller's text that describes these categories, *Sensational Kids*, remains essential reading material today.[145]

- In 2012, the *AAP* recommended that SPD not be given as a stand-alone diagnosis and encouraged caution with its assorted treatments, e.g., OT. Pediatricians at the time were encouraged to promote comprehensive assessment for Autism, ADHD, and other developmental diagnoses that may account for a child's sensory processing issues.[146]

- Despite the work of Miller and others, SPD was not included as a stand-alone diagnosis when the *DSM-V* came out in 2013. Today, it's still not widely recognized as a neurotype, stand-alone medical condition, or mental disorder. Nonetheless, neuroimaging studies support SPD as a valid form of neurodivergence and clinical guidelines for diagnosis and support (usually by an OT) do exist. SPD is currently thought to be at least partially hereditary based on twin studies.[147]

Strength-Based Description

Each SPDer experiences different day-to-day challenges according to the specific way their brain receives, organizes, and evaluates external sensory information and internal sensations. Some SPDers feel chronically overwhelmed to the point that attending school, work, and social functions seem impossible without significant support. Others may cope quite well on their own, only experiencing occasional distress. Whether or not SPD co-occurs with ADHD, Autism, or any other neurotype makes a big difference in this discussion.

Some SPDers have difficulty with only one sensory system in particular, but most will experience difficulty with several systems at once. Additionally, the speed at which sensory processing occurs varies from person to person.

Some SPDers need much more time to process what is going on around them within a multisensory environment than others. A SPDer's personal challenges can fluctuate rapidly based on environmental context, or stay relatively constant over time regardless.

As children, some adult SPDers may have required targeted support to balance their body posture and improve their motor planning skills such that running, writing, and completing multi-step tasks were possible. Others needed support to differentiate between the specific characteristics of stimuli. For example, they may not have been able to automatically distinguish between different types of wet foods; All wet foods were perceived as "yucky." Attending OT may have helped them decipher tasty wet food from that which was genuinely undesirable to eat. Remember, though, that many adult SPDers may have never received support for these kinds of struggles at all. In fact, they may even have been punished for having these challenges. Perhaps this is part of the reason why research indicates adults with high sensory sensitivity tend to display attachment insecurity in their relationships.[148]

SPDers don't always respond to interpersonal or environmental stimuli like the NT majority. Hypersensitivity may result in a SPDer deeming some sensations aversive, even in tiny amounts. Sensory overload can result in any number of defensive behaviors and strong emotions. Hypersensitivity can also be pleasant at times, too. Some SPDers can have exuberant reactions to small measures of positive stimuli! (Indeed, having higher sensitivity to the beauty of music, art, body movements, or tactile sensations can induce unparalleled joy.) On the other hand, hyposensitivity to stimuli may allow a SPDer to tolerate extreme pain, extreme heat, or extreme cold and must be monitored carefully to avoid injury.

Sensory-based motor coordination issues, issues with eating, issues with wearing certain types of clothing, difficulty with touch or sound, and other concerns can linger into adulthood and/or be lifelong. Fortunately, neuroplasticity allows some individuals with SPD to greatly benefit from OT. For kids this usually looks like interventions that resemble play, wherein a clinician actively supports the child while interacting with people and objects in a multisensory environment. For adults, this also may involve interacting with people and objects in a multisensory environment, but in a more age-appropriate way. OT may result in a SPDer forming new neural connections that improve sensory integration, thus reducing distress.

Developing and maintaining a **sensory diet** is an excellent way to cope with SPD challenges. This is especially true when combined with social support. Unlike past eras, a wide variety of sensory coping tools exist in stores today: Weighted blankets, swings, stretchy bands, ear defenders, etc. Whenever possible, using strong self-advocacy skills is crucial (e.g., asking to take a break from a conversation, carefully designing one's own work schedule around sensory needs, seeking appropriate stimulation when understimulated, etc.).

Areas of the Brain Involved

- Neuroimaging reveals SPDers have differences in white matter located in the posterior regions of the brain that perform sensory processing functions.[149]
- A study that looked at *EEG* activity showed brain differences between NT children and children with SPD. Researchers were able to correctly identify a child with SPD based on their *EEG* alone about 86% of the time.[150]

Prevalence

Researchers estimate that between 5% and 16% of American children have SPD.[151]

DSM-V-TR Considerations

At this time, the fact that SPD is still not in the latest version of the *DSM* remains controversial.[152]

Options for Diagnosis

Children in American public schools are not screened for SPD on an individual or group level, nor do children with this diagnosis alone generally qualify for an IEP or 504 Plan. This is because the school system does not consider stand-alone SPD a learning disability, mental health disorder, or medical condition. Although accommodations listed within a child's IEP or 504 Plan may include sensory considerations, they must relate to a child's primary diagnosis of ADHD, Autism, etc.

An OT with specialized training can offer any of the following assessments, along with clinical observation, to provide a diagnosis of SPD: *The Sensory Integration and Praxis Test (SIPT), The Sensory Processing Measure (SPM),* and *The Sensory Profile (SP).* Self, teacher, and parent report questionnaires are also typically used.

Options for Support

- Sensory Integration Therapy (SI).
- Occupational therapy.

Other Considerations

The term **Highly Sensitive Person (HSP)** has recently come into popular use by the general public, clinicians, and researchers. It generally refers to a person who is more attuned to internal and external stimuli than others, who takes more time to think through their own strong emotions than others, and who displays intense empathy. Society casually associates HSPs with female introverts who are "moody" and sometimes codependent. Clinically, however, the moniker focuses more on sensory sensitivity and emotion regulation challenges. Some of these traits can be measured by an assessment called *The Highly Sensitive Person Scale (HSPS)*. Critics of the HSP term argue that its use may cover up what may be really going on, e.g., Autism, ADHD, SPD, etc.

Giftedness

History[153,154]

- *Giftedness* first became associated with high IQ after this quantitative measurement was created in the early 20th century. Society had previously associated *genius* with whatever talent was deemed amazing and useful at the time, or perhaps posthumously.
- American psychologist Dr. Lewis Terman's 1925 book, *Genetic Studies of Genius*, described *Gifted* qualifications very narrowly – an IQ score within the top 1%. Terman's eugenic and racist beliefs emphasized White supremacy and the importance of heredity to intellect. He advocated for selective breeding in society as a whole, and racial segregation within the educational system. Meanwhile, Leta Stetter Hollingworth emphasized the importance of one's educational environment to the development of intellect in her 1926 book, *Gifted Children: Their Nature and Nurture*. She also advocated for American women to be viewed as intelligent as men. In 1935, the work of Dr. Martin Jenkins proved that Black students were just as intelligent as White students.

- Although the definition of Giftedness continued to emphasize IQ for quite some time, there were also attempts to broaden the concept. During the 1950s, for example, Ann F. Isaacs created the *National Association for Gifted Children (NAGC)* to recognize and support Gifted children's varying abilities and needs. To this end, influential works emerged such as Paul Witty's *The Gifted Child* and Virgil S. Ward's *Theory of Differential Education for the Gifted*.
- Between 1964 and 1972, Kazimierz Dabrowski created *The Theory of Positive Disintegration* to explain Gifted development on an individual and societal level.[155,156] He discussed five forms of *overexcitability (OE)* associated with a Gifted person's inner experience: *Physical or Psychomotor OE, Sensual OE, Imaginational OE, Intellectual OE,* and *Emotional OE*. Each of these categories represents a way of responding to stimuli to a higher degree than what is typical. A Gifted individual's OEs were not only thought to contribute to their own success and distress, but also to the potential advancement or detriment of humanity itself.
- In 1971, the United States government defined Giftedness (as it pertains to education) for the first time. While this formally recognized that Gifted learners can benefit from differentiated instruction, it stopped short of mandating Gifted education in all public schools.
- Joseph Renzulli's *Three-Ring Conception of Giftedness*, proposed in 1978, emphasized the interaction between three clusters of skills: Above average ability, creativity, and task commitment.[157]
- The 1980s brought the diversity of Gifted persons, along with their unique needs, into focus. The organization *Supporting Emotional Needs of the Gifted (SENG)* was created in 1981.
- In 1982, Annemarie Roeper chose to highlight the tendency for Gifted persons to experience intense emotions by creating categories of Gifted children that each represent a distinct form of coping: *The Perfectionist, The Child/Adult, The Winner of the Competition, The Self-Critic,* and *The Well-Integrated Child*.[158] Howard Gardner's 1983 *Theory of Multiple Intelligences* also provided greater distance from older notions that centered Giftedness solely around IQ.
- George Betts and Maureen Neihart described six different profiles of young *Gifted and Talented* persons in 1988: *Successful, Challenging, Underground, Dropouts, Double-labeled,* and *Autonomous*.[159] These categories were based on each group's feelings, attitudes, behaviors, and needs while at home and at school.
- *The National Research Center on the Gifted and Talented* was created in 1990. Shortly after, in 1991, *The Columbus Group* established a new definition for

Giftedness inclusive of asynchronous development, advanced cognitive abilities, and overall "intensity." This definition advocated for Gifted students to receive specialized care and instruction.

- From the early 1990s until now, Deirdre Lovecky has brought attention to such issues as the moral and spiritual sensitivity of Gifted children, the peer relationships of Gifted youth, and the needs of Gifted children who may be 2e.[160,161,162,163]

- Today, Gifted education in America remains each state's decision versus a federal mandate. Each state's own Board of Education determines whether Gifted education is mandatory, the definition of a Gifted student, how to test for Giftedness, and what services to provide. The federal government decides what grants, initiatives, and programs to offer funding. The existence and quality of Gifted education services varies widely across geographic regions despite *The National Standards in Gifted and Talented Education* set forth by the NAGC. Minority students, 2e students, and impoverished students generally have the worst opportunities regardless of location. A variety of national studies and advocacy movements have attempted to draw attention to these inequalities.

Strength-Based Description

Gifted persons tend to seek out and create exciting new ideas, learn a lot of new things in a lot of areas very quickly, make interesting connections between historical facts and present or even futuristic concepts, and display an abundance of curiosity. However, they also tend to have very high standards for themselves. They may experience extreme frustration, shame, or self-doubt when something does not come as easily to them as other things have in the past.

Gifted children and adults can experience high intellect or specialized ability in any number of ways. One's Giftedness is not always obvious to others, however. Thankfully, today it is generally understood that Giftedness is not perfectly synonymous with high achievement and/or exceptional performance. Some Gifted children actually underachieve due to low social support, burn out, boredom, lack of specialized learning opportunities in their school environment, or other factors.[164]

A person may be Gifted in one or more areas: Cognitive intelligence, emotional intelligence, athleticism, musicality, artistry, mathematics, writing, languages, etc. All the ways humans may be Gifted are too numerous to list!

When exact quantification is necessary, a loose standard to identify Giftedness may refer to a person's performance within the top 10% (as compared to applicable norms) in whatever specific area is being measured. For scholarly research purposes and some educational purposes, however, Giftedness today is also, at least partially, measured by the Wechsler Intelligence Scale. IQ scores 130 and above are deemed Gifted. This represents the upper end of scores within a population's normal distribution along a bell curve.

Many other quantitative and subjective forms of assessment may be used to define Giftedness. The most comprehensive ones will consider a Gifted person's emotional experience and unique talents in addition to their academic ability. For example, a common characteristic of most Gifted persons is their "intensity." A therapist who is unfamiliar with this Gifted trait, unfortunately, may mistake this for an indicator of ADHD or Bipolar.

Gifted persons tend to display a "spiky" scoring profile when they take a battery of standardized tests. This reflects **asynchronous development**, a term that usually refers to the fact that a Gifted child's overall skill set is highly variable. They usually excel off the charts in a few areas, but score relatively low in others. This term also refers to the observable phenomenon that Gifted kids often present older than their chronological age due to advanced vocabulary and interests. Reminders of their actual age do exist, however, and must be thoughtfully acknowledged. A sweet example of this occurs when a six-year-old Gifted child checks out two books from the library: A college-level textbook on geology, and also a *Curious George* picture book. Validating this child's varied capacities and interests (instead of criticizing them) is important to promoting healthy self-esteem. Sadly, parents who are unfamiliar with Giftedness tend to express chronic confusion or frustration regarding their child's asynchronicity. This can result in demanding more emotional maturity than a child is able to provide.

Gifted persons may experience more **existential depression** than others, or perhaps simply a perpetual sense of being out-of-place.[165] This is often due to a combination of their strong emotions, divergent and fast-paced thoughts, difficulty finding a like-minded set of friends, and a profound and unrelenting awareness of the world's injustices.[166]

Some Gifted persons learn to mask their intellectual ability, vivid imagination, and other talents to escape unwanted attention or bullying. They may also minimize their own achievements to fit in, or perhaps to minimize their own social anxiety.[167] Gifted persons who find a social group wherein all forms of intellect are utilized and appreciated, though, may feel perfectly fine expressing themselves.

Areas of the Brain Involved

- Neuroimaging shows that Gifted brains have high metabolic activity throughout, as well as heightened sensory activation.[168] This may explain why many Gifted persons tend to experience SPD.
- Gifted brains tend to have neural networks that integrate well with each other in flexible, efficient ways.[169,170]
- The brains of Gifted persons tend to have greater volume in the frontal lobes, temporal lobes, parietal lobes, and occipital lobes. They also have increased white and gray matter.[171]

Prevalence

According to the normal distribution of a population's intelligence as measured by IQ score, only 2% will score in the Gifted range of 130 or above. When using various definitions of Giftedness that expand beyond IQ, however, the NAGC estimates between 6% and 10% of American K-12 students may actually be Gifted. This represents between three and five million children. Yet, this updated estimate still may not be accurate because equal access to Gifted assessment is not always provided to minority students. Currently, there is no standardized way to collect prevalence data of Giftedness in America on a national level.[172]

DSM-V-TR Considerations

Giftedness is not listed in the *DSM*. It is, however, recognized to exist at the upper end of a cognitive continuum.

Options for Diagnosis

In the American public school system, schools that offer Gifted classes use standardized tests to determine which students qualify. These tests may be offered equally to all students or only those who perform academically superior. Qualitative tests, such as classroom observation and surveys from parents and teachers, are also usually considered. Depending on the school's unique definition of Giftedness, other forms of assessment (e.g., reviewing a child's art portfolio, athletic performance, musical ability, etc.) may be considered. Some schools also strongly consider a child's level of intrinsic motivation, creativity, and other factors.

Any of the following tests may be used by a school psychologist or other psychologist: *The Comprehensive Test of Nonverbal Intelligence (CTONI-2), The Universal Nonverbal Intelligence Scale (UNIT-2), The Stanford-Binet 5th edition (SB-5), The Wechsler Preschool Primary Scale of Intelligence (WPPSI-IV), The Wechsler Intelligence Scale for Children (WISC-V), The Woodcock-Johnson Tests of Cognitive Abilities (WJ-IV Cog), The Cognitive Abilities Test (CogAT),* or *the Differential Ability Scales (DAS-2).* Regarding nonverbal tests, any of the following may be used: *The Naglieri Nonverbal Ability Test (NNAT-3), The Comprehensive Test of Nonverbal Intelligence (CTONI-2), The Universal Nonverbal Intelligence Scale (UNIT-2),* or *The Otis-Lennon School Ability Test (OLSAT 8).*

There is an urgent need to identify Gifted children who are also 2e or multiexceptional.[173] Once identified, an IEP or 504 Plan may be put in place.

Undiagnosed, potentially Gifted adults seeking personal insight may benefit from a comprehensive evaluation by a psychologist or neuropsychologist.

Options for Support

- Gifted specialists within the school system, e.g., Gifted education teacher, special education teacher, etc.
- School psychologist.
- School guidance counselor.
- National or state-level organizations such as *SENG* or *The Davidson Institute.*
- LPC, LMFT, LCSW, or their equivalent who understands the emotional and intellectual depth of Gifted clients.
- Peer groups and/or enrichment opportunities based on advanced interests and abilities.

Other Considerations

The concept of **Imposter Syndrome** was introduced in 1978 by psychologists Pauline Rose Clance and Suzanne Imes. Many Gifted and/or 2e persons experience a strong sense of inadequacy due to the persistent belief they'll be exposed as a fraud. This chronic self-doubt and insecurity results in an inability to award themselves appropriate credit for both their innate strengths and worldly accomplishments. Persons who struggle with Imposter Syndrome feel they don't actually deserve what they've rightfully achieved. They fear others may find out the shameful "truth" about who they really are. Personal success is often attributed to luck, fate, or another external factor.

Glossary of Bolded Terms

Asynchronous Development   A hallmark of Giftedness. Refers to the noticeable variations between a Gifted child's emotional age, chronological age, and intellectual age. It can also refer to big differences in skill levels across areas, e.g., high achievement in mathematics but very poor hand-eye coordination.

Code-Switching   When a ND person changes aspects of their own expression, style of dress, communication, and behavior as they move between spaces that are predominantly NT versus predominantly ND.

Diathesis-Stress Model   Also known as the Vulnerability-Stress Model. This widely accepted paradigm acknowledges the interplay of nature and nurture. It states that mental and physical disorders develop when genetic predisposition combines with stressful conditions in one's environment.

Epigenetics   The study of how a person's specific context influences the expression (or suppression) of certain genes.

Existential Depression   Also known as Existential Dread. Refers to an overwhelming sense of anxiety about the state of the world, and one's role within it. A person experiencing this may question their identity and purpose, struggle to make meaning of their experiences, and have deep questions about life.

Hyperfocus   The tendency for both ADHDers and Autistics to intensely hone in on a strong interest, for a given period of time, to the exclusion of nearly everything else.

Identity   A complex grouping of personal beliefs, values, characteristics, self-attributions, and other factors that form one's overall sense of personhood. Identity formation is a flexible, ongoing process that unfolds across the lifespan.

Invisible Disabilities   Physical, cognitive, emotional, or neurological challenges that go unseen by the public.

Masking   The conscious or subconscious act of either hiding or minimizing one's ND traits and/or behaviors to conform to NT standards. This defensive strategy may be necessary for safety or the avoidance of negative social consequences.

Multiexceptional Having three or more distinct neurotypes simultaneously.

Neurodevelopmental Disorder The Medical Model dictates this as any physical, psychological, or mental illness affecting a typical growth pattern for the brain. Areas of dysfunction are noted to involve communication, learning, memory, feelings, and impulsivity.

Neurotype The name of a recognized group of co-occurring neural features that function together as the "operating system" of a person's brain.

Neurosubtypes Named subcategories within a particular neurotype category grouped according to features noted through advanced neuroimaging approaches.

Personality A person's unique character traits that distinguish them from others. Some parts of one's personality may be inborn and fixed, and some parts may be flexible.

Sensory Diet Refers to ND person's personal toolbox of coping skills used to identify and maintain their optimal sensory balance.

Temperament A person's inborn, general predisposition.

Twice-Exceptional (2e) Having two neurotypes simultaneously. This is most commonly used to describe Giftedness plus another neurotype such as Autism, ADHD, or Dyslexia.

Unmasking The conscious choice to end the use of masking as a defensive coping skill and reveal one's own ND traits and behaviors that had been previously hidden. Unmasking may or may not be emotionally or physically safe to do; Unmasking is always a personal choice.

Notes

1 Ortug, A., Guo, Y., Feldman, H. A., Ou, Y., Dieuveuil, H., Baumer, N. T., . . . & Takahashi, E. (2022). Human fetal brain magnetic resonance imaging (MRI) tells future emergence of autism spectrum disorders. *The FASEB Journal, 36.*

2 Rudling, M., Nyström, P., Bölte, S., & Falck-Ytter, T. (2022). Larger pupil dilation to nonsocial sounds in infants with subsequent autism diagnosis. *Journal of Child Psychology and Psychiatry, 63*(7), 793–801.

3 Auerbach, J. G., Landau, R., Berger, A., Arbelle, S., Faroy, M., & Karplus, M. (2005). Neonatal behavior of infants at familial risk for ADHD. *Infant Behavior and Development, 28*(2), 220–224.

4 Miller, M., Iosif, A. M., Bell, L. J., Farquhar-Leicester, A., Hatch, B., Hill, A., . . . & Ozonoff, S. (2021). Can familial risk for ADHD be detected in the first two years of life? *Journal of Clinical Child & Adolescent Psychology, 50*(5), 619–631.

5　Xie, S., Karlsson, H., Dalman, C., Widman, L., Rai, D., Gardner, R. M., . . . & Lee, B. K. (2020). The familial risk of autism spectrum disorder with and without intellectual disability. *Autism Research*, *13*(12), 2242–2250.

6　Ijomone, O. M., Olung, N. F., Akingbade, G. T., Okoh, C. O., & Aschner, M. (2020). Environmental influence on neurodevelopmental disorders: Potential association of heavy metal exposure and autism. *Journal of Trace Elements in Medicine and Biology*, *62*, 126638.

7　Moore, S., Paalanen, L., Melymuk, L., Katsonouri, A., Kolossa-Gehring, M., & Tolonen, H. (2022). The association between ADHD and environmental chemicals—A scoping review. *International Journal of Environmental Research and Public Health*, *19*(5), 2849.

8　Tessari, L., Angriman, M., Díaz-Román, A., Zhang, J., Conca, A., & Cortese, S. (2022). Association between exposure to pesticides and ADHD or autism spectrum disorder: A systematic review of the literature. *Journal of Attention Disorders*, *26*(1), 48–71.

9　Gabis, L. V., Attia, O. L., Goldman, M., Barak, N., Tefera, P., Shefer, S., . . . & Lerman-Sagie, T. (2022). The myth of vaccination and autism spectrum. *European Journal of Paediatric Neurology*, *36*, 151–158.

10　Taylor, L. E., Swerdfeger, A. L., & Eslick, G. D. (2014). Vaccines are not associated with autism: An evidence-based meta-analysis of case-control and cohort studies. *Vaccine*, *32*(29), 3623–3629.

11　Sumich, A., Heym, N., Lenzoni, S., & Hunter, K. (2022). Gut microbiome-brain axis and inflammation in temperament, personality and psychopathology. *Current Opinion in Behavioral Sciences*, *44*, 101101.

12　Beck, J. S., Lundwall, R. A., Gabrielsen, T., Cox, J. C., & South, M. (2020). Looking good but feeling bad:"Camouflaging" behaviors and mental health in women with autistic traits. *Autism*, *24*(4), 809–821.

13　Cassidy, S. A., Gould, K., Townsend, E., Pelton, M., Robertson, A. E., & Rodgers, J. (2020). Is camouflaging autistic traits associated with suicidal thoughts and behaviours? Expanding the interpersonal psychological theory of suicide in an undergraduate student sample. *Journal of Autism and Developmental Disorders*, *50*(10), 3638–3648.

14　Al Dahhan, N. Z., Halverson, K., Peek, C. P., Wilmot, D., D'Mello, A., Romeo, R. R., . . . & Christodoulou, J. A. (2022). Dissociating executive function and ADHD influences on reading ability in children with dyslexia. *Cortex*, *153*, 126–142.

15　Serrallach, B., Groß, C., Bernhofs, V., Engelmann, D., Benner, J., Gündert, N., . . . & Seither-Preisler, A. (2016). Neural biomarkers for dyslexia, ADHD, and ADD in the auditory cortex of children. *Frontiers in Neuroscience*, *10*, 324.

16　Hayashi, W., Hanawa, Y., Yuriko, I., Aoyagi, K., Saga, N., Nakamura, D., & Iwanami, A. (2022). ASD symptoms in adults with ADHD: A preliminary study using the ADOS-2. *European Archives of Psychiatry and Clinical Neuroscience*, *272*(2), 217–232.

17　Rommelse, N. N., Franke, B., Geurts, H. M., Hartman, C. A., & Buitelaar, J. K. (2010). Shared heritability of attention-deficit/hyperactivity disorder and autism spectrum disorder. *European Child & Adolescent Psychiatry*, *19*(3), 281–295.

18　Joshi, G., DiSalvo, M., Faraone, S. V., Wozniak, J., Fried, R., Galdo, M., Belser, A., Hoskova, B., Dallenbach, N. T., & De Leon, M. F. (2020). Predictive utility of autistic traits in youth with ADHD: A controlled 10-year longitudinal follow-up study. *European Child & Adolescent Psychiatry*, *29*(6), 791–801.

19 Bethlehem, R. A., Romero-Garcia, R., Mak, E., Bullmore, E. T., & Baron-Cohen, S. (2017). Structural covariance networks in children with autism or ADHD. *Cerebral Cortex*, 27(8), 4267–4276.

20 Antshel, K. M., & Russo, N. (2019). Autism spectrum disorders and ADHD: Overlapping phenomenology, diagnostic issues, and treatment considerations. *Current Psychiatry Reports*, 21(5), 1–11.

21 Ronald, A., Simonoff, E., Kuntsi, J., Asherson, P., & Plomin, R. (2008). Evidence for overlapping genetic influences on autistic and ADHD behaviors in a community twin sample. *Journal of Child Psychology and Psychiatry*, 49(5), 535–542.

22 Aoki, Y., Yoncheva, Y. N., Chen, B., Nath, T., Sharp, D., Lazar, M., . . . & Di Martino, A. (2017). Association of white matter structure with autism spectrum disorder and attention-deficit/hyperactivity disorder. *JAMA Psychiatry*, 74(11), 1120–1128.

23 Hong, S. J., Vogelstein, J. T., Gozzi, A., Bernhardt, B. C., Yeo, B. T., Milham, M. P., & Di Martino, A. (2020). Toward neurosubtypes in autism. *Biological Psychiatry*, 88(1), 111–128.

24 Kotte, A., Joshi, G., Fried, R., Uchida, M., Spencer, A., Woodworth, K. Y., . . . & Biederman, J. (2013). Autistic traits in children with and without ADHD. *Pediatrics*, 132(3).

25 Baron-Cohen, S. (2017). Editorial perspective: Neurodiversity–a revolutionary concept for autism and psychiatry. *Journal of Child Psychology and Psychiatry*, 58(6), 744–747.

26 Chapman, R. (2019, July 30). *Mental Disorder Within the Neurodiversity Paradigm*. Psychology Today. Retrieved January 6, 2023, from https://www.psychologytoday.com.

27 Masuda, A., Qina'au, J., Juberg, M., & Martin, T. (2020). Bias in the Diagnostic and Statistical Manual 5 and psychopathology. In *Prejudice, stigma, privilege, and oppression* (pp. 215–234). Springer, Cham.

28 Burgess, R. (2022, March 31). *Understanding the spectrum – a comic strip explanation*. The Art of Autism. Retrieved January 6, 2023, from https://the-art-of-autism.com.

29 Wolff, S. (2004). The history of autism. *European Child & Adolescent Psychiatry*, 13(4), 201–208.

30 Evans, B. (2013). How autism became autism: The radical transformation of a central concept of child development in Britain. *History of the Human Sciences*, 26(3), 3–31.

31 Rosen, N. E., Lord, C., & Volkmar, F. R. (2021). The diagnosis of autism: From Kanner to DSM-III to DSM-5 and beyond. *Journal of Autism and Developmental Disorders*, 51(12), 4253–4270.

32 Golt, J., & Kana, R. K. (2022). History of autism. *The Neuroscience of Autism*, 1.

33 Silberman, S. (2015). *Neurotribes: The legacy of autism and the future of neurodiversity*.

34 Czech, H. (2018). Hans Asperger, national socialism, and "race hygiene" in Nazi-era Vienna. *Molecular Autism*, 9(1), 1–43.

35 Wing, L., Gould, J., & Gillberg, C. (2011). Autism spectrum disorders in the DSM-V: Better or worse than the DSM-IV?. *Research in Developmental Disabilities*, 32(2), 768–773.

36 First, M. B., Yousif, L. H., Clarke, D. E., Wang, P. S., Gogtay, N., & Appelbaum, P. S. (2022). DSM-5-TR: Overview of what's new and what's changed. *World Psychiatry*, 21(2), 218.

37 Edelson, S. M. (2022). Evidence from characteristics and comorbidities suggesting that Asperger syndrome is a subtype of autism spectrum disorder. *Genes*, 13(2), 274.

38 Coleman, D. M., & Adams, J. B. (2018). Survey of vocational experiences of adults with autism spectrum disorders, and recommendations on improving their employment. *Journal of Vocational Rehabilitation, 49*(1), 67–78.

39 Zeidan, J., Fombonne, E., Scorah, J., Ibrahim, A., Durkin, M. S., Saxena, S., . . . & Elsabbagh, M. (2022). Global prevalence of autism: a systematic review update. *Autism Research, 15*(5), 778–790.

40 Shen, M. D., Swanson, M. R., Wolff, J. J., Elison, J. T., Girault, J. B., Kim, S. H., . . . & IBIS Network. (2022). Subcortical brain development in autism and fragile X syndrome: Evidence for dynamic, age- and disorder-specific trajectories in infancy. *American Journal of Psychiatry*.

41 Lee, J. K., Andrews, D. S., Ozturk, A., Solomon, M., Rogers, S., Amaral, D. G., & Nordahl, C. W. (2022). Altered development of amygdala-connected brain regions in males and females with autism. *Journal of Neuroscience*.

42 Ortug, A., Guo, Y., Feldman, H. A., Ou, Y., Dieuveuil, H., Baumer, N. T., . . . & Takahashi, E. (2022). Human fetal brain magnetic resonance imaging (MRI) tells future emergence of autism spectrum disorders. *The FASEB Journal, 36*.

43 Vakilzadeh, G., Falcone, C., Dufour, B., Hong, T., Noctor, S. C., & Martínez-Cerdeño, V. (2022). Decreased number and increased activation state of astrocytes in gray and white matter of the prefrontal cortex in autism. *Cerebral Cortex*.

44 Dennis, E. L., & Thompson, P. M. (2022). Typical and atypical brain development: A review of neuroimaging studies. *Dialogues in Clinical Neuroscience*.

45 Bloomer, B. F., Morales, J. J., Bolbecker, A. R., Kim, D. J., & Hetrick, W. P. (2022). Cerebellar structure and function in autism spectrum disorder. *Journal of Psychiatry and Brain Science, 7*(3).

46 Ecker, C., Pretzsch, C. M., Bletsch, A., Mann, C., Schaefer, T., Ambrosino, S., . . . & Murphy, D. G. (2022). Interindividual differences in cortical thickness and their genomic underpinnings in autism spectrum disorder. *American Journal of Psychiatry, 179*(3), 242–254.

47 Shen, M. D., & Piven, J. (2022). Brain and behavior development in autism from birth through infancy. *Dialogues in Clinical Neuroscience*.

48 Maier, S., Düppers, A. L., Runge, K., Dacko, M., Lange, T., Fangmeier, T., . . . & Tebartz van Elst, L. (2022). Increased prefrontal GABA concentrations in adults with autism spectrum disorders. *Autism Research*.

49 Zoccante, L., Ciceri, M. L., Gozzi, L. A., Gennaro, G. D., & Zerman, N. (2022). The "connectivome theory": A new model to understand autism spectrum disorders. *Frontiers in Psychiatry, 12*, 794516.

50 Russell, G., Stapley, S., Newlove-Delgado, T., Salmon, A., White, R., Warren, F., . . . & Ford, T. (2022). Time trends in autism diagnosis over 20 years: A UK population-based cohort study. *Journal of Child Psychology and Psychiatry, 63*(6), 674–682.

51 Maenner, M. J., Warren, Z., Williams, A. R. et al. (2023). Prevalence and characteristics of autism spectrum disorder among children aged 8 years—autism and developmental disabilities monitoring network, 11 sites, United States, 2020. *MMWR Surveillance Summaries 2023, 72*(SS-2), 1–14.

52 Zeidan, J., Fombonne, E., Scorah, J., Ibrahim, A., Durkin, M. S., Saxena, S., . . . & Elsabbagh, M. (2022). Global prevalence of autism: A systematic review update. *Autism Research, 15*(5), 778–790.

53 Elsabbagh, M., Divan, G., Koh, Y. J., Kim, Y. S., Kauchali, S., Marcín, C., . . . & Fombonne, E. (2012). Global prevalence of autism and other pervasive developmental disorders. *Autism Research*, *5*(3), 160–179.

54 Sainsbury, W. J., Carrasco, K., Whitehouse, A. J., McNeil, L., & Waddington, H. (2022). Age of diagnosis for co-occurring autism and attention deficit hyperactivity disorder during childhood and adolescence: A systematic review. *Review Journal of Autism and Developmental Disorders*, 1–13.

55 van't Hof, M., Tisseur, C., van Berckelear-Onnes, I., van Nieuwenhuyzen, A., Daniels, A. M., Deen, M., . . . & Ester, W. A. (2021). Age at autism spectrum disorder diagnosis: A systematic review and meta-analysis from 2012 to 2019. *Autism*, *25*(4), 862–873.

56 Centers for Disease Control and Prevention. (2019, August 27). *Spotlight On: Delay Between First Concern to Accessing Services*. CDC. Retrieved from https://www.cdc.gov.

57 Baldwin, S., & Costley, D. (2016). The experiences and needs of female adults with high-functioning autism spectrum disorder. *Autism*, *20*(4), 483–495.

58 Hyman, S. L., Levy, S. E., Myers, S. M., Kuo, D. Z., Apkon, S., Davidson, L. F., . . . & Bridgemohan, C. (2020). Identification, evaluation, and management of children with autism spectrum disorder. *Pediatrics*, *145*(1).

59 Khadem-Reza, Z. K., & Zare, H. (2022). Automatic detection of autism spectrum disorder (ASD) in children using structural magnetic resonance imaging with machine vision system. *Middle East Current Psychiatry*, *29*(1), 1–7.

60 Rehn, A. K., Caruso, V. R., & Kumar, S. (2023). The effectiveness of animal-assisted therapy for children and adolescents with autism spectrum disorder: A systematic review. *Complementary Therapies in Clinical Practice*, *50*, 101719.

61 Hynes, J., & Block, M. (2022). Effects of physical activity on social, behavioral, and cognitive skills in children and young adults with autism spectrum disorder: A systematic review of the literature. *Review Journal of Autism and Developmental Disorders*, 1–22.

62 Newson, E. L. M. K., Le Marechal, K., & David, C. (2003). Pathological demand avoidance syndrome: A necessary distinction within the pervasive developmental disorders. *Archives of Disease in Childhood*, *88*(7), 595–600.

63 Woods, R. (2019). Demand avoidance phenomena: Circularity, integrity and validity–a commentary on the 2018 National Autistic Society PDA Conference. *Good Autism Practice*, *20*(2), 28–40.

64 O'Nions, E., & Eaton, J. (2020). Extreme/'pathological' demand avoidance: An overview. *Paediatrics and Child Health*, *30*(12), 411–415.

65 Green, J., Absoud, M., Grahame, V., Malik, O., Simonoff, E., Le Couteur, A., & Baird, G. (2018). Pathological demand avoidance: Symptoms but not a syndrome. *The Lancet Child & Adolescent Health*, *2*(6), 455–464.

66 Kildahl, A. N., Helverschou, S. B., Rysstad, A. L., Wigaard, E., Hellerud, J. M., Ludvigsen, L. B., & Howlin, P. (2021). Pathological demand avoidance in children and adolescents: A systematic review. *Autism*, *25*(8), 2162–2176.

67 Williams, Z. J., Suzman, E., Bordman, S. L., Markfeld, J. E., Kaiser, S. M., Dunham, K. A., . . . & Woynaroski, T. G. (2022). Characterizing interoceptive differences in autism: A systematic review and meta-analysis of case–control studies. *Journal of Autism and Developmental Disorders*, 1–16.

68 Kinnaird, E., Stewart, C., & Tchanturia, K. (2019). Investigating alexithymia in autism: A systematic review and meta-analysis. *European Psychiatry, 55*, 80–89.

69 Ostrolenk, A., d'Arc, B. F., Jelenic, P., Samson, F., & Mottron, L. (2017). Hyperlexia: Systematic review, neurocognitive modeling, and outcome. *Neuroscience & Biobehavioral Reviews, 79*, 134–149.

70 Wolraich, M. L., Chan, E., Froehlich, T., Lynch, R. L., Bax, A., Redwine, S. T., . . . & Hagan, J. F. (2019). ADHD diagnosis and treatment guidelines: a historical perspective. *Pediatrics, 144*(4).

71 Martinez-Badía, J., & Martinez-Raga, J. (2015). Who says this is a modern disorder? The early history of attention deficit hyperactivity disorder. *World journal of psychiatry, 5*(4), 379.

72 Lange, K. W., Reichl, S., Lange, K. M., Tucha, L., & Tucha, O. (2010). The history of attention deficit hyperactivity disorder. *ADHD Attention Deficit and Hyperactivity Disorders, 2*(4), 241–255.

73 Jendreizik, L. T., von Wirth, E., & Döpfner, M. (2023). Familial factors associated with symptom severity in children and adolescents with ADHD: A meta-analysis and supplemental review. *Journal of Attention Disorders, 27*(2), 124–144.

74 Grinblat, N., & Rosenblum, S. Work participation, sensory processing and sleep quality in adults with attention deficit hyperactive disorder. *Work*, (Preprint), 1–10.

75 Soler-Gutiérrez, A. M., Pérez-González, J. C., & Mayas, J. (2023). Evidence of emotion dysregulation as a core symptom of adult ADHD: A systematic review. *PLoS ONE, 18*(1).

76 Blum, K., Chen, A. L. C., Braverman, E. R., Comings, D. E., Chen, T. J., Arcuri, V., . . . & Oscar-Berman, M. (2008). Attention-deficit-hyperactivity disorder and reward deficiency syndrome. *Neuropsychiatric Disease and Treatment.*

77 Villa, F. M., Crippa, A., Rosi, E., Nobile, M., Brambilla, P., & Delvecchio, G. (2023). ADHD and eating disorders in childhood and adolescence: An updated minireview. *Journal of Affective Disorders, 321*, 265–271.

78 Luderer, M., Quiroga, J. A. R., Faraone, S. V., Zhang-James, Y., & Reif, A. (2021). Alcohol use disorders and ADHD. *Neuroscience & Biobehavioral Reviews, 128*, 648–660.

79 Rohner, H., Gaspar, N., Philipsen, A., & Schulze, M. (2023). Prevalence of attention deficit hyperactivity disorder (ADHD) among substance use disorder (SUD) populations: Meta-analysis. *International Journal of Environmental Research and Public Health, 20*(2), 1275.

80 Krause, K. H., Dresel, S. H., Krause, J., la Fougere, C., & Ackenheil, M. (2003). The dopamine transporter and neuroimaging in attention deficit hyperactivity disorder. *Neuroscience & Biobehavioral Reviews, 27*(7), 605–613.

81 Egan, T. E., Dawson, A. E., & Wymbs, B. T. (2017). Substance use in undergraduate students with histories of attention-deficit/hyperactivity disorder (ADHD): The role of impulsivity. *Substance Use & Misuse, 52*(10), 1375–1386.

82 Haghighatfard, A., Ghaderi, A. H., Mostajabi, P., Kashfi, S. S., Shahrani, M., Mehrasa, M., . . . & Alizadenik, A. (2023). The first genome-wide association study of internet addiction; Revealed substantial shared risk factors with neurodevelopmental psychiatric disorders. *Research in Developmental Disabilities, 133*, 104393.

83 Karaca, S., Saleh, A., Canan, F., & Potenza, M. N. (2017). Comorbidity between behavioral addictions and attention deficit/hyperactivity disorder: A systematic review. *International Journal of Mental Health and Addiction, 15*(3), 701–724.

84 Dekkers, T. J., de Water, E., & Scheres, A. (2022). Impulsive and risky decision-making in adolescents with attention-deficit/hyperactivity disorder (ADHD): The need for a developmental perspective. *Current Opinion in Psychology, 44*, 330–336.

85 Vysniauske, R., Verburgh, L., Oosterlaan, J., & Molendijk, M. L. (2020). The effects of physical exercise on functional outcomes in the treatment of ADHD: A meta-analysis. *Journal of Attention Disorders, 24*(5), 644–654.

86 Tang, Y., Zheng, S., & Tian, Y. (2022). Resting-state fMRI whole brain network function plasticity analysis in attention deficit hyperactivity disorder. *Neural Plasticity, 2022*.

87 Puts, N. A., Ryan, M., Oeltzschner, G., Horska, A., Edden, R. A., & Mahone, E. M. (2020). Reduced striatal GABA in unmedicated children with ADHD at 7T. *Psychiatry Research: Neuroimaging, 301*, 111082.

88 Mehta, T. R., Monegro, A., Nene, Y., Fayyaz, M., & Bollu, P. C. (2019). Neurobiology of ADHD: A review. *Current Developmental Disorders Reports, 6*(4), 235–240.

89 Salavert, J., Ramos-Quiroga, J. A., Moreno-Alcázar, A., Caseras, X., Palomar, G., Radua, J., . . . & Pomarol-Clotet, E. (2018). Functional imaging changes in the medial prefrontal cortex in adult ADHD. *Journal of attention disorders, 22*(7), 679–693.

90 Hoogman, M., Bralten, J., Hibar, D. P., Mennes, M., Zwiers, M. P., Schweren, L. S., . . . & Franke, B. (2017). Subcortical brain volume differences in participants with attention deficit hyperactivity disorder in children and adults: a cross-sectional mega-analysis. *The Lancet Psychiatry, 4*(4), 310–319.

91 Amen, D. G., Hanks, C., & Prunella, J. (2008). Preliminary evidence differentiating ADHD using brain SPECT imaging in older patients. *Journal of Psychoactive Drugs, 40*(2), 139–146.

92 Amen, D. G. (2013). *Healing ADD revised edition: The breakthrough program that allows you to see and heal the 7 types of ADD*. Penguin.

93 Koumbi, L. (2022). The gut microbiota plays a central role in the attention deficit/hyperactivity disorder (ADHD). *Public Health Toxicology, 2*(Supplement 1).

94 Danielson, M. L., Holbrook, J. R., Bitsko, R. H., Newsome, K., Charania, S. N., McCord, R. F., . . . & Blumberg, S. J. (2022). State-level estimates of the prevalence of parent-reported ADHD diagnosis and treatment among US children and adolescents, 2016 to 2019. *Journal of Attention Disorders*.

95 Song, P., Zha, M., Yang, Q., Zhang, Y., Li, X., & Rudan, I. (2021). The prevalence of adult attention-deficit hyperactivity disorder: A global systematic review and meta-analysis. *Journal of Global Health, 11*.

96 Unitt, I. (2022). Autism or ADHD or both in adults: A literature review on the prevalence, issues and challenges. *Good Autism Practice (GAP), 23*(1), 65–75.

97 Morgan, P. L., Woods, A. D., & Wang, Y. (2022). Sociodemographic disparities in attention-deficit/hyperactivity disorder overdiagnosis and overtreatment during elementary school. *Journal of Learning Disabilities*.

98 Kazda, L., Bell, K., Thomas, R., McGeechan, K., Sims, R., & Barratt, A. (2021). Overdiagnosis of attention-deficit/hyperactivity disorder in children and adolescents: A systematic scoping review. *JAMA Network Open, 4*(4).

99 Sainsbury, W. J., Carrasco, K., Whitehouse, A. J., McNeil, L., & Waddington, H. (2022). Age of diagnosis for co-occurring autism and attention deficit hyperactivity disorder during childhood and adolescence: A systematic review. *Review Journal of Autism and Developmental Disorders*, 1–13.

100 Visser, S. N., Danielson, M. L., Bitsko, R. H., Holbrook, J. R., Kogan, M. D., Ghandour, R. M., . . . & Blumberg, S. J. (2014). Trends in the parent-report of health care provider-diagnosed and medicated attention-deficit/hyperactivity disorder: United States, 2003–2011. *Journal of the American Academy of Child & Adolescent Psychiatry*, *53*(1), 34–46.

101 Caye, A., Rocha, T. B. M., Anselmi, L., Murray, J., Menezes, A. M., Barros, F. C., . . . & Rohde, L. A. (2016). Attention-deficit/hyperactivity disorder trajectories from childhood to young adulthood: Evidence from a birth cohort supporting a late-onset syndrome. *JAMA Psychiatry*, *73*(7), 705–712.

102 Agnew-Blais, J. C., Polanczyk, G. V., Danese, A., Wertz, J., Moffitt, T. E., & Arseneault, L. (2016). Evaluation of the persistence, remission, and emergence of attention-deficit/hyperactivity disorder in young adulthood. *JAMA Psychiatry*, *73*(7), 713–720.

103 Taylor, L. E., Kaplan-Kahn, E. A., Lighthall, R. A., & Antshel, K. M. (2021). Adult-onset ADHD: A critical analysis and alternative explanations. *Child Psychiatry & Human Development*, 1–19.

104 Solanto, M. V. (2019). The prevalence of "Late-Onset" ADHD in a clinically referred adult sample. *Journal of Attention Disorders*, *23*(9), 1026–1034.

105 Groenman, A. P., Torenvliet, C., Radhoe, T. A., Agelink van Rentergem, J. A., & Geurts, H. M. (2021). Menstruation and menopause in autistic adults: Periods of importance? *Autism*.

106 Epstein, J. N., Kelleher, K. J., Baum, R., Brinkman, W. B., Peugh, J., Gardner, W., . . . & Langberg, J. (2014). Variability in ADHD care in community-based pediatrics. *Pediatrics*, *134*(6), 1136–1143.

107 Gaba, P., & Giordanengo, M. (2019). FPIN's help desk answers: Attention deficit/hyperactivity disorder: Screening and evaluation. *American Family Physician*, *99*(11), 712.

108 Kemper, A. R., Maslow, G. R., Hill, S., Namdari, B., LaPointe, N. M. A., Goode, A. P., . . . & Sanders, G. D. (2018). Attention deficit hyperactivity disorder: Diagnosis and treatment in children and adolescents. *Comparative Effectiveness Reviews No. 203*.

109 Luo, N., Luo, X., Zheng, S., Yao, D., Zhao, M., Cui, Y., . . . & Sui, J. (2022). Aberrant brain dynamics and spectral power in children with ADHD and its subtypes. *European Child & Adolescent Psychiatry*, 1–12.

110 Kraines, M. A., & Wells, T. T. (2017). Rejection sensitivity and depression: Indirect effects through problem solving. *Psychiatry*, *80*(1), 55–63.

111 Beaton, D. M., Sirois, F., & Milne, E. (2020). Self-compassion and perceived criticism in adults with attention deficit hyperactivity disorder (ADHD). *Mindfulness*, *11*(11), 2506–2518.

112 Beheshti, A., Chavanon, M. L., & Christiansen, H. (2020). Emotion dysregulation in adults with attention deficit hyperactivity disorder: A meta-analysis. *BMC psychiatry*, *20*(1), 1–11.

113 Keluskar, J., Reicher, D., Gorecki, A., Mazefsky, C., & Crowell, J. A. (2021). Understanding, assessing, and intervening with emotion dysregulation in autism spectrum disorder: A developmental perspective. *Child and Adolescent Psychiatric Clinics*, *30*(2), 335–348.

114 Sepanta, M., Abedi, A., Yarmohammadian, A., Ghomrani, A., & Faramarzi, S. (2019). The effect of Fredrickson's positive emotion training program on emotion regulation of students with dyslexia. *Quarterly Journal of Child Mental Health, 5*(4), 94–109.

115 Ptacek, R., Weissenberger, S., Braaten, E., Klicperova-Baker, M., Goetz, M., Raboch, J., . . . & Stefano, G. B. (2019). Clinical implications of the perception of time in attention deficit hyperactivity disorder (ADHD): A review. *Medical Science Monitor: International Medical Journal of Experimental and Clinical Research, 25*, 3918.

116 Vicario, C. M., Nitsche, M. A., Salehinejad, M. A., Avanzino, L., & Martino, G. (2020). Time processing, interoception, and insula activation: A mini-review on clinical disorders. *Frontiers in Psychology, 11*, 1893.

117 La Buissonnière-Ariza, V., Alvaro, J., Cavitt, M., Rudy, B. M., Cepeda, S. L., Schneider, S. C., . . . & Storch, E. A. (2021). Body-focused repetitive behaviors in youth with mental health conditions: A preliminary study on their prevalence and clinical correlates. *International Journal of Mental Health, 50*(1), 33–52.

118 Kirby, P. (2018). A brief history of dyslexia. *Psychologist, 31*(3).

119 Erbeli, F., Rice, M., & Paracchini, S. (2022). Insights into dyslexia genetics research from the last two decades. *Brain Sciences, 12*(1).

120 Eide, B. L., & Eide, F. F. (2012). *The dyslexic advantage: Unlocking the hidden potential of the dyslexic brain.* Penguin.

121 Fawcett, A. J. (2022). Dyslexia world-wide: A view of emerging themes. In *The Routledge International Handbook of Dyslexia in Education* (pp. 371–385). Routledge.

122 Berninger, V. W. (2000). Dyslexia the invisible, treatable disorder: The story of Einstein's ninja turtles. *Learning Disability Quarterly, 23*(3), 175–195.

123 Stoodley, C. J., & Stein, J. F. (2013). Cerebellar function in developmental dyslexia. *The Cerebellum, 12*(2), 267–276.

124 Schwarz, J. (1999). Dyslexic children use nearly five times the brain area. *University Of Washington. [Online].*

125 Wilmot, A., Pizzey, H., Leitão, S., Hasking, P., & Boyes, M. (2022). Growing up with dyslexia: Child and parent perspectives on school struggles, self-esteem, and mental health. *Dyslexia.*

126 Wolff, U., & Lundberg, I. (2002). The prevalence of dyslexia among art students. *Dyslexia, 8*(1), 34–42.

127 Bacon, A. M., & Bennett, S. (2013). Dyslexia in higher education: The decision to study art. *European Journal of Special Needs Education, 28*(1), 19–32.

128 Richlan, F., Kronbichler, M., & Wimmer, H. (2009). Functional abnormalities in the dyslexic brain: A quantitative meta-analysis of neuroimaging studies. *Human Brain Mapping, 30*(10), 3299–3308.

129 Sun, Y. F., Lee, J. S., & Kirby, R. (2010). Brain imaging findings in dyslexia. *Pediatrics & Neonatology, 51*(2), 89–96.

130 Eckert, M. A., Leonard, C. M., Richards, T. L., Aylward, E. H., Thomson, J., & Berninger, V. W. (2003). Anatomical correlates of dyslexia: Frontal and cerebellar findings. *Brain, 126*(2), 482–494.

131 Liebig, J., Friederici, A. D., Neef, N. E., & Consortium, L. (2020). Auditory brainstem measures and genotyping boost the prediction of literacy: A longitudinal study on early markers of dyslexia. *Developmental Cognitive Neuroscience, 46.*

132 Roitsch, J., & Watson, S. M. (2019). An overview of dyslexia: Definition, characteristics, assessment, identification, and intervention. *Science Journal of Education, 7*(4).

133 Shaywitz, S. E., Shaywitz, J. E., & Shaywitz, B. A. (2021). Dyslexia in the 21st century. *Current Opinion in Psychiatry, 34*(2), 80–86.

134 Wagner, R. K., Zirps, F. A., Edwards, A. A., Wood, S. G., Joyner, R. E., Becker, B. J., . . . & Beal, B. (2020). The prevalence of dyslexia: A new approach to its estimation. *Journal of Learning Disabilities, 53*(5), 354–365.

135 Sadusky, A., Berger, E. P., Reupert, A. E., & Freeman, N. C. (2022). Methods used by psychologists for identifying dyslexia: A systematic review. *Dyslexia, 28*(2), 132–148.

136 Solem C. (2021). *A report on practice for the assessment of specific reading and writing difficulties, mathematical difficulties and language difficulties.* Dysleksi Norge.

137 Schelbe, L., Pryce, J., Petscher, Y., Fien, H., Stanley, C., Gearin, B., & Gaab, N. (2022). Dyslexia in the context of social work: Screening and early intervention. *Families in Society, 103*(3), 269–280.

138 Ottosen, H. F., Bønnerup, K. H., Weed, E., & Parrila, R. (2022). Identifying dyslexia at the university: Assessing phonological coding is not enough. *Annals of Dyslexia, 72*(1), 147–170.

139 Nergård-Nilssen, T., & Friborg, O. (2022). The dyslexia marker test for children: Development and validation of a new test. *Assessment for Effective Intervention, 48*(1), 23–33.

140 Carrasco, A., & Carrasco, K. D. (2022). The use of neuronal response signals as early biomarkers of dyslexia. *Advances in Neurodevelopmental Disorders,* 1–8.

141 Jothi Prabha, A., & Bhargavi, R. (2022). Prediction of dyslexia from eye movements using machine learning. *IETE Journal of Research, 68*(2), 814–823.

142 Chung, P., & Patel, D. R. (2015). Dysgraphia. *International Journal of Child and Adolescent Health, 8*(1), 27.

143 Henderson, A. (2013). *Dyslexia, dyscalculia and mathematics: A practical guide.* Routledge.

144 Miller, L. J., Anzalone, M. E., Lane, S. J., Cermak, S. A., & Osten, E. T. (2007). Concept evolution in sensory integration: A proposed nosology for diagnosis. *The American Journal of Occupational Therapy, 61*(2), 135.

145 Miller, L. (2006). *Sensational kids. Hope and help for children with SPD.* NY, A Perigee Book.

146 Zimmer, M., Desch, L., Rosen, L. D., Bailey, M. L., . . . & Wiley, S. E. (2012). Sensory integration therapies for children with developmental and behavioral disorders. *Pediatrics, 129*(6), 1186–1189.

147 Goldsmith, H. H., Van Hulle, C. A., Arneson, C. L., Schreiber, J. E., & Gernsbacher, M. (2006). A population-based twin study of parentally reported tactile and auditory defensiveness in young children. *Journal of Abnormal Child Psychology, 34*(3), 378–392.

148 Kerley, L. J., Meredith, P. J., & Harnett, P. H. (2022). The relationship between sensory processing and attachment patterns: A scoping review. *Canadian Journal of Occupational Therapy.*

149 Owen, J. P., Marco, E. J., Desai, S., Fourie, E., Harris, J., Hill, S. S., . . . & Mukherjee, P. (2013). Abnormal white matter microstructure in children with sensory processing disorders. *Neuroimage: Clinical, 2*, 844–853.

150 Davies, P. L., & Gavin, W. J. (2007). Validating the diagnosis of sensory processing disorders using EEG technology. *The American Journal of Occupational Therapy, 61*(2), 176–189.

151 Crasta, J. E., Salzinger, E., Lin, M. H., Gavin, W. J., & Davies, P. L. (2020). Sensory processing and attention profiles among children with sensory processing disorders and autism spectrum disorders. *Frontiers in Integrative Neuroscience, 14*, 22.

152 McArthur, A. L. H. (2022). The debate over sensory processing disorder. *American Journal of Psychiatry Residents' Journal.*

153 Robinson, A., & Clinkenbeard, P. R. (2008). History of giftedness: Perspectives from the past presage modern scholarship. *Handbook of giftedness in children* (pp. 13–31). Springer.

154 Dai, D. Y. (2018). A century of quest for identity: A history of giftedness. *The APA handbook on giftedness and talent, 3*–23.

155 Dabrowski, K. (1964). *Positive disintegration.* Boston: Little, Brown, & Company.

156 Dabrowski, K. (1972). *Psychoneurosis is not an illness: Neuroses and psychoneuroses from the perspective of positive disintegration.* London: Gryf Publications.

157 Renzulli, J. S. (1978). What makes giftedness? Reexamining a definition. *Phi delta kappan, 60*(3), 180.

158 Roeper, A. (1982). How the gifted cope with their emotions. *Roeper Review, 5*(2), 21–24.

159 Betts, G. T., & Neihart, M. (1988). Profiles of the gifted and talented. *Gifted Child Quarterly, 32*(2), 248–253.

160 Lovecky, D. V. (1997). Identity development in gifted children: Moral sensitivity. *Roeper Review, 20*(2), 90–94.

161 Lovecky, D. V. (1995). Highly gifted children and peer relationships. *Counseling and Guidance Newsletter, 5*(3), 2.

162 Lovecky, D. V. (1998). Spiritual sensitivity in gifted children. *Roeper Review, 20*(3), 178–183.

163 Gilman, B. J., Lovecky, D. V., Kearney, K., Peters, D. B., Wasserman, J. D., Silverman, L. K., . . . & Rimm, S. B. (2013). Critical issues in the identification of gifted students with co-existing disabilities: The twice-exceptional. *Sage Open, 3*(3).

164 Ramos, A., Lavrijsen, J., Linnenbrink-Garcia, L., Soenens, B., Vansteenkiste, M., Sypré, S., . . . & Verschueren, K. (2022). Motivational pathways underlying gifted underachievement: Trajectory classes, longitudinal outcomes, and predicting factors. *Gifted Child Quarterly.*

165 Guthrie, S. L., & Gurskyj, C. L. (2022). Gifted and talented: Not always a gift. In *Best practices for trauma-informed school counseling* (pp. 138–157). IGI Global.

166 Lovecky, D. V. (1986). Can you hear the flowers sing? Issues for gifted adults. *Journal of Counseling and Development, 64*(9), 572–575.

167 Ngieng, D. F., Abd Razak, A. Z., & Amran, A. N. S. (2022). Social Anxiety Level Among Gifted and Talented Students. Conference Proceeding.

168 Eide, B., & Eide, F. (2004). Brains on fire: The multimodality of gifted thinkers. *New Horizons for Learning.*

169 Solé-Casals, J., Serra-Grabulosa, J. M., Romero-Garcia, R., Vilaseca, G., Adan, A., Vilaró, N., . . . & Bullmore, E. T. (2019). Structural brain network of gifted children has a more integrated and versatile topology. *Brain Structure and Function, 224*(7), 2373–2383.

170 Jin, S. H., Kwon, Y. J., Jeong, J. S., Kwon, S. W., & Shin, D. H. (2006). Differences in brain information transmission between gifted and normal children during scientific hypothesis generation. *Brain and Cognition, 62*(3), 191–197.

171 Tetreault, N., Haase, J., & Duncan, S. (2016). The gifted brain. *Gifted Research and Outreach*, *17*.

172 McIntyre, E. (2016). Identifying gifted and talented students with equity proves difficult. *Education Dive*.

173 Arnstein, K. B. (2022). The intersectionality of twice-exceptionality: Historic, current, and future perspectives. *Critical issues in servicing twiceeExceptional students* (pp. 3–18). Springer.

Section II
Best Practices

Exploring the Relationship with Your Own Brain

4

Just as strongly as they emphasize the fundamentals of couple therapy, traditional graduate programs tend to encourage counseling students to think deeply about their own lives. Helping to develop each pre-professional into an appropriately introspective, differentiated therapist is a worthwhile goal, as a self-aware therapist tends to be a good therapist. Accordingly, the best schools promote exposure to learning materials and hands-on experiences that invite inquiry in deeply personal areas. Trauma, spirituality, gender, sexuality, relationships, culture, and race seem to be the areas most often explored.

Over the span of one's graduate school experience, there are usually numerous opportunities to work alone or alongside other students on introspection-based assignments. Some examples include personal reflection papers, group discussions, interactive projects within the community, and more. Additionally, students usually complete one or more standardized personality inventories (or similar assessments) and attend mandatory case supervision sessions to process countertransference. Some schools even require attendance at individual therapy or professional mentoring sessions. Trauma is given special attention as nuanced aspects of each student's personality, abilities, and interpersonal dynamics are explored. It's encouraging that many clinical training programs are currently known to be quite comprehensive in their development of both therapy skills and personal growth.

The vast majority of therapy training programs repeatedly fall short, however, regarding neurodiversity. They do not provide opportunities for

DOI: 10.4324/9781003351337-7

students to explore their own brain features, the relationship they have with their own brain, and the significance of neurodiversity to their personal life and professional practices. Regarding couple therapy programs, many overt invitations to examine one's own relationship dynamics exist, but neurotypes are rarely given proper attention. This trend continues after graduation; There are almost no professional development seminars or continuing education classes available on these topics. Is this due to the pervasive effects of ableism? Or, does it simply represent an unfortunate lack of awareness?

Regardless of the reasons for this problem, implementing solutions does not have to be difficult.

Research points to successful outcomes from therapy training styles that emphasize students' uniqueness. Harry Joseph Aponte's *Person of the Therapist (POTT)* model is a wonderful example of this.[1] His framework seeks to actively nurture counseling students towards greater knowledge, access, and management of their innate selves. The POTT model has been used positively within at least one graduate program to effectively foster students' self-insight and clinical efficacy during therapeutic discussions of race and ethnicity, gender, sexuality, religion, and politics.[2] Awareness of these Person of the Therapist issues has been suggested to contribute positively to couple therapy.[3] Adding the explicit exploration of brain wiring to the scope of this model seems an enhancement that is easily implemented. This could be as simple as inviting students to participate in confidential, free assessments. This is already done, after all, in many programs concerning a variety of other topics! *The Big Five Personality Test, The Enneagram Test, The Myers–Briggs Type Indicator (MBTI)*, or the *Dominance, Influence, Steadiness and Compliance (DISC) Assessment* are just some popular examples. Revealing one's own results, of course, should always remain a matter of personal choice.

Why would a therapist <u>not</u> seek to learn about their own neurotype? Knowing how one mentally operates and physiologically experiences the world is important to the stewardship of two important professional qualities: Authenticity and presence. The therapeutic alliance relies upon these qualities in the therapist to be effective. A therapist cannot be present when dysregulated, of course, so it can be extremely eye-opening to explore how one's own brain-based strengths and challenges relate to self-regulation. Learning about one's neurotype can also help prevent compassion fatigue, professional burnout, ethical blunders, and even bias. Any of these issues can hinder or destroy therapeutic relationships – and may even cost a therapist their license.

When a therapist's own brain wiring is not considered at either the systemic or individual level, valuable opportunities for professional development can be missed. For one, a therapist's knowledge gaps will always limit their capacity to serve others. Education can bring a fresh perspective to increase the depth of compassion one has available to themselves and their clients. Additionally, when a therapist does not know their own neurotype, they are unable to make a fully-informed decision about whether or not to utilize and/or disclose this aspect of their personhood with clients. This eliminates a potential connection point for neurodiverse populations. (Many partners in neurodiverse relationships tend to view a therapist's brain wiring as an important factor when selecting a professional with whom to work.) Of course, personal disclosure of one's own neurotype is not always safe, possible, or desirable in some professional settings. The benefits and risks to a therapist's personal disclosures should always be carefully weighed.

Regardless of a therapist's own disclosure choices, at least some level of private, personal insight regarding their own neurotype, their own neurodiverse relationship experiences, and their own brain-based self-identifications is essential. In fact, it is a central component to the effective practice of neurodiverse couple therapy. This type of work requires it! Neurodiverse couple therapy intentionally brings brain features and brain-based relationship dynamics into focus, affording many opportunities for the therapist to experience countertransference on a dimension they're probably not used to working through. Neurodiverse couple sessions may trigger a distinct kind of physiological and/or emotional dysregulation. The customized introspection exercises presented later in this text may help a therapist identify areas of their own vulnerability. They are also intended to promote a more holistic sense of self and greater clinical competence when interacting with neurodiverse populations.

Some students and professionals may find exploring their brain wiring and brain-based interpersonal dynamics particularly empowering. Others may find this incredibly draining. It's certainly ok to alternate between the two feelings, or to simply feel a bit unsettled when pursuing accurate information and insight regarding one's own neurodivergence or neurotypicality. Taking a fresh look at one's life experiences, including past and present relationships with caregivers, intimate partners, relatives, and children, can be daunting. Learning new things about oneself or loved ones, remembering past scenarios, and processing complex social dynamics is not always a positive experience. The emergence of denial, grief, anger, hurt, or other negative feelings is always a possibility. This is not unlike the inherent risks of any other type of personal inquiry process that counseling students already undertake, however. All feelings that come up should be acknowledged. It's never too late to start a personal **neurodiscovery** journey, which should unfold at one's own pace and without undue pressure.

The first step in neurodiscovery is to recognize that no person can ever "opt out" of a relationship with their own brain. Humans are innately and unequivocally relational, not only with other humans, but also within themselves. The concepts of body image and self-esteem easily illustrate this point. In simple terms, one's body image represents a relationship with the appearance and mechanics of their own body. Self-esteem represents the entirety of one's relationship with themselves as a multidimensional being. Therapists and clients readily discuss these constructs, usually with ease. For example, relational language is often used when a client seeks to build a healthier connection to their own rapidly changing body during pregnancy, or during recovery from disordered eating patterns.

Truly, each client's *relationships* with their body, food, money, the church, etc. and the way this impacts self-esteem is constantly being discussed in therapy. This can be meaningful, because these relationships are recognized to exist and exert influence over one's thoughts, feelings, and behaviors – whether or not they are consciously acknowledged. Intentionally bringing these relationships to light can lead to insight, healing, and growth. Why not talk about the relationship each client has with their own brain? Talking about this invites invaluable discussion. Currently, though, even if a therapist encourages a client to consider how "having" their neurotype, (e.g., "having Dyslexia" or "having Autism") impacts their self-esteem, they usually stop there. Not many therapists provide overt guidance to help a ND client explore their relationship with their own brain, let alone promote insight about how this may impact interactions with an intimate partner. Systemic therapists tend to be more concerned about overall relationship dynamics than the ways each partner's brain-based self-identifications factor in.

The concept of **brain-esteem**, or one's relationship with their own brain, has equal importance as self-esteem or body image. As such, it's hugely relevant. The fact that couple therapists are not used to speaking about the brain in relational terms can be changed with time and practice. The following explanations, terminology, and visual representations may help.

Brain-esteem can be categorized as either *positive, neutral,* or *negative* based on how one feels about their relationship with their own brain at any given time. Overall, though, this *sentiment* is largely formed through the internalization of poignant messages gleaned from the accumulation of social experiences to date. Interactions with caregivers, bosses, past or present romantic partners, peers, and more all contribute. Cultural considerations, gender expectations, and environmental conditions also play a role. Ultimately, the way one feels about their own brain is sculpted by the actual (or perceived) rewards and consequences garnered from others' reactions to their brain-based features. Witnessing consequences happen to others, either in person or via the media, may be equally impactful. One's emotional and physiological responses to these first- or second-hand social dynamics matter greatly in the formation of feelings about their own brain, as does their level of education regarding brain anatomy, physiology, psychology, etc.

Brain-esteem is not static, as it can fluctuate due to external circumstances (e.g., being either denied or granted helpful accommodations) or physical conditions (e.g., losing a previously-held ability due to brain injury). This leads to the notion of one's relational *stance* regarding their own brain at any given time. A person may stand *aligned with, alongside,* or *against* their own brain. The relational stance a person takes with their own brain tends to be a product of all the factors mentioned above regarding sentiment, but it also considers the degree to which one recognizes and accepts their neurotype as a part of their overall identity framework.

What does negative brain-esteem look like visually?
Usually, a person who has a *negative* sentiment about their own brain also embodies a relational stance *against* it. Persons in a negative relationship with

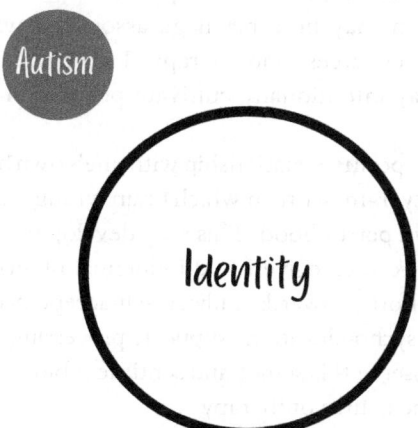

Figure 4.1 One example of negative brain-esteem

their brain tend to distance their identity from the struggles they perceive their brain causes, to oppose their diagnostic labels, and to define themselves by <u>anything but</u> brain-based features.

This position may result from the accumulation of traumatic, critical, rejecting, or ableist experiences within one's family and/or society in general. It may also directly relate to a person's experience with the diagnostic process, such as when a diagnosis is weaponized against them in some way or results in any other form of unsafety.

A person with negative brain-esteem may blame their brain for their life's painful experiences and resent "being the way they are." They tend to view their neurotype as a defect to be cured, a handicap to overcome, or an enemy to conquer. Low self-esteem and depression can easily co-occur with this stance and sentiment. These individuals tend to frequently compare themselves to an idealized, NT version of themselves that simply does not exist. If they are in a neurodiverse relationship, they may believe the myth: "If I was NT like my partner, my relationship would automatically be easier/ better." They may or may not spend a lot of energy maintaining the outward appearance of neurotypicality in order to defend themselves from actual or perceived harm.

What does positive brain-esteem look like visually?
Those with a *positive* sentiment toward their brain tend to stand *aligned with* it. Individuals with positive brain-esteem have learned to respect their brain for its strengths and uniqueness. They are also generally skilled at acknowledging their own brain-based challenges and tend to reach out for support when needed. (That is, if support is available.) In some cases, positive brain-esteem may be a privilege associated with socioeconomic stability, access to resources, and therapy. However, there are certainly individuals who may intentionally cultivate positive brain-esteem despite hardship.

Usually, being in a positive relationship with one's own brain tends to reflect an integrated identity framework in which brain wiring is considered valuable and inextricable from personhood. This may develop from the experience of unconditional love from caregivers and influential others, or perhaps solely from one's own efforts towards radical self-acceptance. Therapists who provide unbiased psychoeducation, support, processing space, and healthy coping skills may observe this stance and sentiment blossom and grow within some clients over the course of therapy.

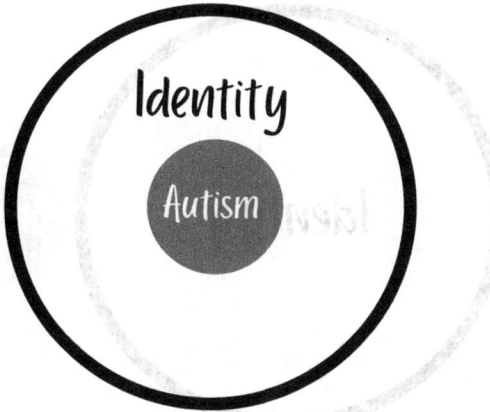

Figure 4.2 One example of positive brain-esteem

It's also possible for a person to enjoy positive brain-esteem <u>without</u> choosing to emphasize their neurotype as central to who they are.

Figure 4.3 Another example of positive brain-esteem

What does neutral brain-esteem look like visually?
A person who feels a *neutral* sentiment toward their own brain can usually be thought of as standing *alongside* it. These individuals may or may not choose to integrate their neurotype within their personal identity framework. Regardless, brain neutrality is akin to a peaceful coexistence where one's neurotype simply "is what it is."

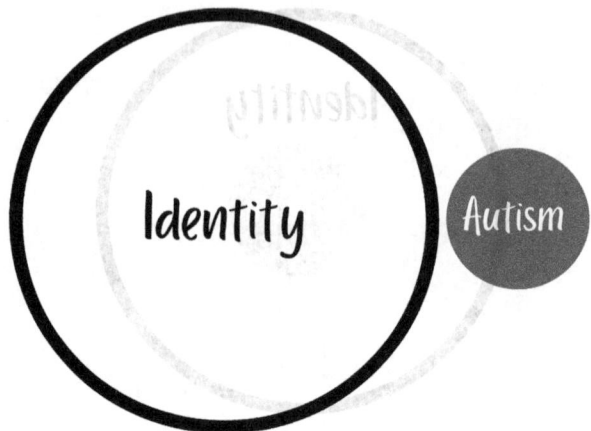

Figure 4.4 One example of neutral brain-esteem

Individuals who embrace brain neutrality tend to recognize their brain-based labels and characteristics as just some of many aspects of what makes up who they are as a person.

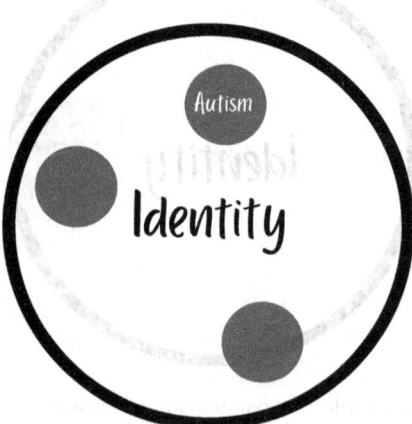

Figure 4.5 Another example of neutral brain-esteem

Brain neutrality may exist because life experiences, sociocultural factors, media exposures, and other influences have not imparted any particularly loaded messaging. Sometimes, though, a person will choose to intentionally work their way up to a position of brain neutrality in order to heal from negative brain-esteem. They may or may not continue towards positive brain-esteem after this. And, they don't have to. Positive brain-esteem is not necessarily everyone's goal. It can be perfectly healthy for a person to simply exist in a neutral relationship with their own brain.

How does this discussion relate to Person of the Therapist issues?
A therapist who has a *positive* relationship with their own brain . . .

- Likely has pursued differential self-diagnosis of either neurotypicality or neurodivergence. May also have pursued formal diagnosis, if it was safe and wise to do so.
- May or may not have internalized loaded messages regarding their own brain features, good and bad, from life situations or media exposure. May or may not have either witnessed or directly experienced negative consequences involving their neurotype. (If they have, they may have actively worked towards healing.)
- Intentionally stands *aligned with* their own brain by working with it instead of against it (e.g., by utilizing specific brain-based coping skills).
- May or may not choose to ethically disclose their neurotype within the practice of neurodiverse couple therapy or other professional endeavors.
- Likely integrates their neurotype within their overall identity framework. The degree to which they do so may vary.
- Displays gratitude for their brain, attributing certain strengths to their neurotype while avoiding toxic positivity.
- May be a self-advocate and ally for ND persons in their personal and/or professional life.
- May easily and intentionally create space in the therapy room for neurodiverse couples to explore emerging ND or NT identity narratives.

A therapist with positive brain-esteem wastes zero energy operating against their own innate and unchangeable brain qualities. Doing so can free up valuable capacity to clarify their own brain-based strengths and creatively utilize them within the counseling room. Although this can be a particularly healthy position for a neurodiverse couple therapist, it is not a requirement. In fact, these therapists in a positive relationship with their own brain need to exercise caution in order to avoid unintentionally promoting toxic positivity. They should also use caution to not assert that this is the one correct way for any client to exist. (Remember, healthy brain-esteem can also look like maintaining a neutral relationship with one's own brain.) Each therapist, as well as each client, deserves the right to choose their own personal stance and sentiment – which can fluctuate.

A therapist who has a *neutral* relationship with their own brain . . .

- May or may not have pursued differential self-diagnosis of either neurotypicality or neurodivergence. May or may not have pursued formal diagnosis if it was safe and wise to do so.
- May or may not have internalized loaded messages regarding their own brain features, good and bad, from life situations or media exposure. May or may not have either witnessed or directly experienced negative consequences involving their neurotype. (If they have, they may have actively worked towards healing.)
- Views their own brain as neither a friend nor foe. They walk *alongside* their brain in peaceful coexistence.
- May or may not choose to ethically disclose their neurotype within the practice of neurodiverse couple therapy or other professional endeavors.
- May or may not integrate their neurotype within their overall identity framework.
- May or may not be an ally to ND persons in their personal or professional life.
- May or may not find it easy to create space in the therapy room for neurodiverse couples to explore emerging ND or NT identity narratives.

Maintaining a neutral relationship with one's own brain represents a suggested minimum standard for any therapist seeking to offer *Brain-Informed Neurodiverse Couple Therapy (BINCT)*. This is because it's extremely difficult to have enough energy to effectively guide neurodiverse couples through the kinds of complex issues they face while harboring negative brain-esteem.

A therapist who has a *negative* relationship with their own brain . . .

- May or may not have pursued differential self-diagnosis of neurodivergence or neurotypicality, and are unlikely to pursue a formal diagnostic process. If they have experienced a formal diagnostic process, however, they may associate their brain-based labels with shame, anxiety, inferiority, brokenness, or fear/danger.
- Has likely internalized negative messages from others regarding their brain, and also experienced negative social consequences or trauma based on their brain-based features.

- Stands *against* their own brain qualities in an adversarial position: Attempts to deny, camouflage, or eradicate that which makes them neurologically different from others.
- Unlikely to disclose their neurotype within the practice of neurodiverse couple therapy or other professional endeavors.
- Purposely chooses to exclude their brain-based features from their overall identity framework.
- Utilizes coping mechanisms that do not consider their own brain-based needs.
- Unlikely to be an ally to ND persons in their personal or professional life. Knowingly or unknowingly, may promote neurotypical standards.
- Unlikely to create space in the therapy room for neurodiverse couples to explore emerging ND or NT identity narratives. May experience significant countertransference when working with neurodiverse couples.

Remember that almost everyone feels like their own brain is an enemy sometimes, and neurodiverse couple therapists are no exception. A therapist in a negative relationship with their brain for too long or too often, however, is unlikely to conduct good neurodiverse couple therapy. Consistently resenting one's brain is incredibly exhausting. And although therapists should always have the right to mask and unmask any part of themselves as they see fit, the act of continual masking can interfere with the power of therapist authenticity.

Neurodiverse couple therapists who are prone to this stance and sentiment should actively self-monitor to ensure they do not unintentionally express bias against neurodivergence, promote ableism, react inappropriately to countertransference, or experience professional burnout. It may be necessary to pause working with neurodiverse clients for a time or to choose to serve a different client population all together.

Some professionals can continue to serve clients well via the thoughtful use of coping skills and social support during temporary periods of negativity towards their own brain. This is not unlike when therapists experience bouts of intense spiritual or existential contemplation, relational pain, grief, or illness over the span of their career. Some professionals can continue practicing empathy, genuineness, and other clinical skills while going through their own dark times. Others will find their clinical skills become compromised. It's more than okay to take a pause and reach out for help with negative brain-esteem. Therapists are allowed to be human.

Are there any practical exercises to help me explore the relationship I have with my own brain?

The relationship one has with their own brain does not form in a vacuum. It's dynamically shaped by life experiences, cultural assumptions, myths, family mottos, spiritual beliefs, educational opportunities, media influences, and much more. Reading the descriptions in this chapter can help determine one's stance and sentiment towards their own brain, but a more comprehensive way to assess brain-esteem may involve the following exercises. *Brain Branching* and *Writing a NeuroNarrative* explore the intersectionality of sociocultural factors with one's own physiological, neurological, and emotional experiences. *Individual Circle Mapping* considers the ways brain features may or may not fit into one's holistic identity framework. *The Masking Exercise* examines one's own masking or unmasking patterns across various social settings.

These exercises carry some risk, as brand-new information about oneself may rise to the surface (e.g., genetic information, diagnostic labels, traumatic memories). Slowing down to consider one's life experiences can be especially jarring if there is a history of systemic injustice or if family members have historically denied, camouflaged, mislabeled, vilified, or otherwise distorted neurodiversity topics. Of course, it's also possible to uncover personal data that is neuroaffirming! Neurodiverse couple therapists are encouraged to first complete these introspection-based exercises on their own, or together with their own personal therapist, before attempting to use them with clients. Both ND and NT persons may stand to benefit.

Brain Branching

Brain Branching is an accessible activity designed to be flexible enough to promote personal insight regardless of a participant's social boundaries, learning style, or neurotype. Presented as a sort of neurological genogram, its main purpose is to list and examine the brain attributes of one's family members (and associated interpersonal dynamics) across three generations. It also considers what noteworthy messages regarding physical wellness, mental health, disability, and brain wiring the participant may have internalized.

The first step is data collection. Although answers to the questions below may be gathered solely from personal reflection, whenever appropriate, valuable data collection may also result from family interviews. (Auditory learners, in particular, may find these types of in-person or virtual conversations beneficial.) Of course, interviewing one's family requires a level of access and safety that simply may not exist. This should never be done if unsafe or otherwise unwise. A therapist who uses *Brain Branching* with clients should help each participant carefully consider their interpersonal dynamics, preferences, and boundaries regarding how to collect data. They should also encourage clients to think through any potential psychological impacts and/ or unexpected social consequences of this exercise.

The second step of *Brain Branching* involves formatting one's findings into a loose sketch. The act of sketching is encouraged, especially for kinesthetic and visual learners, but not mandatory. The point is to simply arrange one's data in any way that allows analysis.

Last, inferences can be made from one's answers.

The exercises in this chapter will include examples based on a fictional 29-year-old female of Korean descent named Amy. She is not a therapy professional.

Step 1: Data Collection

Across three generations, list your own name and the names of your family members. Also include those related by adoption or marriage, as well as anyone you've considered especially influential in your life (e.g., a coach, best friend, or mentor).

For yourself and each person on your list, note the following:

- Medical conditions.
- Head injuries.
- Physical disabilities.
- Cognitive/Intellectual disabilities.
- Mental health concerns.
- Sensory challenges (e.g., "Uncle Jack had an aversion to loud noises, strong smells, and desperately avoided being in crowds.")

List any specific support needs regarding the above issues. Were these needs validated by others?

Are there any formally diagnosed, self-diagnosed, or highly-suspected neurodivergent (ND) people on your list? If so, write each person's actual or suspected neurotype(s) by their name (e.g., Autistic, ADHD, Dyslexic, Gifted, 2e).

Society has not always accurately identified or respected neurodivergence, especially in past generations. Even today, ND features and their associated behaviors are often misunderstood or mischaracterized. Have any of these descriptors ever been applied to you directly? To anyone on your list?

- "Retarded."
- "Lazy."
- "Odd."
- "Socially awkward."
- "Genius."
- "Quirky."
- "Slow."

If so, how might these labels relate to actual or suspected brain differences?

Both for yourself and each person on your list, note any of the following life experiences:

- Incarceration.
- Being denied acceptance into school, the military, etc. or being kicked out.
- Experiencing prejudice and/or bullying.
- Abusing others.
- Being the target of abuse.
- Chronic unemployment.
- Addiction.
- Psychiatric institutionalization.
- Being "sent away" to be raised elsewhere and/or living in an adult group home.
- Failing out of academic or vocational programs.
- Skipping a grade or being held back a grade.
- Attempting suicide.
- Attending college at a young age.

Is it possible that some of these experiences may relate to actual or suspected brain differences?

How have the known (or suspected) ND persons on your list acted over time, in general? If you've ever had direct interactions with these persons, what have those interactions been like?

In general, how have you and/or others treated the known (or suspected) ND persons on your list?

Step 2: Sketching

Look over your answers. Sketch your most important data points onto one large piece of paper, however you'd like. This can look like an actual family tree with branches, a genogram, a series of stick figures, a chart, a graph, or something else entirely.

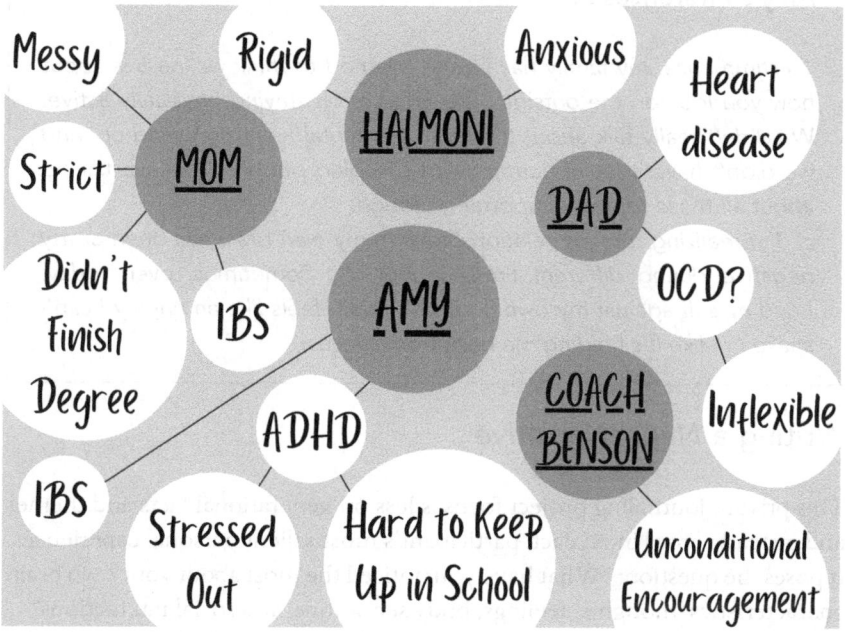

Figure 4.6 Amy's sketch

Step 3: Making Inferences

What do the people on your list seem to believe about the following topics:

- Physical wellness.
- Mental health.
- Disability.
- Brain wiring.

What do you believe about these topics?

Each person's beliefs and experiences influence the relationship they form with their own brain. This relationship can be either *positive*, *negative*, or *neutral* at any given time. Currently, how would you describe the relationship you have with your own brain?

Additionally, at any given time, one can either stand *aligned with, against,* or *alongside* their own brain. How would you describe your current relational stance toward your brain?

Amy's Inferences . . .

To summarize, my family has always seemed to think wellness is about how you look on the outside. The focus is on staying physically active. We didn't really talk about the brain or mental health growing up, and we didn't have a lot of contact with Disabled people. I believe talking about all these topics is important, though.

I'm realizing that my relationship with my own brain has been pretty negative during different times in my life. Sometimes, even today, I find myself against my own brain. My brain feels like an enemy I can't shake . . . like it's holding me back from success.

Writing a *NeuroNarrative*

This private journaling project focuses less on generational facts and themes and instead zeroes in on each participant's most salient personal experiences. It poses the question: "What have you noticed the most about your own brain characteristics, thoughts, feelings, body sensations, and social interactions?"

Writing a *NeuroNarrative* invites participants to recall their own brain-centric details from different developmental periods and to explore how they may relate to their current view of themselves. Memories of trauma, discrimination, bullying, exploitation, or invalidation are especially important to note. However, this exercise does not focus exclusively on painful memories. It also highlights neuroaffirming moments and joyous times.

Persons of any neurotype can participate in this exercise, as exploring one's life story from a neurological perspective can offer a unique insight. For known or suspected ND participants, though, writing a *NeuroNarrative* can carry special significance. This is because it can be particularly beneficial to talk through any formal, informal, or self-diagnostic processes. These areas hardly ever receive proper attention in therapy despite the fact they involve complex feelings, relationship dynamics, identity concerns, etc.!

Regarding late discovery of one's own neurodivergence, or that of a partner, in adulthood, common reactions can involve intense relief, anger, happiness, disgust, grief, and more. No two ND people will react the exact same way to finding out they are ND. Additionally, no two NT people will react the exact same way to finding out their partner is ND. Generational differences, as well as cultural and gender-based differences, deserve proper recognition when discussing this or any other aspect of a participant's *NeuroNarrative*.

For late-identified ND adults in America, some version of the following mental and emotional processes tends to take place upon realization of their own neurodivergence:

Validation Elation . . .

"Everything in my life makes so much more sense now!"
"I'm not broken, I'm ND!"

Dismay . . .

"How could I have not known this about myself until now?"
"Why didn't someone see this in me sooner and offer support?"

Anger . . .

"Why have others in my family mistreated/miscategorized/invalidated me?"
"Why is the world the way it is, systemically?"
"Why am I the way I am?"

Identity Exploration . . .

"What does my neurodivergence mean to me?"
"How does my neurodivergence fit into my overall identity framework?"
"How does my neurodivergence impact my intimate relationship?"

Grief . . .

"The world just doesn't seem built for people like me."
"Others have never/may never fully understand me."
"It's really hard being me sometimes."

Acceptance . . .

"I'm ok with all the parts of me, including my neurodivergence."
"My neurodivergence affords me a unique lens by which I experience Earth's sensory multiverse."
"I know how neurodivergence fits into my overall identity framework."
"I know how neurodivergence fits into my intimate relationship."

Pride . . .

"I like myself."
"My neurodivergence imparts certain strengths that I wouldn't otherwise have."
"I don't have to change myself into someone I'm not to be more palatable to the NT majority."
"I'm learning healthy ways to cope with the challenges associated with my neurodivergence."

Current societal trends lean towards ND people in America discovering their own neurotype earlier and earlier. One reason for this is because each new generation has better access to information and resources. But, "late" diagnosis will likely always exist to some degree.

Step 1: Completing a Questionnaire

The following prompts are meant for independent introspection. (Family interviews aren't encouraged here, as the *NeuroNarrative* prioritizes each participant's own experiences from their own perspective.) Jot down your answers, type them out, speak them into a voice recorder, or draw them out in pictures. Please consider discussing any traumatic memories or intense feelings with a therapy professional.

Your Everyday Life from Preschool to Age 12

What were your preferred ways to play?

Describe your eating habits. Were you ever referred to as a picky eater? Would you ever put non-food items in your mouth? If you had challenges regarding feeding, did you receive support?

Describe your sleeping habits. If you had challenges regarding sleep, did you receive support?

How did your communication skills develop? Did you receive any services (e.g., speech therapy)? If so, what did you think of those sessions?

Describe your experience with toilet training. Did you ever experience bed-wetting, soiling your clothes in public, or other challenges? If so, did you receive appropriate support?

Did you ever have frequent headaches, stomach aches, constipation, or other uncomfortable body sensations? Did they seem related to anxiety, sensory issues, or any other reason?

Did you have any unsafe behaviors? If so, did you receive support for them?

Describe your emotional and physical experience of puberty. Did you receive support if you needed it? Did you receive any form of sexual education in school or from caregivers?

What is your favorite memory during this time period, and does it relate to your brain wiring at all? (For example, enjoying playground swings may relate to your sensory system's wiring.)

Your Interactions with Others from Preschool to Age 12

How were you disciplined, and for what reasons?

What behaviors were you most rewarded for by others?

How did you interact with your peers, and how did they respond to you?

Did you have an IEP and/or receive Gifted services, Special Education services, etc.? If so, what was your experience of this?

Overall, did you feel like you "belonged" at home and within the world? Why or why not?

Your Brain from Preschool to Age 12

Did you receive any formal or informal brain-based labels? If so, how did you become aware of them? Did they affect your view of yourself?

If you received a formal brain assessment at a doctor's office, school, or other location, what was this process like for you? Was your participation voluntary or forced?

Did you receive any services such as behavioral therapy, occupational therapy, or counseling? If so, was participation voluntary or forced? What was your experience of those sessions?

Were you prescribed medication for any brain-based concern? If so, how did this come about? Was the medication explained to you? What did you think about it? What were the medication's effects on your mind and body?

Did you experience any type of head trauma? If so, what was your experience with the incident itself? Did you receive treatment? If so, what was your experience of this? Were there any lingering effects of either the incident or its treatment?

Your "Ways of Being" from Preschool to Age 12

Were you especially drawn to, or repelled by, any specific body sensations, e.g., feeling cold, putting things in your mouth, spinning or swinging, having a full bladder, the feeling of firm pressure on your skin?

Did you experience intense emotions? If so, how would you try to cope with them? How did your caregivers, teachers, and peers respond to your feelings?

How did you learn best during Elementary School and Middle School? Was this learning style understood and supported by caregivers and teachers?

Did you engage in any repetitive behaviors like echolalia or stimming? If so, what did this behavior do for you on both a physical and emotional level? How did others react?

Did you have any strong interests? If so, were you able/allowed to engage with these interests?

Did your caregivers or anyone else try to "cure" you of any brain-based label? If so, were you subjected to any special diets, exercises, religious rituals, or other interventions? What was your experience of this, and how did it affect you?

Did anyone really "see" the real you at this age? Why or why not?

Your NeuroNeeds* from Preschool to Age 12

List your brain-based joys, aversions, and challenges from Preschool to age 12 in the following categories.

Table 4.1

Seeing	Hearing	Tasting	Touching	Smelling	Moving My Own Body Around	Interoception (My Internal Body Sensations)	Learning

*The term *NeuroNeed* is shorthand for any brain-based need related to sensory processing, emotion regulation, learning, communication, etc.

Your Everyday Life from Age 13 to Age 18

Describe your eating and sleeping patterns.

Did you have any dating experiences? If so, what were these relationships like?

Did you have a job? If so, how did you balance work with school, friends, hobbies, self-care, etc.?

Did you ever experience self-harm or suicidal thoughts, food restriction, binge eating, or running away? If so, did you receive appropriate support?

Did you experiment with drugs or alcohol? If so, what was the outcome?

What is your favorite memory during this time period, and does it relate to your brain wiring at all?

Your Interactions with Others from Age 13 to Age 18

How did you interact with peers, and how did they respond to you?

Did you experience bullying, either in person or via social media?

Did you experience criticism and/or discrimination by caregivers, teachers, or other adults?

Was your learning style identified and supported by your High School teachers? Did you have an IEP and/or receive Gifted services, Special Education services, etc.? If so, what was your experience of this?

What behaviors were rewarded and punished by others, and how?

Overall, did you feel you "belonged" within your family, school, work environment, place of worship, and society in general? Why or why not?

Did anyone really "see" the real you at this age? Why or why not?

Your Brain from Age 13 to Age 18

Did you receive any brain-based labels during a formal or informal diagnostic process? If so, what was your experience of this like? (Alternatively, did you self-diagnose any brain-based label?)

If applicable, how were your brain-based labels used by others? Were any brain-based labels ever used against you?

Did you have the option to attend any kind of therapy or supportive service such as speech therapy, occupational therapy, social skill groups, etc.? If so, what was your experience like? Was anything like this ever forced upon you?

Were your brain characteristics ever specifically discussed with you regarding your grades, extracurricular activities, friendships, future plans, etc.?

Were you prescribed medication for any brain-based concern? If so, how did this come about? Did you have a choice? How did you feel about taking medication? What were its effects?

Did you experience any type of head trauma? If so, what was your experience with the incident itself? Did you receive treatment? If so, what was your experience of it? Were there any lingering effects of either the incident or its treatment?

Your "Ways of Being" from Age 13 to Age 18

Did you choose to adopt (or reject) any brain-based label as a <u>self-identification</u> as a teenager? Why or why not?

What role did various media sources, including social media, play in your life? Do you remember seeing anyone who had a brain like yours on TV, in the movies, or on the internet?

Did you experience times of intense emotions and/or physiological overload? If so, how did this feel on a physical and mental level? What would cause it? How did you attempt to cope? Did others ever support you?

Did you ever use stimming as a coping skill, a form of personal expression or communication, or just for fun? If so, what were your preferred stims?

Did you have any strong interests? If so, were you able/allowed to engage with them?

Did your caregivers or anyone else try to "cure" you of any brain-based label? If so, were you subjected to any special diets, exercises, religious rituals, or other interventions? (Alternatively, did you seek out anything like this on your own behalf?) How did this affect you?

Did anyone really "see" the real you at this age? Why or why not?

Your NeuroNeeds from Age 13 to Age 18

List your brain-based joys, aversions, and challenges from age 13 to age 18 in the following categories.

Table 4.2

Seeing	Hearing	Tasting	Touching	Smelling	Moving My Own Body Around	Interoception (My Internal Body Sensations)	Learning

Your Everyday Life from Age 18 Until Now

What role did/do various media sources, including social media, play in your life?

Have you ever had (or do you currently have) any reasonable accommodations at school or work due to any of your specific brain features? If so, how did these come about? Are they helpful?

Have you experienced times of self-harm or suicidal thoughts, food restriction, binging, or purging?

Have you or a loved one been concerned about your use of alcohol, drugs, sex, gambling, or gaming?

Have you quit a job or school pursuit? If so, why?

Have you experienced rejection by a school, job, or other pursuit? Have you had difficulty obtaining or maintaining employment?

What is your favorite memory from this time period, and does it relate to your brain wiring at all?

Your Interactions with Others from Age 18 Until Now

How would you describe your romantic pursuits, if any?

How would you characterize your friendships?

Has your brain wiring ever been used against you by a person in power, a friend, a coworker, a family member, or an intimate partner?

Has anyone really "seen" the real you as an adult? If so, who?

Your Brain from Age 18 Until Now

Have you sought out any brain-based labels, for the first time, as an adult? If so, where did they come from? (Alternatively, have you self-diagnosed any brain-based label?)

Have you taken medication for any brain-based concern? If so, how did this come about? What were/are its effects?

Your "Ways of Being" from Age 18 Until Now

Have you chosen to adopt any brain-based label as an intentional self-identification? Why or why not?

Have you experienced/do you experience times of emotional overwhelm and/or physiological overload as an adult? If so, what triggers these times? How have you felt on an emotional and physical level when they happen? How do you attempt to cope? Have others been supportive?

Have you used/do you use stimming as a coping skill, a form of personal expression or communication, or maybe just for fun as an adult? If so, what were/are your preferred stims?

Have you identified any of your own sensory joys or aversions? If you're a parent, do any of your children seem to share any similarities to you regarding their sensory processing?

If you're a parent, do any of your children seem to think, emote, learn, behave, or respond to stress similarly to you?

Your NeuroNeeds from Age 18 Until Now

List your brain-based joys, aversions, and challenges from age 18 until now in the following categories.

Table 4.3

Seeing	Hearing	Tasting	Touching	Smelling	Moving My Own Body Around	Interoception (My Internal Body Sensations)	Learning

Your Internalized Messages

Have you received any loaded messages about your own brain features from others? This chart has some examples that pertain specifically to neurodivergence. However, neurotypical persons can also be bombarded with messages.

Table 4.4

Messages from Others about Your Own Neurodivergent Brain:

Positive Messages	Negative Messages
I accept that you're an ADHDer.	You're too high-functioning to really have ADHD.
ADHD is your superpower!*	Don't let ADHD define you.
Your brain is not diseased.	Your brain is diseased.
You're not a broken neurotypical, you're a typical neurodivergent person.	Why can't you just be like everyone else/work harder to fit in?
Your emotions and sensory experiences deserve validation.	You're exaggerating or lying about your emotions and sensory experiences; You're too dramatic, too sensitive, etc.
Your brain challenges are real and deserve to be seen and supported.	Sensory challenges and executive functioning challenges aren't real. Don't make excuses. Get over it.
It's ok to have intense interests and pursue them.	Your intense interests are too odd, too intense, etc. Stop engaging with them and try to fit in with others better.
You're not too much for this family or this world.	You're too much for this family and the world.
You have inherent value.	You're worthless.
The way your brain works is: • Ok. • Unique. • Worthy.	The way your brain works is: • Wrong. • Childish/Immature. • Sinful.

*This may represent toxic positivity.

In summary, the <u>main message</u> I've learned from others about my own brain is:

_____

_____

_____

_____

The *sentiment* I currently have toward my own brain is (circle one):

Positive

Neutral

Negative

The *stance* I currently have toward my own brain is (circle one):

Aligned with

Alongside

Against

Step 2: Telling Your Story

Compile your answers from the above questionnaire into a single *NeuroNarrative*. Use any format you'd like: A voice recording, a written story, a piece of artwork, a song, etc. It can be as long or short as you like.

Amy's *NeuroNarrative* . . .

I had a pretty good childhood with no trauma. My brain differences made me feel different at school, though, despite the fact that most kids were nice. I always had friends, but sometimes I was teased for asking questions in class after they'd already been answered. I also couldn't seem to keep track of my homework, my jacket, or my toys. I got in trouble for losing things. Fifth grade was when I first heard the word "ADHD" from a doctor. I think my parents considered this some kind of excuse, though. No one talked about it, and nothing changed.

I worked hard in school, yet this was never good enough. My parents used to argue with me and each other about my grades a lot. My dad

---

called me "spacey" and "too stressed out" to focus properly. He'd say that this reminded him of his mother, whom I know he resents. Those talks made me feel like a failure. When my parents asked my teacher to sit me at the front of the classroom, I got embarrassed. I didn't really understand what my NeuroNeeds were from Preschool to age 12, and my parents didn't either.

My parents divorced when I was 11. I lived with my mom and saw my dad every other weekend. They both never stopped putting pressure on me to pay more attention in school and to bring home good grades. My mom was such a hypocrite! She was messy herself, but expected me to be really neat. And, my little brother could always get away with anything – but not me! Thank God for my soccer coach and my teammates who gave me unconditional acceptance and support. Soccer was my escape. I was the life of the party on the field and at school functions, even though I was a disappointment at home. When I started going to a Christian youth group around this time, I learned that God created me and loved me . . . this kept me from getting too down on myself.

From 13 to 18, I didn't really think about ADHD too much. I was more interested in maintaining a social life and staying out of my parents' houses. There were a few characters on TV that reminded me of things I struggled with in school, but I didn't like how they were portrayed as dumb and ditsy. That wasn't me. I worked extremely hard to keep up with my classes, and I know I'm a very smart person. I just couldn't seem to juggle everything like everyone else. It was internally exhausting to pretend like I could do it all. When I broke down to my mom at age 15 about how hard school truly was for me, she finally gave me the option to take ADHD medication. This was a huge relief at first. But, soon the medication's side effects made me feel really weird physically. My primary care doctor didn't give me any good options for other medications to try, so I just stopped taking it. Things went back to baseline pretty quickly after that. Thankfully, I had a great group of friends that kept me moving forward. I kept playing soccer and somehow managed to graduate with a decent GPA. I took some risks with marijuana and boyfriends, but nothing too serious. I still went to church, which kept me grounded. What I learned about my NeuroNeeds from age 13 to age 18 was that they probably weren't that important if I was able to do ok in school by working hard and leaning heavily on my social group.

In college I only took ADHD medication prescribed by the campus doctor if I needed to study for a major test. The doctor told me this was fine because I was too successful to be severely ADHD. She said there wasn't a need for me to take medication on a daily basis. This doctor blamed my difficulty keeping up at school, managing my emotions, and staying organized on anxiety. It's true that I was always stressed out when I talked to her, but I think there was more going on than just anxiety. There was just so much that came at me all at once when I went away to school. My friends seemed to have it all together, but not me! I was drowning, but I hid it from others. I couldn't seem to balance my assignments with my social life, and I would get really mad at myself (and my brain) when I fell short. I'd try to shame myself into succeeding by working harder, staying up later, etc. Around this time, the vocational counselor on campus sounded just like my parents . . . she pushed me to "just apply myself more" when I went to her for advice. This made me so angry. Why did no one believe how hard I was working just to break even? After I failed an important class in my major, enough was enough. I ended up impulsively dropping out of college altogether.

Fortunately, it wasn't long before I landed a job that paid well and that I was great at doing. I started feeling good about myself. I even got really excited to make my own path in life instead of doing what was expected of me. Plus, even though I never went back to finish my degree, this new company didn't care – I kept getting promotions. After a while, my parents stopped lecturing me about going back to finish my education. They couldn't deny the fact I was making good money. They even actually started being proud of me. When I was 29 I met an amazing guy and we moved in together. I got pregnant unexpectedly, so we decided to get married.

Our son is two years old now. I have a good life. Underneath my smile, though, I still feel broken and messy. My mind wanders a lot, and I can't seem to get things done the way I used to before the baby. Would getting back on ADHD medication help, or do I need an antidepressant? My husband keeps begging me to figure out an answer. I just can't seem to keep up with everything since the baby was born. It feels like I'm back in college, drowning all over again. Our house is an embarrassing disaster. We end up arguing about chores a lot. He says I'm no fun anymore. I miss being fun, too! But when all my *brain-power each day goes to my job and parenting, there's nothing left over for chores, time for myself, or time together – let alone fun! How do other moms juggle it all? My eating and sleeping patterns are all messed up because I haven't been able to exercise in ages. We try to go to church together as a family, but sometimes it's just too hard to get out the door.*

I wonder how much my brain wiring is a factor in my life these days. ADHD has always been this nagging thing to me that I've never understood. Do I need to just stop whining and pull myself together? Do I need to work harder? Do I need to have more faith in Jesus? Do I need medication? I'm still learning about what having ADHD means to me.

I'm encouraged that our neurodiverse couple therapist is here to help my husband and I sort this all out. Now that I'm an adult, I'd also like to get an official ADHD evaluation.

I don't exactly know my NeuroNeeds from childhood, but I think my current NeuroNeeds chart looks like this:

Table 4.5

Seeing	Hearing	Tasting	Touching	Smelling	Moving My Own Body Around	Interoception (My Own Body Sensations)	Learning
All the clutter in my house makes me feel ashamed and anxious.	I work best when listening to music. I always have my headphones in.	I can't stand slimy textures of some foods.	I feel "touched out" by the end of every single day. I don't want my husband to ask for sex right now.	I love the smell of lavender. I gag at the smell of cinnamon.	I feel best when I'm able to exercise regularly. If I don't exercise, I get restless and down on myself.	When I'm stressed out I feel tension in my neck and lower back	I learn by doing.

Individual Circle Mapping

Individual Circle Mapping is meant to quickly draw upon the personal insights discovered via the *Brain Branching* and *Writing a NeuroNarrative* exercises. Just like any of the exercises in this chapter, however, it can also be used as a stand-alone exercise.

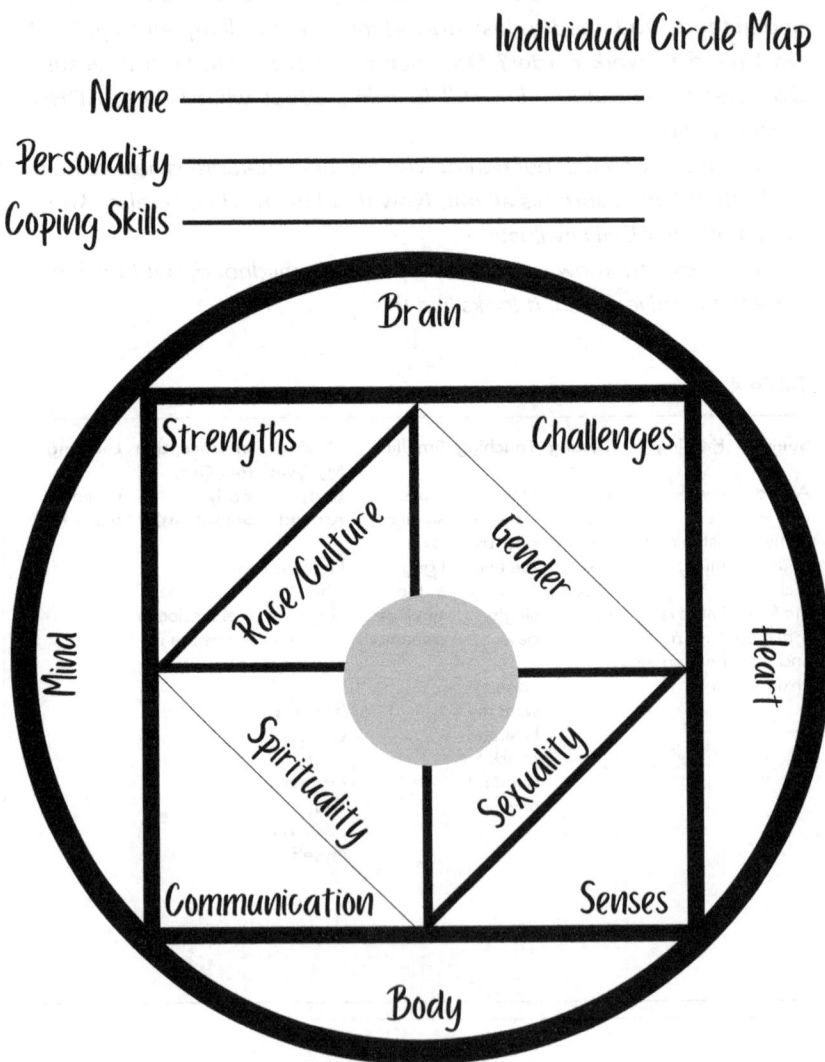

Figure 4.7 Blank template for an *Individual Circle Map*

Jot down answers about yourself onto a blank *Individual Circle Map* template. Place an asterisk (*) beside any category that represents an area you are currently exploring. The end result will be an infographic that represents a visual snapshot of your holistic identity framework as it now stands.

Your Core Features

Write in your **Name**. If desired, include the meaning of your name and/or its personal significance.

Fill in any known **Personality** data about yourself i.e., *Myers–Briggs Typology* results, *Enneagram* results, *DISC* results, etc. If you do not have this information, simply write in a few key words to describe your personality.

Write in your top three **Coping Skills** in response to stress (e.g., journaling, listening to music, taking a walk, stimming, etc.).

What is most central to who you are as a person? This may be your identity in Christ, your life calling or vocation, a personal value, or something else. Represent this with a symbol, word, or phrase inside the innermost circle.

Your Self-Identifications

List your **Racial/Cultural**, **Gender**, **Sexual**, and **Spiritual** self-identifications. Feel free to use whatever language that feels most appropriate to you.

Your Brain, Body, Heart, and Mind

In the **Brain** area, list your known or suspected neurotype(s). Also list any brain-related injuries, medical conditions, or mental health diagnoses.

In the **Body** section, list any chronic physical health conditions and/or disabling physical attributes. You may also wish to write in any body part that is especially significant to your identity. For example, a professional musician may wish to list their hands or voice, or a Black individual who embraces their natural hair may wish to list their hair, etc. Additionally, persons with symbolic tattoos or piercings on their body may wish to include those here.

In the **Heart** section, list your *Love Language(s)*. The concept of *Love Languages* was introduced by Gary Chapman.[4] They are: *Acts of Service, Physical Touch, Quality Time, Words of Affirmation*, and *Gifts*.

In the **Mind** section, list your preferred style of <u>taking in</u> information from the outside world. Is this from *seeing*, *hearing*, or *touching*? Also list your style of <u>processing</u> incoming information. Is this *internal* or *external*? *Internal Processors* need time alone to think and reflect on new material, whereas *External Processors* need time with others to think out loud and talk things out.

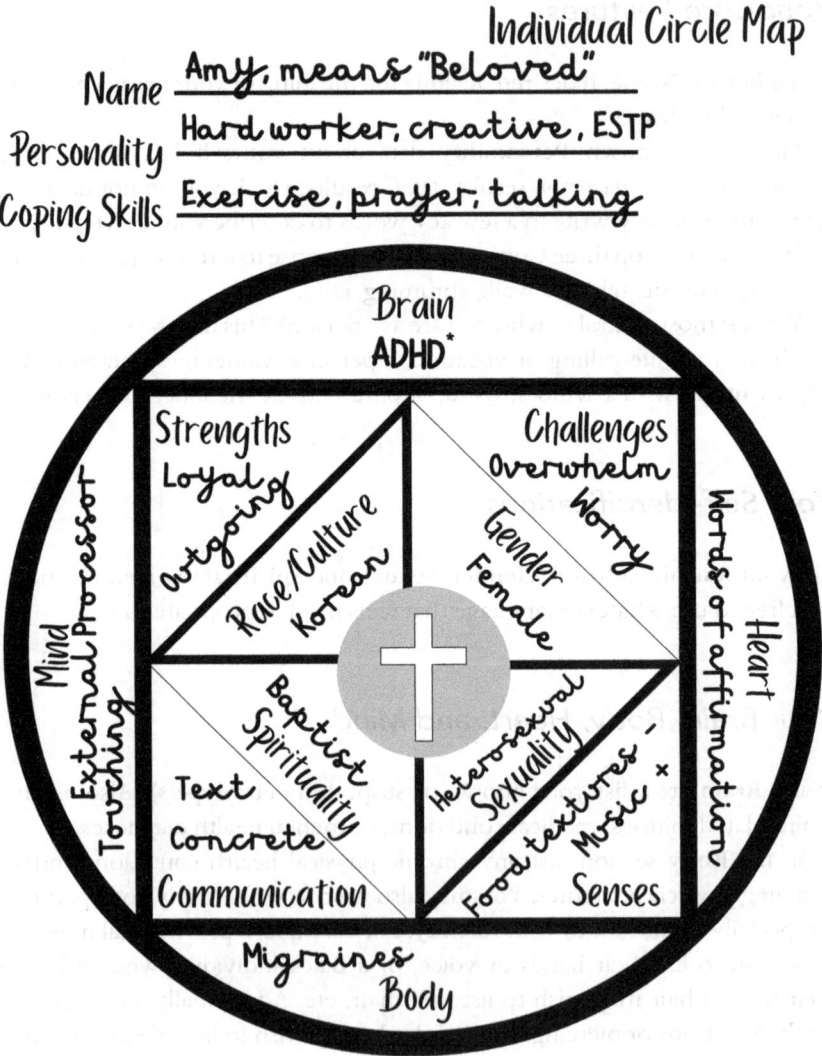

Figure 4.8 Amy's *Individual Circle Map*

Your Other Unique Features

List your top **Strengths.**

List your top **Challenges.**

In the **Senses** section, list your sensory joys (marked with a "+" sign) and sensory aversions (marked with a "−" sign).

List your preferred **Communication Style** (e.g., *In-person, Via Text, Assertive, Passive, Harmony-Seeking, Challenge-Provoking, Concrete, Indirect, etc.*).

The Masking Exercise

The final activity in this chapter is called the *Masking Exercise*. It was designed to draw upon a participant's completed *NeuroNarrative* and *Individual Circle Map*, but can also stand alone. This free-form journaling project poses the question: "What parts of yourself are you free to express around others, should you wish to do so?" Your answers may be written, spoken into a recorder, or drawn out in pictures.

- Which parts of your identity are currently visible to others, and which are invisible? Do you have a choice in this visibility?
- What parts of yourself are you <u>proud</u> to have others notice? Are there any parts of yourself that you wished others noticed more often?
- Is there anything about yourself that is embarrassing, shameful, vulnerable, or even dangerous, when others notice it? What tends to happen in these situations?
- Do you ever intentionally minimize parts of yourself for safety or any other reason? If so, which parts and why? In what personal and/or professional settings does this currently take place? When did this start?
- Do you ever find yourself suppressing any of your identified *NeuroNeeds* in public and/or in private? If so, how? When did this start? Who or what taught you these needs are too much, don't matter, aren't even real, etc.?
- Have you ever felt free to be totally "you" when alone, or in the presence of others? If so, when? What specifically made you feel safe and seen? After the fact, were/are there any social consequences, good or bad, to being totally "you?"

Amy's *Masking Exercise* . . .

I've always been an open book emotionally compared to most of my family members. What's invisible, though, is how jammed up my brain gets sometimes and how hard I work to keep my life organized. Part of me wishes this struggle could be seen and supported by the world, but at the end of the day I prefer to keep the details of my struggle private. Sure, I talk about being frustrated and overwhelmed with my close friends, but I leave out a lot. No one needs to know how messy my closet and pantry really are, or that I can't get even myself together enough to write out a grocery list. That kind of choice to mask probably started when I was very young. My parents made me feel like a burden whenever I needed help. I learned to "suck it up" and work harder. Plus, I learned the way to get ahead was to show only the best parts of myself to others. Thank God that soccer practice was the one place I always felt freedom to be me.

As a kid, I was embarrassed about being labeled with ADHD only because it meant sitting at the front of the classroom. That's all I really knew about the diagnosis back then – it gets you seated in front of the class to help you pay attention. It was (and still is) exhausting to work so hard to keep up with everyone else while wearing the mask of having it all together while everyone is watching you.

These days, I don't really know what to think about my ADHD. I know it's a part of me, I guess, but is that a good or bad thing? Both? No one except my parents and my husband knows that I was diagnosed as a kid with ADHD. In fact, I hope my boss <u>never</u> *finds out. I'm afraid she may see me as less capable and limit my career opportunities. So, I definitely put a lot of energy into masking at work. At church I tend to put on a happy face, too.*

Glossary of Bolded Terms

Brain-Esteem   One's level of acceptance and confidence regarding their own neurotype, inclusive of the ways their brain wiring manifests within everyday interactions and their overall identity framework.

Neurodiscovery   The process of learning about one's own brain-based features and/or those of a loved one.

NeuroNeed   Any brain-based need regarding sensory processing, emotion regulation, learning, communication, executive functioning, etc.

Notes

1 Aponte, H. J. (2016). The person-of-the-therapist model on the use of self in therapy: The training philosophy. In *The Person of the Therapist Training Model* (pp. 1–13). Routledge.

2 Pennant, A., & Shamoon, Z. (2022). Reflections on implementing the POTT program in a Master's clinical program. *Australian and New Zealand Journal of Family Therapy*.

3 Oral, S., Zeytinoğlu-Saydam, S., Söylemez, Y., Akmehmet-Şekerler, S., & Aponte, H. J. (2022). Developing the person of the therapist when working with couples. *Contemporary Family Therapy*, 1–14.

4 Chapman, G. (2010). *The five love languages: The secret to love that lasts*. Chicago, IL.

Respecting Neurodivergence from First Contact

5

Can any relationship therapist learn how to support neurodiverse couples, even if they don't intend to specialize in neurodiversity topics? Absolutely! This can be as simple as implementing a few key habits, or as profound as taking steps towards whatever level of advocacy or allyship feels appropriate. Professional readers are strongly encouraged to use this text as a springboard to seek out more education and training opportunities to help them decide exactly *how* and *why* they'll serve neurodiverse couples. There are numerous ways to practice at least some degree of *Brain-Informed Care (BIC)*. These include, but are not limited to, offering virtual or in-person therapy sessions for neurodiverse couples, writing, speaking, conducting research, and more. Even just maintaining an accessible, informative online presence can make a positive impact. Deciding the degree to which one will integrate neurodiversity topics within their career boils down to personal preference. One's strengths, capacities, goals, and contextual factors are important considerations.

An obvious starting point regarding the support of neurodiverse couples involves the notion of genuineness. Above all, therapists must sincerely believe in the innate value of all ND persons and desire to promote their wellbeing and that of their NT partners. It should go without saying, then, that any helping professional who hones in neurodiversity topics merely because doing so can quickly distinguish them as an expert within an emerging field represents a huge red flag. Deciding to specialize in neurodiverse couples just because this guarantees a full appointment calendar is unethical. Sadly, it's necessary to discuss the potential for this

DOI: 10.4324/9781003351337-8

kind of exploitative practice across many professions – not just the therapy field. In fact, this controversy is currently being discussed within some business circles in which *neurodiversity* has recently emerged as a hot new buzzword impacting hiring practices.

The disproportionately high unemployment rate of ND individuals versus NT individuals is currently juxtaposed onto a few interesting trends. First is a notable increase in the number of scientific studies that focus on previously ignored, positive attributes of ND brain wiring.[1] Additionally, escalating around the time *The Harvard Business Review* and others began to publish popular articles about the benefits of hiring Autistic, ADHD, and Dyslexic workers, some industries have started campaigns to attract persons of certain neurotypes deemed especially beneficial to their bottom line.[2] These systemic shifts have both pros and cons.

On the surface it seems exciting for some researchers to move away from itemizing and bemoaning the ways ND people are burdensome to society. It also seems encouraging that some employers are offering ND persons new vocational opportunities. Focusing on the positive aspects of having ND employees on staff (with some companies even offering ongoing inclusion programs) can be a very good thing. Yet, the question of genuineness comes to mind. While any positive changes that are the result of actual pro-neurodiversity sentiment are cause for celebration, it's probably naive to think that every participant within these trends has entirely pure motives. Just like it's problematic for any person of any neurotype to be undervalued, it's equally unfortunate to overinflate any person's value. True respect for ND persons means far more than searching out their hidden strengths and mining for undiscovered talent.

The imperative to carefully consider one's own personal and professional motivations is universal across all fields, but is especially important within the helping professions. Doing so not only protects the public from exploitation, but also protects therapy professionals themselves. This is because taking time to ensure a good fit between a therapist's own motivations, personhood, and value system is a protective factor against professional burnout. As an added bonus, doing this type of introspective work provides great preparation for those times a client directly asks *why* you serve. While most therapists' private reasons for serving may not be considered important to all clients, they may actually be critically meaningful to some neurodiverse couples. Sometimes neurodiverse couple therapists can experience greater scrutiny, something that is understandable given the fact that ND persons and their partners tend to report a history of negative experiences and/or invalidation at the hands of helping professionals.

Show Respect Online

How a therapist represents themselves online matters, especially because a client's first contact is usually via the internet. This is largely a sign of the times. But, it's also significant to note that some ND persons experience a high degree of social anxiety regarding telephone communication. Some may prefer (or even require) electronic forms of communication to interact. First impressions regarding a therapist's perceived level of accessibility, competence, and compassion are very important.

Know that the difference between a prospective client scheduling an initial appointment versus abandoning their pursuit of therapy all together can sometimes come down to small, but meaningful, details. Before choosing to reach out to a relationship therapist, for instance, American couples who embrace the descriptor *neurodiverse* to describe their dynamic tend to scan a professional website for two main things:

1. The use of inclusive language.
2. The therapist's personal connection to neurodivergence, i.e., is the therapist ND themselves? Are they NT but in a partnership with a ND person? Are they raising one or more ND children?

This type of screening may or may not originate from a reasonable level of defensiveness based on past experience. Regardless, though, it reflects the question: "Can this therapist truly understand me/us and what we go through as a neurodiverse couple?" Human nature tends to steer people towards those with whom they can readily identify with. A wise professor once taught that what really underlies the level of specificity behind a client's search for a therapist is the vulnerable question: "Can this person really help?" This anxiety mirrors the exact same concerns some prospective clients may have regarding the marital status, gender, race, age, culture, religion, or other personal characteristics they deem important within a potential therapist.

Just like a Christian couple may look for a therapist who is a fellow believer in Christ, a neurodiverse couple may seek out a therapist who describes their own immediate family as neurodiverse and/or perhaps their own brain as neurodivergent. Yet, if both these fictional couples embark on an online search for a therapist with those specific qualities (i.e., Christianity or neurodivergence), they will likely experience two very different outcomes. A Christian couple who seeks a Christian therapist is very likely to find one through a simple online search, especially in geographical regions such as the American South. This is because many Christian therapists overtly advertise themselves as believers. Even if a therapist does not list their religious affiliation on their website, they may still provide clues about their beliefs such as listing a graduation date from a well-known Christian school. A neurodiverse couple seeking a ND counselor, or one in a neurodiverse relationship, however, may not be so lucky. It's currently uncommon in almost every part of the world for therapists to publicly list whether they are NT or ND. Therapists are even less likely to list whether or not they're in a neurodiverse relationship. Furthermore, there are usually no clues about this within a therapist's professional biography, as it's virtually unheard of for any school to be popularly known for its focus on neurodiversity.

Each client has the right to choose the right therapist for their needs, and each therapist has the right to choose how to describe themselves (and their partner or children, if applicable) online. A partner and children's consent is a must, of course, prior to making any disclosures about them. Likewise, personal disclosure of any kind deserves a thoughtful approach. A therapist's personal online disclosures should always be a matter of discretion after careful consideration of one's own motivations, intentions, and context. Even unintended consequences need to be thought through. Consider, for instance, the potential impact of a therapist's public blog or social media post that references themselves as Autistic. In some areas of the world, a professional's choice to share this kind of personal information may be normative, encouraged, and even celebrated. This may quickly endear some clients to this therapist. In other areas, however, a similar move may be professionally disastrous and even personally dangerous. The social, cultural, political, and professional climate matters greatly in this discussion. Stigma against neurodivergence varies widely, as do norms regarding what types of therapist disclosures constitute a breach of ethics or social propriety.

Avoid Unintentional Disrespect Online

Therapists who are genuinely interested in welcoming neurodiverse couples to their private practice should strongly consider removing potential barriers to treatment. Particularly in Western countries, clients may actively look for signs of disrespect towards neurodiverse populations within a therapist's online presence and overall body of work. This includes websites, biography pages, public social media pages, books or articles, public blog entries, and anything else easily searchable online.

What may be Considered Offensive?

A clinician's use of certain outdated or noninclusive terms will almost always be considered offensive. Furthermore, this can convey that a therapist may be too out of touch to be able to provide clients effective support. The use of certain images, symbols, or catch phrases associated with specific groups or ideologies that tend to be nearly universally disliked by ND populations may also be considered insensitive. Perhaps what matters most, however, is whether or not a therapist chooses to use IFL or PFL. Not all, but some, prospective neurodiverse couples will automatically distrust a therapist who uses PFL due to its association with the Medical Model.

Each of the following additional points is typically of little to no concern for most NT couples, yet may represent a huge red flag for some neurodiverse couples who search for support online:

- Using "cure" or deficit-based language.
- Using phrases like "suffering from" or "battling" ADHD, Autism, etc.
- Using functioning labels.
- Posting **inspiration porn** or similar content.

A neurodiverse couple therapist should cultivate an online presence that reflects sensitivity to the types of hurts that are frequently expressed by ND self-advocates. Thankfully, guidelines for how to use inclusive language have been created by both neurodivergent-led organizations and the *American Psychological Association (APA)*.[3,4] As helpful as these resources are, though, they cannot always provide the level of detail needed to consider this topic fully. There will always be nuances to consider. For instance, even the simple act of participation within the popular trend of adding a temporary banner to one's professional social media profile picture in support of a certain ideology or cause requires careful discernment. What may seem like a show of allyship may actually convey the opposite! This is because many ND self-advocates consider *awareness* campaigns (versus *acceptance* campaigns) highly problematic. The best example of this concerns the United Nations' declaration of April 2nd as an annual Autism Awareness Day. For some, this has ushered in an annual season of mental exhaustion each April due to its bombardment of public conversation that may or may not center around actual ND lived experience. They find the corresponding necessity to advocate for actual inclusion for themselves and their neurokin quite draining. Willingness to acknowledge distinctions between awareness-based efforts versus efforts to promote systemic change is a valuable professional quality.

Be Exceptionally Clear

Neurodiverse couples tend to have a wider variety of needs than NT couples. They may also require more direct support to help articulate their challenges and clarify their goals. A therapist who intentionally works to provide clients accurate, clear information can be a breath of fresh air.

Specifically, most neurodiverse couples tend to inquire about any combination of the following services or topics upon initial contact or during the course of treatment:

- Whether or not to pursue a formal diagnosis of neurodivergence, if desired, and how to do so.
- How to obtain sufficient documentation, if desired, to apply for work or school accommodations, insurance benefits, government benefits, etc.
- Medication assessment and management.
- Nutritional advice or guidance regarding over-the-counter supplements.
- Vocational coaching or life coaching.
- Telehealth within state lines, across state lines, or even internationally.
- Family therapy (which may include one or more ND children).

Depending on training, some of these are well beyond a therapist's scope of practice! The involvement of multiple practitioners across several disciplines is sometimes needed to support a neurodiverse couple's needs. Remember, though, that the general public does not usually understand the exact job description and limitations of the multiple providers they may need to contact. And, why would this be expected of them? Providing clear, courteous psychoeducation about the exact nature of one's own professional services is vital, as is making appropriate referrals when necessary. Any therapist who works with neurodiverse couples should offer compassionate care without violating their professional boundaries.

One's own professional abilities and limitations must be explicitly stated from the moment of first contact onward. There are numerous opportunities to do so, such as:

- On a professional website, blog, biography listing, social media page, etc.
- During an initial client consultation.
- During an Intake session.
- Within an Informed Consent document.
- Throughout the course of therapy, as needed.

Be Informative

Some couples will contact a neurodiverse couple therapist after failed attempts at traditional relationship counseling. These clients are acutely aware of their need to pursue a different therapy strategy, and elated to find a professional who may finally be the right fit. Other couples, however, may be new to relationship therapy and/or unsure about basic neurodiversity concepts – particularly, whether or not their relationship "qualifies" as neurodiverse in the first place.

Creating informative website content to provide basic definitions, answer common questions, speak to neurodiverse couples' pain points, and offer an easy path to a free consultation can be extremely helpful. The general public deserves an accessible way to learn more about neurodiversity and how brain-wiring can impact relationship dynamics. They also deserve the chance to understand what neurodiverse couple therapy *is* and *is not*.

The following scripts may be adapted for use on a private practice therapist's website. Or, they may be utilized by an administrative professional who manages private practice Intake procedures. The talking points listed can also be useful to keep in mind during free consultations.

"What's a neurodiverse couple?"
"When one partner is neurotypical (NT) and one partner is neurodivergent (ND), this couple is called neurodiverse.

Being NT means that your brain operates similarly to the majority of other people: You <u>do not</u> have characteristics associated with Autism, ADHD, Giftedness, Dyslexia, etc.

Being ND means that your brain operates differently from the majority of other people: You <u>do</u> have characteristics associated with Autism, ADHD, Giftedness, Dyslexia, etc."

"Neither of us has a formal diagnosis. Do we still qualify for neurodiverse couple therapy?"
"Having a formal diagnosis of neurodivergence is not required to attend neurodiverse couple therapy! Self-diagnosis is valid. It's also perfectly ok to be unsure about what your neurotypes may be.

Whether or not to pursue a formal diagnosis is always your choice. You're welcome to discuss with your therapist the pros and cons of doing so. But, remember, you can always attend neurodiverse couple therapy no matter what you decide.

Note that it's generally beyond the scope of neurodiverse couple therapy for the counselor themselves to provide you with a formal diagnosis, should you desire one. It's your therapist's responsibility to clarify right away whether or not they can ethically offer this service based on their level of training. Usually a referral to a psychologist, psychiatrist, neurologist, or other qualified professional is needed."

"What makes neurodiverse couple therapy different from regular couple therapy?"
"Traditional counselors understand that each person thinks and feels differently, of course, but they don't usually consider the significance of each partner's specific neurology to their relationship dynamics. Neurodiverse couple therapy is talk therapy that explores how each partner's brain wiring directly impacts their experience of the world, themselves, their partner, and their relationship."

Be Efficient

Gathering detailed, brain-based data from the point of initial contact is an important starting point for neurodiverse couple therapy. Without taking up too much additional time during an initial contact, the following checklist may be used to bolster conversations that already take place whenever prospective clients reach out.

Therapists who employ an administrative assistant to manage their Intake procedures should provide appropriate training regarding how to maintain confidentiality, compassion, boundaries, and brevity when using this checklist. They should also know how to provide an appropriate referral should a prospective client request any service that is beyond the therapist's scope of practice.

Initial Contact Checklist

Do you or your partner identify as neurodivergent?
Yes
No
Unsure

Do you or your partner have any formal diagnosis, self-diagnosis, or suspected diagnosis that involves the brain?
Yes (please list): _____
No

Do you or your partner have a history of concussions or other head injuries?
Yes
No

Do you or your partner identify as Disabled?
Yes
No
Unsure

Would you or your partner like extra support to complete the Intake Forms needed prior to attending your first therapy session?
Yes
No

Would you or your partner like extra support during the therapy appointments themselves?
For example: "Our appointment day of the week and time of day always needs to be the same because this helps me remember it" or "I'd like to bring a non-traditional animal with me to each session for emotional support."
Yes (please list): _____
No

Know Some Important Dos and Don'ts

Do:

Ease clients' executive functioning load by streamlining the routine business aspects of therapy, as well as the therapy experience itself, as much as possible.
Fully explain any electronic systems used for billing, scheduling, completing forms, and sending automated messages such as appointment reminders. Provide a printed summary page, or an electronic link to one, that includes step-by-step instructions for how to use these systems. Also provide a short

troubleshooting guide for technical issues, as well as a short list of any relevant boundaries (e.g., do not communicate crises via text or email). For virtual therapy, offer a brief trial run prior to any initial therapy session if clients would like to practice handling any technical issues that may arise or just to become familiar with the virtual therapy experience.

Only within the limits of confidentiality and with clients' explicit permission, it can be helpful to provide neurodiverse couples quick and easy access to information relevant to their ongoing treatment. This information should be brief and accessible. For example, some ND clients with executive functioning challenges find being provided a short, written, summary of their visit after each session is a huge relief. (Personal details should always be excluded from these summaries.) Rather than enabling clients to lack initiative or accountability for their own growth, these efforts may energize some ND clients' work in between therapy visits. Not having to recall multistep directions, track down resources, or contact the therapist for clarification on something can remove barriers to couple success that have absolutely nothing to do with relationship dynamics and everything to do with executive functioning capacity.

Very short session summaries that exclude personal details can be provided via email after obtaining proper client consent. Infographics that explain new concepts may be attached as .pdf documents, and hyperlinks to specific resources can be included:

Session Summary

Skill(s):
_____

Resource(s):
_____

Homework:
_____

Ensure your own communication style is accessible during sessions.
This means keeping your lips visible to the clients at all times, as some clients may benefit from lip reading. It also means speaking at a reasonable volume.

For times when verbal communication may become challenging for a client, or is simply non-preferred, a therapist should be prepared to make reasonable accommodations. This can include offering a white board to temporarily write on back and forth during an in-person session, or pausing verbal conversation in favor of using the secure chat option in one's telehealth software to communicate during a virtual therapy visit.

Whenever possible, answer questions from clients in a direct manner.
Neurodiverse couple therapists should avoid communicating in ways that
ND persons may find vague. For instance, don't assume all clients will readily
interpret the meaning of common metaphors, idioms, facial expressions,
and hand gestures. Many ND clients tend to appreciate, and some even may
require, a higher degree of concreteness to everyday speech than most NT
clients. If a client's question cannot be answered or does not have a simple
answer, just say so.

*Give both partners explicit permission to ask for clarification from you, and each
other, whenever needed.*
When a client asks you for clarification, it can be healing to both normalize
their need for better understanding and praise their choice to display
vulnerability and assertiveness by asking – instead of masking their confusion.
(This ingrained defense mechanism can prolong misunderstandings.)

Therapists should provide the necessary clarification promptly and without
judgment or defensiveness. This is valuable modeling, as partners can then be
coached on how to ask each other for clarification when needed, and how to
provide it. They can be given opportunities to practice these interpersonal
skills during couple sessions. The resulting corrective emotional experiences
may be especially important for clients who have experienced criticism,
ridicule, or other forms of invalidation in the past due to asking questions
when they've become lost in a conversation or unclear about whatever social
dynamics may be occurring.

*Recognize that a neurodiverse couple therapy session may be akin to "relational
cardio" for some ND persons (i.e., participation may feel like strenuous exercise).*
Each couple therapy session will affect both partner's body, mind, and heart
differently. Many NT people's tolerance for social interaction and other
therapy demands, however, tend to be higher than that of many ND persons.
This is not always true, of course, but is something to keep in mind when
working with ND persons and even highly introverted NT persons.

A neurodiverse couple therapist can easily check in with each partner
at the start of every visit regarding the level of "relational cardio" they feel
capable and desirous of experiencing during the day's session. Then, they can
collaboratively set the session's agenda together. As needed, the therapist can
check in with each client regarding the pace of the session as it unfolds and its
physiological effects. Making process comments pertaining to either individual
or the couple dynamic itself in the here-and-now can be helpful in this effort. At
the end of each session, clients can be asked if they felt their agenda topics were

addressed. If not already discussed, the therapist should also inquire about any coping methods either client may have used to promote self-regulation during the visit. If applicable, they can discuss what may have triggered dysregulation. Were their self-regulation efforts visible or invisible? Effective or ineffective? Any of the clients' unresolved concerns, as well as new concerns, can be added to the list of topics to cover during their next session.

Be prepared to tap into your most creative and authentic "ways of being" in order to best serve neurodiverse couples.
A neurodiverse couple therapist must be equally prepared to keep things consistent and predictable for those clients who thrive on sameness, and also quickly adaptable for those clients who require customized interventions on the fly. Like all therapists, they have the opportunity to utilize their own brain features in order to meet these challenges . . . especially creativity! Remaining flexible and discerning about how to lend parts of yourself (within healthy boundaries) to face various clinical situations is key.

Don'ts:

Don't be rigid about the length of each neurodiverse couple therapy session.
This does not mean to throw away all professional boundaries regarding scheduling and fees, of course. However, it may mean that a neurodiverse couple therapist occasionally offers to shorten a couple therapy visit (and only bill for the time the clients actually received support) in certain scenarios. For example, this may occur when a ND partner expresses they've reached their capacity for social interaction midway during a couple session and needs to stop therapy early. The therapist's compassionate recognition of this client's display of interoceptive awareness and assertiveness can provide a corrective emotional experience. Note that providing the reasonable accommodation to end a couple session early should occur without any hint of criticism or disappointment from the therapist. Should this become an ongoing pattern, the therapist can easily suggest scheduling shorter sessions together.

Normanda is a 26-year-old ND female married to Kenneth, a 29-year-old NT male. After attending neurodiverse couple therapy biweekly for about a month, the following interaction occurs about 20 minutes into a session together.

Normanda, while visibly stimming with her hands:

"I was so close to not coming to couple therapy tonight, even though I do want to work on our marriage. My job was awful today, again, and I'm super burned out in general. It's taking all my energy just to focus on these interactions happening right now between all of us. I don't want to fail Kenneth, because I always feel like I'm failing him, but I just don't know how to give this session my full attention. My heart is racing even though I'm exhausted, and I'm just so upset I can't think straight. I want to be here because I want to work on our marriage, but I also just want to go home."

Kenneth:

"I hate to hear that you had another rough day, but it seems like all your days are rough lately. It's like there's always something getting in the way of facing our marriage issues, and I'm getting resentful and impatient for change. Why run away from dealing with things?"

In this example, it's honorable that Normanda showed up to the couple session with what little energy she felt capable of giving to the therapy process that day. However, it would not be honorable for her, or anyone else, to push beyond her own limits. Her expression of overwhelm deserves respect and careful attention.

A healthy response by the therapist would be to express gratitude for Normanda's self-awareness, her use of stimming for self-regulation, and her choice to share her thoughts and feelings versus suppressing them. The therapist should also validate Kenneth's desire to engage together toward problem-solving their relationship issues. But, what should happen next?

Obviously, a therapist's choice to plow through a neurodiverse couple therapy session despite a ND partner's expression of physiological, cognitive, or emotional overload does not generally yield good results. For one, it invalidates this person's self-awareness and self-advocacy efforts. Second, it usually reinforces the very relationship dynamics responsible for maintaining couple distress. Lastly . . . it's just plain disrespectful.

There's a big difference, of course, between a ND client's expression of a firm boundary regarding their overwhelm (e.g., "I need the therapy session to stop right now") and simply expressing overwhelm in and of itself. Here, Normanda reports physiological dysregulation and uncertainty about whether or not she can continue the session despite her sincere desire to do so.

After validating both partners, inviting them to unite around the fact they both want to see their relationship improve is a good next step. The therapist can then thoughtfully present two options:

1.   To immediately respect Normanda's sentiment that she'd prefer to go home, ending the session without further questions. (Ideally, if possible, the session would not actually end before briefly helping each partner create a coping plan for the rest of the day and scheduling a future appointment to pick up where they left off.)

2.   To empathetically explore Normanda's current experience of overwhelm in the here-and-now, proceeding with the session for whatever length of time is desirable, at her pace. It should be emphasized that this option does not require the couple to finish the entire session. Just as any other therapy visit, Normanda can participate for whatever duration she deems possible. This option offers the chance for both partners to have a better understanding of what triggers personal and interpersonal dysregulation, what each of their internal sensations are when this happens, the way each partner attempts to cope, and how this all relates to their stated marital problems.

Neither the therapist nor Kenneth should push either option; It's Normanda's choice.

Don't enforce traditional therapy schemas.
Until the COVID-19 pandemic normalized telehealth, the typical American **schema** for a private practice couple therapy appointment involved each client traveling to an office building, sitting in a waiting room, sitting in the therapist's office for about an hour of face-to-face interactions, paying for the session, scheduling another session, and exiting. One of the problems with this format is that it relies on NT standards for executive functioning, sensory processing, and emotion regulation . . . which tend to not fluctuate to the same degree most ND persons experience. A ND person who struggles in any or all of these areas may find it very difficult to preserve enough mental, emotional, and physiological capacity for participation within therapy. This is exacerbated by the fact that the therapist's own capacities, including their appointment schedule, always take priority over the clients' fluctuating capacities on any given day. A therapist's availability may or may not coincide with the times a ND client is capable of self-regulating to the degree that traveling and/or participating with the level of social interaction required for couple therapy is possible.

Virtual counseling has evolved its own schema, one that may especially benefit some ND persons, and therefore neurodiverse couples. As previously discussed, having access to therapy that takes place within one's home environment can impart an unmatched degree of sensory security. Next, executive functioning strain may be greatly reduced when clients don't have to plan to get out the door on time for an upcoming appointment, navigate transportation-related anxieties, overcome social anxiety, etc. There also may be far more flexibility regarding session type and length. For instance, offering the accommodation of multiple, short check-in sessions per week (instead of one long 50-minute session per week) would not be practical if the couple had to drive back and forth to the therapist's office.

Don't make automatic, negative assumptions about a ND partner's quietness and/or lack of participation during a session.
All therapists should acknowledge the potential to interpret client behavior with some degree of conscious or subconscious bias. In particular, though, neurodiverse couple therapists should avoid jumping to conclusions based on any assumptions made by viewing ND behaviors through a NT lens.

ND persons can be easily invalidated in the couple therapy room if their observable behavior is misinterpreted. For example, while it may be tempting to associate a ND partner's quietness and/or lack of participation during a session as a sign of the couple's overall dynamic . . . this may actually have nothing to do with that! A person's quietness doesn't necessarily indicate disinterest, disrespect, or therapeutic resistance. Rather, it could represent a logical and physiologically-based response to something totally unrelated to the session. Maybe the person did not get enough sleep the night before and then experienced a lot of traffic on the way to the office, leaving them too drained for social interaction. Or, they could be experiencing troubling physical sensations such as a flare-up of chronic illness.

Frequently, but not always, a ND person who appears outwardly quiet, unitnterested, bored, or "disengaged" with their NT partner or the couple therapy session may actually be very engaged in their own way. They may be quite mentally busy and potentially even utilizing invisible strategies. For example, they could be caught up in their own racing thoughts. Using cognitive stimming (e.g., replaying information inside one's own mind) or visual stimming (e.g., looking out the window at the details of the falling leaves) to cope with this may not be easily understood by others.

There's also a possibility a quiet ND client is simply taking time to ponder something that was said earlier during the session. Some ND people need more time to process incoming social content and formulate their response than what is typically expected (and allowed) by the NT majority. Therapists need to learn how to allow long pauses in the flow of conversation within neurodiverse couple therapy when necessary, and to avoid jumping in too soon with their own thoughts and interventions. This is a best practice that can offer targeted support to ND clients while providing valuable modeling to the NT partner.

If a therapist wishes to properly understand and interpret a person's quietness and/or lack of participation during a neurodiverse couple therapy session, they should first use a process comment. Then, they should invite discussion. This allows the ND partner to practice sharing their internal experiences, and the therapist and NT partner to practice hearing about them. Importantly, both partners can practice giving and receiving feedback about how they tend to interpret each other's outward mannerisms and reduce negative automatic assumptions back and forth.

Don't be afraid to say the wrong thing regarding neurodiversity.
No clinician says the right thing all the time, as it can be difficult to keep up with how rapidly accepted terminology sometimes changes. What matters is not a therapist's level of perfection, but rather the willingness to attempt respectful engagement with neurodiversity topics. Owning up to one's mistakes and being teachable is key. This involves overcoming the fear that you may unintentionally offend someone along the way.

Don't be intimidated or otherwise put off by forms of personal expression sometimes associated with neurodivergence.
In conversation, for example, some ND persons can display bluntness, firm black-and-white thinking, and extreme sensitivity to actual or perceived injustice. Others may display out-of-the box creativity, lightning-fast mental processing, and emotional intensity. All ND persons are different, yet tend to share at least some degree of unconventionality (when measured by NT standards) when socializing in majority NT spaces. Of course, this may be totally undetectible for persons who utilize a high degree of masking.

Some ND clients display so-called eccentric or bizarre, yet totally benign, mannerisms. Clothing and hairstyles can range from total gender nonconformity to total gender conformity, or may not even relate to gender whatsoever (e.g., when a person styles their hair to match a favorite fictional character). Personal style as a whole can range from having a singular focus on sensory comfort and practicality, to portraying extreme fashion-forwardness. This may not match the weather outside.

These kinds of variations in personal expression exist within all client populations regardless of neurotype. As a population, though, ND persons' general propensity towards unconventionality tends to make noticeable variations more frequently observable in a neurodiverse couple therapist's office. Some self-advocates argue that "unconventional personal expression" represents a distinct and meaningful aspect of ND culture.

Don't redirect a neurodiverse couple away from "odd" mutual interests or nontraditional ways of connecting to one another.
Some neurodiverse couples form intense bonds over their shared interests in niche topics. A therapist should demonstrate unconditional acceptance of any of the ways clients connect to one another that do not represent a safety hazard, moral or legal issue, or interpersonal boundary violation.

Actively incorporating a couples' shared interests is a great way to unite them towards their stated goals. Stereotypically, hobbies that tend to be associated with neurodivergence involve such interesting categories as: LEGO, computer or video-based games, animation, collectibles, fantasy or sci-fi, strategy-based games, cosplay, exotic pets, historical time periods, and more. Therapists should seek to recognize whether or not they have any negative biases regarding any so-called "odd," "immature," or "obsessive" special interests.

Don't downplay your own intellect.
Some Gifted or 2e individuals report, without a hint of arrogance, a fruitless search for a therapist who can meet them on an intellectual level. Why? This may be partially due to an unfortunate myth within some clinical circles. Some schools of thought presume a therapist who allows their own intellect to shine in the therapy room, for any reason, exacerbates the imbalance of power between the professional and their clients. In an effort to promote an equal balance of power in the therapy room, many Gifted or 2e counselors thus automatically and intentionally downplay this personal quality – regardless of whether or not it's therapeutically appropriate to do so. How potentially degrading for all parties!

First, the underlying assumption that a therapist will always be more intelligent than their clients is problematic. Some clients are far more intelligent than their therapist. Second, the belief that a therapist's demonstration of their own intelligence always equates to inaccessibility is also problematic. While it's clear that a therapist should never embody a condescending expert in the room, are there not instances where utilizing one's full intellectual ability *increases* client accessibility?

Joining with certain ND clients, and their NT partners, on an intellectual level early on in the therapeutic relationship can be powerful. Some ways to explore this type of connection with clients, when appropriate, are:

- Asking partners how they experience **intellectual intimacy** together, collaboratively brainstorming ways that they may increase this. Note that some neurodiverse couples may prioritize their intellectual bond over sexual attraction.
- Engaging in complex discussion (or even lively debate) that thoroughly analyzes diverse theories, research-based evidence, historical context, popular opinions, and other data only as it relates to clients' immediate therapy goals.
- Demonstrating one's own familiarity or expertise regarding clients' niche interests.

Don't shy away from illustrating psychological concepts or relationship dynamics in unique ways.

A neurodiverse couple therapist should be ready and able to switch up the kinds of word pictures they may be accustomed to using with NT couples. Sometimes, for instance, utilizing terms and principles found in science or math may be a better way to communicate psychological constructs and relationship dynamics. A therapist's flexible efforts to respect ND and NT brain-based differences related to the use of **social language** may make a huge difference.

Therapist:

"Let's say Partner A solves an equation like this . . .

$$2(3 + 4) = 2(7) = 14$$

. . . while Partner B solves the same equation like this:

$$2(3 + 4) = 6 + 8 = 14$$

Which person has solved the equation the 'right' way? Although each person uses a different approach, the *Distributive Property* allows them to arrive at the same correct answer.

Each partner in a couple will view their relationship challenges differently. And, human nature indicates we will each see our own view as the best view! This means we have to put forth effort to be more open to our partner's perspective."

Glossary of Bolded Terms

Inspiration Porn   Media features that overinflate the actions of Non-Disabled persons toward Disabled persons (e.g., when a NT student's "promposal"* to their Autistic classmate is recorded and shown on the evening news). Also refers to media features that celebrate Disabled achievements in infantilizing ways or use Disabled persons as props.

* A "promposal" is a new slang word . . . it's not a proposal of marriage . . . but it's a combination of the words "prom" and "proposal." It's when High Schoolers ask each other to prom in elaborate ways, like making signs and carrying balloons or doing a choreographed group dance. It's always a spectacle and always recorded for social media. It only becomes inspiration porn when this involves a NT / Non-Disabled person recording themselves "promposing" to a ND / Disabled person. It reads like an act of pity and self-glorification.

Intellectual Intimacy The mutually-satisfying mental stimulation two partners share together in their relationship.

Social Language The verbal and nonverbal skills people use in everyday conversation and other kinds of informal interactions.

Notes

1 Colzato, L. S., Beste, C., & Hommel, B. (2022). Focusing on cognitive potential as the bright side of mental atypicality. *Communications Biology, 5*(1), 1–6.
2 Austin, R. D., & Pisano, G. P. (2017). Neurodiversity as a competitive advantage. *Harvard Business Review, 95*(3), 96–103.
3 American Psychological Association. (2019). *Publication manual of the American Psychological Association, (2020)*. American Psychological Association.
4 Bottema-Beutel, K., Kapp, S. K., Lester, J. N., Sasson, N. J., & Hand, B. N. (2021). Avoiding ableist language: Suggestions for autism researchers. *Autism in Adulthood.'*

Understanding the Issues Neurodiverse Couples Face

6

Is it possible for a neurodiverse couple to achieve a healthy, mutually-satisfying relationship? Yes! Neurodiverse partners who describe their intimate relationship using positive terms tend to say things like:

- "We're never bored! Our brain differences keep things exciting."
- "We've learned to respect each other's way of experiencing life."
- "Having opposite skills balances us out as a couple."
- "We connect intellectually."
- "We've learned to fully accept ourselves and each other."

Every couple needs a little relationship guidance from time to time. Unfortunately, though, neurodiverse couples may encounter much more difficulty than neurotypical couples when they attempt to locate professional support. They may visit multiple therapy providers before finally receiving appropriate treatment, if they find effective help at all.[1] This is sometimes due to the fact that their brain wiring differences, and corresponding dilemmas, are often unfamiliar to clinicians who are used to primarily serving neurotypical populations. As previously discussed, otherwise excellent clinicians can lack the right education, experience, and skills to meet the specific needs of ND clients and their NT partners – and sometimes they're even unfamiliar with the Neurodiversity Paradigm all together.[2]

Neurodiverse couples tend to face complicated issues above and beyond the nearly universal problems that most couples bring to therapy already.

DOI: 10.4324/9781003351337-9

Just as when a therapist chooses to work closely with any unique population, this places a specific load on the professional's shoulders. Specifically, a neurodiverse couple therapist must be prepared to offer unbiased and up-to-date psychoeducation about the biological mechanisms that underlie a variety of neurotypes. They may also be called upon to help clients consider the pros and cons of pursuing certain brain-based evaluations and supportive services, or to explore their emerging identity narratives. Neurodiverse couples also tend to appreciate support as they discern for themselves whether or not it's safe and desirable to unmask at work, school, church, or other social settings. They may need to process trauma that directly relates to their own neurodivergence, or that of a partner or child(ren). Other concerns can include, but are not limited to: Facing past or present societal discrimination, setting healthy interpersonal boundaries, learning self-advocacy strategies, healing from burnout, exploring sensory-based sexual issues, and working through a whole host of stressful parenting scenarios. These topics, and more, can be consolidated into six broad categories. Almost every neurodiverse couple tends to face these issues, to some degree:

1. Trauma or hardship.
2. Identity dimensionality.
3. Communication challenges.
4. Emotion regulation differences.
5. Executive functioning differences.
6. Sensory processing differences.
7. Sexual challenges.
8. Parenting stress.

The need to address these concerns within a private practice setting may be immediate, such as when a couple mentions them during the Intake process. Or, discussions on these topics may unfold organically over the course of therapy. Neurodiverse couple therapists should broach these topics with compassion and respect, at the clients' pace . . . without losing sight of the clients' original reasons for seeking therapy in the first place.

Issue #1: Trauma or Hardship

The therapy room provides a safe environment in which painful life experiences can be processed by each partner, regardless of neurotype. Couple therapists know that the effects of unhealed trauma or hardship may either be consistently intense enough to affect daily life, or perhaps lay just under the surface until activated by an interpersonal or environmental trigger. Most mild to moderate trauma that stems from the clients' current relationship and/or either partner's personal history may be effectively supported in neurodiverse couple therapy. Sometimes, though, a referral for individual therapy or a higher level of care is required. Neurodiverse couple therapy is <u>not</u> appropriate for couples with a recent history of abuse or who are a danger to themselves or one another. An ongoing safety assessment during the course of treatment is paramount. All existing private practice protocols regarding physical abuse, sexual abuse, suicidality, self-harm, and other urgent concerns must be followed.

Some ND partners report a history of negative scenarios rooted in social inequalities or systemic issues. This is not to imply that NT persons are immune to similar wounds. However, ND persons may recall poignant negative experiences with educational systems, the medical profession, mental health counselors or psychiatrists, or abusers more often than NT persons. Furthermore, when a NT person and a ND person each experience the same terrible circumstance, they will each process it from a fundamentally different neurological home base. This is just one reason why it's completely understandable that partners in a neurodiverse coupling may feel deeply misunderstood by each other – even if they have similar backgrounds.

The fictional voices in the following example should not be taken as representative of all NT people or all ND people. They're merely used to illustrate how brain wiring differences can affect two peoples' experience of the exact same situation.

Getting lost and almost abducted at a sporting event as a child (NT perspective):

"I had lost sight of my dad in the crowd, so I felt really scared. I ran around calling his name until a lady stopped to help. She looked like a nice person, so I trusted her when she said she'd take me to the Information Desk. Instead, though, she grabbed my hand and tried to force me out of the stadium with her. I wrestled my hand out of her grip and ran away from her as fast as I could. Thankfully, I saw my Dad running toward me at that exact moment. I was so relieved! I remember we both cried but ended up staying for the rest of the game. Dad let me sit on his lap. This helped me feel safe again. When we went to another game together the next week, I was sure to hold onto my dad's hand more tightly. I didn't really think about it too much after it happened."

Getting lost and almost abducted at a sporting event as a child (ND perspective):
   "I had stopped to watch an ant with wings crawling on the brick wall outside the stadium. When I looked up, I didn't see my Dad. I remember there was a huge crowd of people and everything was loud. I got super panicky; My heart was beating out of my chest and I got tunnel vision. It was like my brain was scrambled and I couldn't even think straight. I was frozen in place until a lady stopped to help me – or so I thought. When she grabbed my hand and tried to force me out of the stadium, I knew something was wrong but I didn't know how to react. I ended up wrestling my hand away from her just as I saw my Dad running towards me. By that point, I was crying so hard I couldn't breathe. I clung to my dad and begged to go home, so we did. I didn't sleep a wink that night. I hated baseball after that. It took me so long to even think about baseball positively again, and I avoided any kind of crowd for years."

It may seem tempting to conclude the ND voice here simply has a better memory for details or is more sensitive to trauma than the NT voice. It's also tempting to chalk up their differences to the obvious fact that a similar traumatic event can affect two people of any neurotype (including those with the same neurotype) in very different ways. But, these premature conclusions miss the point.

From what neurological home base does each voice experience a similar event?
The ND voice describes getting lost at the stadium from a sensory-based, physiological perspective – because this is exactly how their brain and body experienced it! Their brain's stress response is more intense and lasts for a longer duration than the NT voice reports. Meanwhile, the NT voice describes getting lost by using a few feeling words, but mostly by listing the facts of the story in chronological order. This is because their brain and body experienced a lesser degree of physiological activation, as evidenced by a quicker return to baseline functioning.

Neurodiverse couple therapists must take the time to comprehensively explore how each client has mentally and somatically experienced the trauma and hardships in their life. Many ND persons experience negative life events, and even certain aspects of everyday life, more intensely than most NT persons. Remember, though, that the opposite can also be true. Some ND persons experience hyporeactivity due to brain injury or simply because this is how their brain processes events. Additionally, some NT people respond to trauma with hypervigilance due to PTSD, brain injury, their innate temperament, interpersonal factors, etc. Some NT persons may also respond with hyporeactivity.

Although it can certainly be difficult for persons of any neurotype to explore their trauma during therapy, ND partners may have more marked difficulty doing so. For one, discovering an appropriate pace for their self-disclosures from session to session can be an issue. Some find themselves providing too many painful details too soon, leaving them feeling overexposed. Others lament they do not seem to be physically able to articulate themselves at the pace they desire to address their issues (reasonable accommodations can help this).

It's important to coach the NT partner towards patience if their ND partner experiences serious challenges with communicating about their own personal pain. The therapist should never enforce NT standards for intimate partner communication during these times, such as via insisting on the use of verbal communication or eye contact. Instead, offering a ND client free use of a white board and a dry erase marker may be a helpful option. Or, the client can type out their thoughts on their own time outside of therapy for the therapist and NT partner to read during a session. Of course, these exact same tips can also benefit any NT partner in need of extra support. It's normal for all clients to have fluctuating communication capacities and preferences.

Sometimes a ND partner is best able to articulate complex feelings when expectations regarding verbal speech are completely eliminated. Fictional client Charley, who has Autistic traits and co-occurring anxiety, brought the following paragraphs to a couple session with their NT wife, Sam. They requested for the therapist to read aloud the following:

"When Sam raises her voice at me it's like her negative energy sends a jolt straight into my system. It makes the hairs stand up on my arms. I even get queasy sometimes. Arguments have always been hard for me to handle because my parents did a lot of yelling at each other when I was younger. I learned to block out their chaos by going to my room and hiding under a blanket. When I was older, I listened to loud music instead. Or, I'd leave the house. If it seems like I'm not listening to Sam during an argument, it's often because she's started to raise her voice. Sometimes even if she's not yelling there's just something in her tone of voice that freaks me out. I can't explain it, but it makes me feel like a terrified kid again. My insides get all twisted up. I don't want her to think I don't care, so I stay in the interaction . . . but I lock up. Inevitably, when she walks away from me in tears, I feel like a complete failure for not being able to say anything."

Allowing Charley to express their thoughts in writing helps their childhood trauma narrative to safely rise to the surface, along with how it's currently affecting their intimate relationship.

Toxic messages abound during hardship and trauma, which then tend to be internalized. Both identifying and unlearning these messages is crucial to individual and relational health. Consider the following fictional scenarios which each highlight a different pain point sometimes associated with ND lived experience: Invalidation by close family members, discrimination, and sexual trauma. The toxic messages within each experience will be explored.

Quentin is a recently diagnosed Autistic male married to Leona, a NT female. He shares the following story during neurodiverse couple therapy:

"My family went to a big theme park for the first time in the late 1980s. I was around ten years old. I remember completely losing my cool by the end of the day. So much stress had built up inside me from the heat and activity. I was overwhelmed, but my family wasn't slowing down to listen. I ended up screaming at them over and over again that I needed to leave. My family was embarrassed, so they tried to shame me into being quiet. 'You're much too old to be having these fits,' they said.

I just couldn't get a hold of myself. Everything was too much, and no one was helping me. Someone in the crowd called for security after I pushed my dad and knocked over a big trash can in the process. I was just trying to get him to listen to me! But since I was a 120-lb Black kid who stood about 5' tall, I think the people watching this happen must have gotten scared. Everyone always thought I was older and stronger than what I actually was. Come on, I wasn't a threat. I was just a kid having a hard time.

Security came and told me and my family that I was having a panic attack and offered help. I wasn't sure I trusted them, so I just kept on pacing back and forth trying to calm down on my own. They talked calmly to my family for a while, and I started to feel better. Looking back, the park staff was actually pretty nice about the whole thing – it was my parents and aunts who made things worse. After security left, my mom and dad scared me half to death by going on and on about how this kind of behavior could have gotten me killed. 'What if someone had judged you to be a real danger? You could've gotten shot.' My aunts accused me of ruining the day for my younger siblings and cousins.

I felt awful for getting so overwhelmed and acting the way I did, but I just couldn't help it. I couldn't explain what was going on inside me at the time like I can now, so I was just really quiet on the long drive home. My family never understood me. Things like this happened from time to time when I was a kid, and it was always my fault for 'having a fit.' I also always got the safety lecture. Pretty soon I just learned to keep everything to myself by exploding quietly on the inside. When I got older I started pouring a few drinks whenever I felt overloaded."

Toxic messages:

- Getting overwhelmed is shameful and immature. If it happens in public, it may even be dangerous.*
- The only way to deal with being overwhelmed is to stay quiet and get over it alone: No one else will help you.
- Drinking can take the edge off long enough to calm down and move on.

*This may not represent a toxic message in and of itself, as studies show unarmed Black men can sometimes be at a higher risk of being fatally shot by police.[3] However, the manner in which this message is delivered can be experienced as negative.

This affects Quentin and Leona's current relationship because Leona complains her husband becomes emotionless during their most important discussions. She also expresses concern about Quentin's occasional bouts of binge drinking in response to parenting stress.

Jorge is a late-diagnosed Dyslexic male married to Ginnifer, a NT female. During couple therapy, he recounts the following past experience with discrimination:

"I've always felt stupid on the inside, even though I know I'm a very smart person. This started when teachers at elementary school scolded me relentlessly for making crooked letters and having bad spelling. Thankfully, my mom helped me with all my lessons after school. We also had an English-speaking nanny who was patient and kind.

After we moved to America from Ecuador for my dad's new job, I remember how badly he wanted my sisters and I to attend this one particular private Middle School. He always told us that being bilingual would give us a huge advantage in the job market and that going to the right schools before then could help us succeed.

Although my sisters got accepted into this school right away, I didn't. My parents fought hard to get me in by convincing the school that my challenges with reading, writing, and spelling were simply due to English being my second language. My parents promised that I would improve with hard work, just like I had always done in Ecuador.

I was finally accepted into school, which made my parents so proud, but some of the teachers clearly didn't want me there. I know for a fact that they graded me harsher than the other kids in order to fail me out. Because of this, I became obsessed with doing things like trying to spell things perfectly every single time so that I could prove that I belonged. I was just as smart as my classmates, maybe even smarter, but I really struggled in class at times due to my undiagnosed Dyslexia.

My parents were my biggest fans and stood up for me whenever people like Mrs. Simpson treated me badly at school. Well, the joke's on her! I made it through that first year of school and beyond with extra tutoring. I have a great life now with a family of my own and endless career possibilities. I know my parents are looking down on me from heaven with pride."

Toxic messages:

- You don't belong; You have to work harder than other people to prove your intelligence and worth.
- Others are watching and waiting for you to fail.

Jorge's current struggle with work-life balance negatively affects his relationship with his wife Ginnifer. She states his chronic perfectionism and long work hours makes it feel like she and their children are less of a priority to him than advancing his career.

Cynthia is the AuADHD female partner to Brian, a NT male. Their presenting concern for couple therapy is a desire to address Brian's mounting sexual discontent. Cynthia tells the following story of past sexual trauma:

"I floundered my way socially through college in the early 2000s in southern California, feeling like I was from another planet . . . even though I'd grown up nearby. This wasn't a new feeling. Ever since I was a kid, I was always trying to figure myself out. I always felt different. Interacting with people I didn't know was always tough. I learned how to study others before talking to them. My strategy was to find something we had in common and then strike up a conversation about that. For a while we'd hang out all the time and obsess over that 'thing' together until, eventually, they'd make up excuses to stop hanging out.

I felt lonely since my closest High School friends had all gone away to different schools, and I just couldn't seem to make other friends. I knew being diagnosed Autistic and ADHD when I was younger had something to do with the ups and downs of all this, but my college psychiatrist downplayed those labels and said I was probably Bipolar instead. That diagnosis never sat right with me. I never took the medications he recommended.

After I started dyeing my hair different colors and trying on different looks for myself, I started getting sexual attention from random cute girls and guys. This was a brand new, and exciting, feeling. People started approaching <u>me</u> for a change, which took the pressure off me to make the first move. I started making friends that then became more than friends. I started branching out sexually, and this became confusing. It was hard to be someone's friend one minute and naked in bed with them the next. I soon realized that all I really wanted was to hang out, nonsexually, with friends who were interested in the real me that I was finally starting to figure out.

There were so many times I had sex, even when I didn't want to, just to be able to talk and play video games together afterwards. I couldn't figure out how to say no to sex since I'd already said yes so many times already. I'm still not sure how this happened, but I went from having no friends at college to three or four 'friends with benefits' simultaneously. Finally, though, enough was enough. During sex with one of these guy friends, I said I wanted to stop. He pressured me to keep going. It was awful. When I told him later how that wasn't ok, he never talked to me again. Weirdly, word got around and the other guy and girl who I'd had a thing going with also stopped talking to me. Things got too weird for everyone, I guess. It was so hurtful to realize no one wanted to just be with me for me; They all valued the sexual time over the nonsexual time.

The icing on the cake that year was that I ended up getting sexually assaulted at a sleepover by a brand-new girlfriend I thought was safe enough to confide in about all this."

Toxic messages:

- Sex can be a commodity to ensure companionship, at least temporarily, but it also can be used against you.
- You're only worth what you can offer others sexually.
- You're not neurodivergent, you're mentally ill.

The effects of this trauma affect Cynthia and Brians' current relationship. Although they report deep love for each other and a mutual desire to be an exclusive couple for the long term, Brain states he struggles with feeling deceived. He laments that Cynthia seemed to have a very high sex drive when they first met, yet now appears to have none at all. He finds this hard to understand and wonders if she'll ever desire sex with him the way she used to.

Issue #2: Identity Dimensionality

Many aspects of each client's unique personhood are essential to explore early on during neurodiverse couple therapy, provided that the relationship is stable enough to do so. As they specifically relate to the relationship concerns clients bring to therapy, it can be meaningful to define the psychological constructs of *temperament, personality, neurotype,* and *identity* along with their biological underpinnings. Using clear and accessible verbiage, each partner's brain characteristics can be discussed in terms of how they may manifest in each of these categories. A therapist can then help the couple discuss how these constructs impact their couple dynamics, and also their **couple identity**. These rich discussions are a distinct offering of good neurodiverse couple therapy. Hopefully they provide invaluable insight as clients learn more about themselves and each other, which can help them determine realistic goals as individuals and partners.

To begin, a ND partner's overall self-concept and level of self-esteem are important considerations when exploring identity dimensionality at both the individual and couple level. This is because (similar to what can occur after a person of any neurotype suffers sexual abuse) some ND individuals have internalized a pervasive sense that *who they are* is fundamentally wrong. A therapist may also notice signs of **learned helplessness**. These effects are often the logical result of chronic invalidation, trauma, or hardship.

On top of this, or as a standalone issue, some ND persons can experience an especially intense form of *Imposter Syndrome*. These persons question whether their own personal neurological, physiological, and cognitive characteristics are "enough" to claim neurodivergent status. They wonder, "Am I really different enough from others to warrant the brain-based label I'm considering for myself, or have been given by a professional . . . or is this just all in my head?" It's quite common for ND persons to doubt whether or not they "deserve" to self-identify with a particular neurotype, or whether they "belong" within ND and/or Disabled spaces. This specific form of identity insecurity seems to affect females more often than males, and may result from chronic invalidation or gaslighting by others – including professionals.

ND *Imposter Syndrome* may also result from internalized ableism, anxiety, and/or a lack of accurate ND media representation. Some ND clients have never actually met someone who experiences the world similarly to the way they do, nor have they seen someone represented in popular culture who thinks, feels, or acts similarly! Instead, they have a stereotypical image in mind about how someone with their potential neurotype should be. Older generations and those in certain cultural or socio-economic groups may be most susceptible to this line of thought. (It's encouraging that a recent spike in ND representation on social media platforms is starting to make neurodivergence more visible to young people who have access to the internet in places such as America, England, and Australia.)

Regarding gender and sexuality, some neurodiverse couples may benefit from professional support as a ND partner explores these dimensions of their own identity and the corresponding affects to couple identity. Research shows that ND populations tend to report more complexity in gender and sexuality than NT populations. For example, one study noticed its adult participants with Autistic characteristics reported **gender dysphoria** six times more than its non-Autistic participants.[4] Interestingly, similar statistics were reported in a 2014 study that reviewed parent reports of both Autistic children and ADHD children's behavioral expressions of gender variance. The Autistics were about 7.5 times more likely to express gender nonconformity than the children in control groups, and the ADHDers were about 6.6 times more likely to do so.[5] To summarize all these results, important clinical considerations concerning gender were found to exist in approximately 1–2% of the NT persons studied versus 6–7% of the ND persons studied. More recent scholarly literature also confirms overrepresentation of gender-dysphoric traits among Autistic adults versus NT adults, as well as higher rates of homosexuality, asexuality, and bisexuality.[6,7,8]

Therapists tend to lack appropriate nuance when discussing the above data amongst themselves and with clients. (That is, a person's **gender identity** can be different from their **gender expression**, and both of these concepts are distinct from **sexual identity** and **sexual expression**.) There also tends to be a lack of comprehensive sex education aimed at ND populations.[9]

ND clients and their NT partners deserve unbiased support when seeking therapy to explore such sensitive aspects of personhood and partnership. Therapists are also encouraged to recognize the intersectionality of these topics with spirituality, race, and culture. Additional resources on each specific dimension mentioned above exist in order to keep these discussions complex, nondiscriminatory, and ongoing.[10,11]

Issue #3: Communication Challenges

Every couple therapist knows that issues with communication and conflict resolution are the most frequent problems clients list on their Intake paperwork. Neurodiverse couples are no different in this regard, but are far more likely to need support with such things as learning how to accurately interpret each other's tone, volume, and gestures. This is important to address because the ability to interpret nonverbal communication back and forth, and to nondefensively clarify any misunderstandings that may occur, is vital for any two sighted partners.

A common pitfall of applying traditional couple therapy modalities with neurodiverse couples is an unequal focus on improving the ND partner's interpersonal skills. This is an incomplete intervention at best, and ableist at worst, as research shows communication difficulties between ND and NT people are bidirectional. Communication is always a reciprocal experience; Improving communication takes work on both sides! For instance, NT persons tend to have just as much difficulty understanding Autistic persons as Autistic persons have understanding them. This is partly because NT and Autistic persons have been found to use facial expressions and body movements in ways that can confuse one another.[12,13] Additionally, one study found that NT persons tend to overestimate the level of their Autistic family member's egocentrism and cognitive rigidity – factors which can easily affect their interpretation of communication.[14] Milton called the whole of these kinds of struggles the **Double Empathy Problem**.[15]

It's no surprise that neurodiverse partners often report chronic, mutual invalidation when speaking to each other. Through no fault of their own, their neurological home bases are different. They tend to have difficulty demonstrating empathy and support to each other in ways they both can easily recognize. Each partner needs help to grasp how the other person feels inside as their brain responds to stimuli and process information. Then, they need help to find the best way to offer their partner validation. Effective conflict resolution can only take place after these steps happen first.

Giving clients psychoeducation about ND versus NT stylistic differences during communication (and connecting these to neurology) can be highly beneficial. Without this, neurodiverse partners can easily misconstrue each other's behaviors and intentions. For example, clients are often unaware that most NT persons tend to attribute a much higher value than most ND persons on posture, attentiveness, eye contact, and physical appearance while communicating. Learning more about how this may show up within their relationship can shed new light on some aspects of their interpersonal conflict.

Generally, ND persons tend to prefer more overt and specific forms of communication than NT persons. Some are prone to taking things quite literally. In response to a NT partner saying they are feeling worn out, for instance, some ND partners may be more naturally inclined to go to the medicine cabinet and bring over a bottle of vitamin C tablets than to infer their partner is referring to mental exhaustion. Contrastingly, the majority of NT persons tend to use a lot of ambiguous language, subtext, or unspoken rules as they communicate. They can be prone to wanting a ND partner to accurately surmise these nuances and getting frustrated when they don't. Thus, it's common for NT partners to lament "having to spell things out" to their partner, while ND partners lament "having to figure out how to read between the lines" in their relationship.

It can be helpful to discuss together how a lack of representation within the media has likely exacerbated clients' patterns of mutual invalidation. There are very few examples of neurodiverse couples communicating well together! Futhermore, accurate representations of ND communication tendencies don't really exist within popular music, books, television, and movies. Naturally, NT partners can be a bit clueless about how to send and receive messages the way their ND partner prefers. And while ND persons have no shortage of exposure to neurotypicality in real life situations and the media, they can still find it exceptionally difficult to match their brain-wiring and personal style with NT standards for communication.

Many neurodiverse couples benefit from reviewing concrete examples of healthy versus unhealthy forms of communication between neurodiverse partners . . . especially when these examples explore and explain brain-based tendencies. A therapist may play audio or visual clips from the media, if available, or simply come up with their own fictional examples as needed. Providing clients plenty of opportunity during sessions to practice role-playing both types of interactions (i.e., healthy versus unhealthy) can be eye-opening. This tends to be far better than assigning communication exercises as homework, as increased support is often needed. This can easily be provided by the therapist via in vivo scaffolding.

A therapist's efforts, in particular, can help NT partners critically examine any of the following underlying negative assumptions regarding communication in their relationship . . .

- "My ND partner doesn't want to talk to me."
- "My ND partner doesn't like to talk to me."
- "My ND partner doesn't want to open up to me."

. . . and potentially replace them with a more accurate perspective on their situation:

- "My ND partner wants to talk to me, and likes to talk to me, but we don't always know the best ways to communicate back and forth yet."
- "We're both learning about our communication tendencies, which often relate to our brain wiring."
- "We both want to connect on a deep level and are learning the skills to help us do so."

Both partners in a neurodiverse relationship deserve unbiased support to learn about their own communication style and that of their partner, inclusive of what they're most likely to misinterpret back and forth. They deserve specific opportunities during couple sessions to practice recognizing when these misunderstandings occur and learn how to choose healthy responses. Of course, the therapist should also recognize the intersectionality between each partner's personality, culture, and gender in regards to communication. Sometimes, too, promoting insight about how a partner's concurrent physical disability affects couple communication can play a pivotal role in therapy.

Consider the following fictional story in which Raina (a middle-aged Autistic female) is married to Dae (a NT male five years her senior). They've just transferred to a Brain-Informed therapist after six months of traditional couple therapy with another private practice therapy provider.

Raina:

"Dae always thinks I'm yelling. He polices the way I speak to him and others, especially in public, and I can't take it anymore. I need him to do less micromanaging of me and to do more listening. We used to talk so much better before we had kids, but now life is busy and full of misunderstandings. We've read a lot of marriage books and tried a lot of their suggestions, but nothing helps. We've even attended couple therapy a few times together. Those efforts did lead to my choice to pursue an Autism diagnosis for myself recently, but our communication hasn't improved. Why can't Dae see that I'm doing the best I can when I speak? My tone or volume is <u>not</u> always something I seem to be able to control, especially when I'm tired or stressed."

Dae:

"Let me just say, first, that I'm not mad at Raina for being Autistic. It actually explains a lot, and I accept this about her. I'm just more and more frustrated these days because she doesn't want to admit that she often speaks very loudly and aggressively to me and the kids. Her tone is often too harsh for the situation, and this can be embarrassing when it happens in public. It really bothers me that when I try to point this out as it's happening, she gets defensive. Everyone in the family notices this harshness except her! It's upsetting that she and I don't seem to get anywhere anymore when we talk about this or other subjects. I don't know why this is happening. When we first met things were so much easier to talk about and I didn't really notice this issue."

Traditional couple therapy may attempt to offer this couple a chance at relief by coaching NT-biased communication and conflict resolution skills from the start, but at what cost? Doing so may be invalidating and ineffective in the long run. It also perpetuates the very cycle of ableism that underlies their communication problems. A neurodiverse couple therapist, on the other hand, can offer a totally different approach.

A Brain-Informed therapist first carefully considers what is actually *changeable* about a couple's communication issues (versus *unchangeable*) <u>before</u> attempting to teach any new skills. In doing so, they seek to join and collaborate with each partner to properly assess their innate communication capacities, preferences, habits, and tendencies. Importantly, the therapist also provides psychoeducation that communication style differences do not always represent deficits.

Upon starting neurodiverse couple therapy, Raina and Dae's new therapist notices right away that Raina's style of speech subtly reflects pronunciation, volume, and vocal inflection differences from the majority that are often associated with Deaf culture. Even though no auditory Disabilities were indicated on her Intake Form, the therapist respectfully asks Raina about her hearing. Surprised at this question, Raina states she was born with mild hearing impairment in both ears and wears removable hearing aids in certain environments as needed. She states no other therapist has ever implied her hearing may be a factor in their marital communication dynamics, and that this possibility was also never mentioned in the relationship self-help books they've read.

Learning more about how each partner processes incoming sounds and produces outgoing sounds can impart powerful insight. In this example, being Autistic and partially Deaf causes Raina's verbal speech to frequently deviate from the NT communication standards Dae craves – despite her best efforts to conform. (It's particularly difficult to mask when she's tired or stressed.) Although Dae says he accepts Raina as an Autistic person, he does not seem to understand Autistics sometimes have brain-based challenges with modulating their vocal tone and volume. He also seems conflicted about how to understand her inborn Deaf mannerisms. It's perhaps most problematic, though, that he assumes these characteristics are totally within her control to change at whim.

Other points of discussion:

- The couple was probably better able to cope with their communication differences earlier in their relationship due to a few important factors. For one, grace is high at the start of any relationship relative to later years when parenting demands and other life stressors usually increase. The effects of aging on each partner's physical and physiological processes probably also plays a role now, as do cultural factors (e.g., extended family expectations). Lastly, it may also be important to consider masking. If masking is physically possible for Raina, she may have had more energy at the start of their relationship to intentionally (or subconsciously) utilize this to conform to NT communication standards. She may have less energy or physical capacity mask now . . . or maybe she just does not wish to do so!

- Dae's frustration with Raina's communication style, especially in public settings, may be rooted in unmet NT expectations, cultural expectations, and gender expectations. Tone policing could be his attempt to cope with his own uncomfortable physiological response to disappointment and embarrassment regarding the situation. Of course, his frustration could also simply indicate a strong preference for NT styles of communication.
- Some aspects of Raina's communication style may unintentionally convey confrontation to Dae and other NT persons, especially when combined with atypical volume and/or tone. For example, she tends to position her body directly in front of another person during conversation because seeing their lips move is helpful to her auditory processing. NT conversational standards may deem this an "aggressive" stance.

Psychoeducation will be very important within this couple's treatment. It's also important for the therapist to ask each client, "What are your interoceptive experiences in response to your partner's communication style?" Identifying and discussing the way each partner experiences (on both an emotional and physiological level) not only the content of their partner's communication, but more importantly the style of their communication is vital. This is a great start towards coaching increased interoceptive awareness and reduced defensiveness.

It's also important for the therapist to ask each client, "What is changeable versus unchangeable about your respective communication styles?" Specifically, Dae may not be able to change the fact he tends to become physiologically agitated in response to Raina's high volume or atypical tone. But, he can probably learn how to recognize internal signs that he's becoming agitated and learn to cope in a better manner than using tone policing. Raina's vocal tone and volume modulation differences may be permanent. Nonetheless, she can probably learn to validate Dae's concerns should he learn how to provide healthier feedback about her mannerisms and his communication preferences (versus tone policing).

All of these interventions seek to promote increased education and empathy regarding neurodiverse communication dynamics, which lays a great foundation for more effective problem-solving and skill-building. For instance, the couple may discuss whether or not a different style of hearing aid could better support Raina and whether she is willing to explore this option. Dae may decide he is willing to practice the proactive act of positioning his body closer (and in direct view of Raina) when they are speaking together.

This could allow her a better view of his lips, freeing her up to focus more energy and attention towards whatever level of modulation of her own vocal tone and volume may be possible. The couple could role-play various communication skills in session.

Ultimately, good neurodiverse couple therapy can help clients determine whether or not they desire to understand, accept, and work through the communication challenges inherent to their relationship. Normalizing ND-NT communication styles and coaching self-regulation techniques to use during and after inevitable communication misunderstandings is probably the most important intervention of all.

Issue #4: Emotion Regulation Challenges

Neurodiverse couples frequently report high stress due to one, or both, partner's difficulties with regulating their emotions. Sometimes a NT partner reports feeling they're at the mercy of their ND partner's over or under-reactivity. Things can also be the other way around, however. Although ND partners may be more biologically predisposed to emotional unsteadiness, some NT partners are also vulnerable. This is especially true when a NT person has a trauma background, mental health concerns, medical conditions or chronic health issues, substance abuse issues, or simply lacks coping skills. Certain culture and gender norms regarding the identification and expression of one's own feelings can also play a significant role in a person's struggle to regulate their emotions, regardless of neurotype.

Neurodiverse couples who attend therapy in a private practice setting may report any of the following concerns, and more, related to emotional dysregulation:

- Mild to moderate self-harm, without suicidal ideation.*
- **Autistic burnout.**
- Compassion fatigue or caregiver fatigue.
- Anger management issues.
- Frequent fight, flight, or freeze responses.
- Emotional eating or food restriction.
- Mild, moderate, or severe mood swings.
- Going emotionally numb, shutting others out, and/or disassociating.
- Substance abuse issues.
- Codependent behavior.

- Difficulty attending school, maintaining employment, or keeping commitments.
- Difficulty making friends or maintaining friendships.
- Impulsive or compulsive risk behaviors (e.g., gambling, sex, etc.).
- Depression.
- Anxiety with or without panic attacks.

*Regarding self-injury without suicidal intent, a 2020 meta-analysis found that 42% of Autistic persons studied had experienced self-injury. This was most often by hitting themselves with their own hands.[16] (Other forms of self-harm can be biting, scratching, cutting, burning, skin-picking, hair-pulling, etc.) In comparison, research estimates between about 5% and 17% of NT participants experience this type of self-harm tendency.[17]

Any client who is willing to self-reflect, learn, and grow can be coached towards some degree of improvement in their ability to recognize and regulate their emotions – even those who are alexithymic. In particular, some elements of *Dialectical Behavior Therapy (DBT)* can offer effective support. Its succinct, direct, skill-building approach towards increased self-insight, interoceptive skills, and physiological self-regulation can be appealing to ND persons. This is especially true now that classic DBT has been adapted to better suit the needs of ND populations.[18,19] Designed for Autistic adults, a form of therapy called *Aligning Dimensions of Interoceptive Experience (ADIE)*, may also reduce the frequency of meltdowns over time because it teaches participants how to cope with overwhelm.[20]

Note that there may be times during a neurodiverse couple session when the ND partner experiences emotional and/or physiological dysregulation to a very significant degree. This may be due to a combination of sensory insecurity, interpersonal stress, and other considerations like the topics being discussed or the effects of past trauma. It's even possible for the sympathetic mode of a client's autonomic nervous system to become activated in the therapy roomn. Every therapist should have an understanding of the biological mechanisms that underlie a client's experience when this happens.

What happens when a client experiences an intense overwhelm?

This means the client's amygdala, part of the limbic system in the brain's temporal lobe, has perceived something in their sensory environment as an *external* threat via messenger neurons connecting the eyes, ears, nose, or taste buds to the thalamus. (The thalamus relays sensory-based data to both the amygdala and prefrontal cortex.) Or, perhaps the client's interoception system has perceived an *internal* threat inside their own body. Both types of threats may actually occur simultaneously, and seriously overload the person's capacity for resilience. For example, let's say a certain ND client prone to intense overwlem hears a loud siren from the street outside a therapy room window. This may amplify the simultaneous sensations of their current stomach ache and their experience of mounting emotional pressure from the session. If this happens, the client's prefrontal cortex will inform their amygdala about conclusions it draws from analyzing data about the current situation – using help from memories stored in the hippocampus. Whereas a NT amygdala can usually determine the actual threat level of this kind of situation and rely on the prefrontal cortex to choose how to effectively cope, a chronically stressed, damaged, or ND amygdala sometimes cannot. The prefrontal cortex may be rendered largely inaccessible, and the brain will defensively plunge into a *Fight* or *Flight* state. Alternately, the *Fawn* and *Freeze* brain states are two other self-protective responses. The *Fawn* state involves the sympathetic mode, while the *Freeze* state relies on both the sympathetic nervous system as well as activation of the back side of the vagus nerve – known as dorsal vagal activation – via the parasympathetic nervous system. Both *Fawning* and *Freezing* utilize varying levels of psychological numbness, depersonalization, or dissociation to mentally detach from the threat. *Freezing* can involve emotional and physical shut down, while *Fawning* involves mostly emotional shutdown. One's ability to "go through the motions" with outward behaviors remains during *Fawning* in order to survive via placating others. This is not usually possible in a *Frozen*, *Fighting*, or *Fleeing* brain state. Stephen Porges' Polyvagal Theory supplies greater detail about each of the above brain responses, while other researchers explore the biological specifics of the microbiota-gut-brain axis in order to inform future counseling techniques.[21,22]

Extreme dysregulation is often quite recognizable to a therapist when it occurs in a NT person during a session. Highly distressed ND persons who are good at masking, however, may not be as easily spotted. (Rest assured, while a neurodiverse couple therapist may miss this, the NT partner in the room almost never does! They tend to draw attention to their ND partner's dysregulation as it happens, usually in a critical manner.)

Thankfully, many counselors have received training about how to support clients who experience distress in their presence. This training typically highlights NT responses and support strategies, however. How many counselors are aware and prepared for dysregulation to occur more frequently in ND persons than NT persons during neurodiverse couple therapy? Are counselors ready and able to thoughtfully explain to a neurodiverse couple how an Autistic person's amygdala may be biologically wired to be more hyperactive or inconsistently reactive?[23] Therapists who can provide psychoeducation about what happens in most NT brains when overwhelmed versus what happens in most ND brains can provide invaluable insight, perspective, and care.

How would you break down the following information into layman's terms?

- In response to a trigger, the *Fight* or *Flight* response occurs in all people once the amygdala alerts the hypothalamus to signal the adrenal glands to release adrenaline, a.k.a. epinephrine. The skeletal system also releases the hormone osteocalcin into the bloodstream.[24] Pupils enlarge and metabolism shifts to give more blood glucose availability to the brain and muscles. The heart beats faster and blood pressure rises in order to push blood to the muscles, while breathing is quickened to bring more oxygen to the brain. Digestion, sexual arousal, and logic go offline. The brain goes on heightened alert, prioritizing the body's most basic needs to best equip it for survival. Some ND persons may be triggered more easily and more frequently.
- Ironically, one of the brain's tactics in response to overwhelm involves increasing sensory sensitivity! In a NT person, this advanced environmental awareness may allow them to find an escape path more quickly, design a more strategic fight plan, etc. For a ND person, however, increased sensory sensitivity can just add to overall sensory overload . . . and even keep them reacting to the original "threat" for a long period of time.
- The HPA Axis (the hypothalamus, pituitary gland, and adrenal glands) sends out various hormonal signals to maintain physiological hypervigilance and metabolic control until the "threat" is neutralized and the brain decides to drop its defenses. One such signal involves cortisol, which is problematic when it occurs in excess. Too much cortisol over too long can cause adrenal fatigue, high blood pressure, low serotonin, high blood sugar, and increased inflammatory processes throughout the body. The HPA Axis stays on high alert until the parasympathetic nervous system slows down the stress response. Eventually, the brain and body returns to baseline. It takes most ND people longer to return to baseline than most NT people.

For Autistics, an extended and particularly intense episode of the *Fight, Flight, Freeze,* or *Fawn* response is referred to as an **Autistic meltdown**.[25] (Note that this is currently the term used in most scholarly and self-advocacy circles. Those who find this language infantilizing may prefer to use the term

neurological emergency instead.) A meltdown may result from the brain's response to a single highly aversive sensory trigger, from the inability to process many things at once, from the accumulation of stress over time, or a combination of any/all of the above. As stated above, meltdowns can also occur in response to acute or chronic neurodiverse partnership dynamics. Yet, meltdowns are not necessarily a hallmark of being Autistic! Someone who is rarely in a socially toxic or physically unsafe environment, is highly skilled at using coping skills, and who is surrounded by healthy social support may actually rarely experience this type of brain-based defense. This is because it generally only occurs as an automatic physiological response to situations that induce overwhelming stress, unbearable sensory sensations, emotional overload, physical danger, and/or interpersonal anxiety.

Therapists can conceptualize an Autistic meltdown as the brain's activation of a protective state because the required internal processing demands overwhelm its capacity. These experiences <u>cannot</u> be minimized as merely a "behavioral" concern. There is always an underlying neurological context! Furthermore, a client's behaviors during a meltdown are logically in proportion to the level of physiological and emotional overload they're experiencing. Understandably, these situations can feel exceptionally intense to both Autistic persons and any outside observers. Few in general society know how to properly recognize and support an Autistic person during a meltdown. Tragically, certain situations may even be life-threatening if someone experiencing a neurological emergency is wrongly deemed a threat to themselves or others.

A neurodiverse couple therapist may observe a client have an Autistic meltdown during a session, or perhaps simply hear about those that have occurred in between sessions or at some point in the past. When discussing past meltdowns, the therapist can ask, "What were its triggers?" "What helped?" "What made things worse?" A self-care plan should be made in advance of any future overwhelm that takes into account the person's personal history, level of access to resources, physiological self-soothing preferences, desired degree of NT partner involvement, location(s) where the meltdown may occur, etc.

If an Autistic meltdown occurs during a couple session, the therapist may respond in the following ways:

1.   Immediately shift away from big-picture therapy goals. The safety and self-regulation of all parties now becomes top priority. If

applicable, follow the self-care plan collaboratively made earlier for this type of occurrence.

2. Reduce environmental stimuli, including interpersonal demand. Remove potentially aversive sensory aspects of the therapy environment (e.g. dim bright lights, quiet the NT partner). Remove any expectation for the ND client to participate in back-and-forth communication.

3. Without using too many words, encourage the ND client to use their preferred self-regulation strategies. Keep a variety of stim toys, a weighted blanket, sensory putty, or other therapeutic supplies easily accessible for this purpose.

4. Offer a co-regulation strategy by coaching everyone in the room towards diaphragmatic breathing. If the ND client is unable to participate and/or does not wish to participate, do not press them to do so.

5. When in doubt, simply maintain calm silence. Less is more! It's well-intentioned, but entirely unhelpful, for a therapist to try to talk a client through a true meltdown. Reciprocal communication is only possible when the brain and body re-approach physiological baseline.

Issue #5: Executive Functioning Differences

The neural connections between one's prefrontal cortex and other brain regions are a major factor in working memory, task initiation, planning, organization, cognitive flexibility, self-monitoring, impulse control, and emotion regulation. These higher-level brain processes are called executive functioning skills, which are more sophisticated than more basic processes that focus on survival. Executive functioning skills help clients perceive a problem, think through possible solutions, and work towards a desired outcome – all while monitoring their own feelings and physical sensations. These skills also allow humans to recognize and adapt to all the changing stimuli going on around them within their external environment. Importantly, they also allow organization and interpretation of one's own internal environment (e.g., body, mind, and heart.)

Existing research usually emphasizes deficits in ND executive functioning relative to NT baselines without giving proper attention to strengths. It's encouraging, though, that a recent review of literature has recognized that Autistics without co-occurring intellectual disability tend to display strong planning and decision-making skills. These individuals were noted to be weak in working memory and cognitive flexibility when compared to NT persons, however.[26]

The sum of each client's inborn and learned skills regarding executive functioning matters to their everyday life, including their interpersonal dynamics. This is especially true when skill sets vary widely between partners in a neurodiverse relationship. Unfortunately, though, these partners are unlikely to have ever received education about the science behind executive functioning. They also have usually never been taught how to identify their own strengths and weaknesses in these areas. But it's not just partners with different neurotypes who miss the fact that executive functioning differences may be contributing to some of their interpersonal problems . . . traditional therapists usually miss this, too!

In the early stages of illuminating the dynamics that may be fueled by executive functioning differences, certain unfair misattributions can be uncovered. For example, NT partners tend to presume that their ND partner's repetition of frustrating behaviors occurs due to intentional malice. They have not usually considered that innate brain wiring, the result of brain injury or illness, or simply underdeveloped executive functioning skills may play a role. As such, NT partners tend to spend a lot of time expressing hurt, anger, confusion, and exasperation regarding their ND partner's problematic (but not unsafe) behaviors. These behaviors often trigger something related to their own attachment wounds, and couple therapy discussions can be very emotionally-charged as a result. It can be a difficult tightrope for a therapist to walk when trying to both validate the NT partner's concerns while providing psychoeducation about executive functioning.

In the following fictional story, both partners are certainly allowed to feel upset. The NT partner's emotional reactivity is understandable based on her past. The ND partner's frustration with himself, and also in response to his partner's invalidation, is also reasonable. Yet, their mutual defensiveness is bound to prove relationally destructive if this pattern continues.

Jen (NT):

"Why are you home empty-handed again? Don't you remember you agreed to stop by the store and grab that missing ingredient we need to make dinner tonight? The store is right by your work! You've been saying you were going to get it all week."

Jack (ADHDer):

"I forgot again, sorry. I can't believe I didn't remember, actually, because I even put a sticky note in my car this time and also set a reminder on my phone. Give me a little credit, ok? Can't you see how hard I tried?"

Jen (NT):

"It's not that hard. Just do what you say you're going to do. Why can't I count on you to do basic stuff? We've talked so much about how your forgetfulness hurts me. Don't you dare blame this on your ADHD again. It's not just about a missing ingredient for dinner, you know. Every time you forget something, it feels like I'm 12 years old again waiting for my Mom to show up to my soccer games . . . but she never came to a single one. My husband should be different. I shouldn't have to put up with your empty promises. If you're too lazy to remember getting a lousy can of beans from the store when we need one, how can I trust you with anything else?"

Like so many other neurodiverse couples, Jen and Jack need help processing their hurt and viewing their situation from a neurological perspective. Only then can they collaborate towards lasting change, if desired. A therapist can provide psychoeducation about executive functioning while helping these clients set reasonable, flexible expectations for themselves and each other as they learn the new skills each need to heal from the past and avoid perpetuating this dynamic going forward.

In this example, it's unclear how long this particular pattern of disappointment has been going on. What's very clear, however, is a critical assumption by the NT partner. Jen mistakenly equates Jack's executive functioning challenges with a character flaw (i.e., laziness). Even though there are definitely times when ADHDers can be lazy, that doesn't appear to be the case here. In fact, many ADHDers are actually very hard-working people due to having to learn creative ways to overcompensate for their challenges! This is tiring and unsustainable, though. There may be many ups and downs before an ADHDer learns the kinds of support they need to bolster and maintain their executive functioning skills.

NT assumptions are often unfair when they don't take into account ND executive functioning challenges.

Table 6.1

NT Partner's Assumption	ND Partner's Underlying Executive Skill Challenge(s)
They don't respect my time because they're always running late.	*Planning, Self-Monitoring, Organization*
I can't count on them to finish anything they start.	*Planning, Impulse Control*
They're irresponsible, always losing things.	*Organization*
I can't trust them. They make positive changes for a little while then end up right back where they were before.	*Self-Monitoring, Impulse Control*
They give up before they start, avoid doing hard things, or procrastinate.	*Task Initiation*
They don't care enough to remember what I say. I have to repeat myself over and over.	*Working Memory*
They disrespect me and our shared living space by being messy.	*Organization*
They make decisions on the fly or by gut feelings.	*Impulse Control, Emotion Regulation*
They're too stubborn about having to do things their own way.	*Cognitive Flexibility*

It can be helpful to normalize a few things, too, regarding executive functioning differences. For one, these differences usually only become problematic after being a couple for some length of time or reaching a major relationship transition (e.g., moving in together, getting married, getting a dog, having a child). This is because the early days of dating typically represent a low-stress, high-grace period characterized by minimal interpersonal demand. As time goes on, stress and interpersonal demand increase. Brain differences regarding NT and ND executive functioning are far more likely to become noticeable at this point. Additionally, it can be very normal for opposites to attract regarding executive functioning capacities. For example, one partner may excel in task initiation while the other struggles to even get started. Sometimes, certain stereotypes can actually play out in real life: An ADHDer may marry a professional organizer, an alexithymic person may marry a counselor, etc.

Studies show that very specific trends exist between groups of ND persons as compared to groups of NT persons regarding executive functioning. However, since no group is ever homogenous, therapists should avoid generalization. Do not assume that a NT clients will not struggle with executive functioning at times, or that ND clients will struggle in every single area of executive functioning. An ADHDer may actually be extremely neat, for instance. (Perhaps this particular ADHDer's personality gravitates towards neatness, so they've put forth great effort to learn coping skills to combat their brain-based difficulties with organization. Maybe, too, they've had a lot of support and opportunities to practice these coping skills in a low-demand environment.)

Research shows that repeat exposure to skill-building opportunities can improve the executive functioning skills of both NT and ND persons who do not have physical brain damage, certain medical conditions, anatomical limitations, or cognitive issues. Formal or informal tests may be used, when appropriate, to help therapists plan interventions accordingly. Rigid NT standards for executive functioning skills should not be enforced; Each client should be supported towards their own unique best in this area.

Issue #6: Sensory Processing Differences

ND clients can report ongoing periods of sensory overload, difficulty regulating physiological and emotional responses to stimuli, sensory-seeking or avoiding behaviors, or even difficulty discriminating between sensations. ND clients may also recall salient memories in which their attempts to seek help for sensory-based concerns were dismissed or punished by others, events which can easily have a negative impact on self-concept.[27, 28] Sadly, this is usually because the mechanics of sensory processing are not well understood by the general public . . . let alone NT-ND sensory processing differences.

Pain tolerance or intolerance is an example of a common area of sensory processing variability that can be easily misunderstood.[29] Tolerance or intolerance to heat or cold is another common example. Regardless of what it is, though, invalidating a person's sensory experience can be a special form of gaslighting:

- "The sun is out, so you can't possibly feel cold. Take off that jacket."
- "I cooked the chicken the same way that I always do. There's nothing wrong with its texture."
- "Stop crying, there's no way that little scratch hurts you so much."

An additional consideration on the topic of sensory processing is that research shows Autistic brains may not *habituate* to incoming sensory information in a typical way.[30] This means that the Autistic brain can continue to hone in on a stimulus, and react to it, long after a NT person has totally processed the same stimulus and moved on from it. Take the high volume of an unexpected fire alarm at school or work, for example. Both ND and NT persons are usually bothered by this kind of interruption at first. Most NT people, though, will react with less upset, quickly tune out the sound (even sometimes while it's still occurring), and return to their physiological baseline without much effort. Some Autistic persons, on the other hand, may experience multiple levels of dysregulation in this situation. The initial intensity of both the interruption to their day's plans and the volume of the alarm's sound may cause them to feel very physiologically and/or emotionally upset. They may feel the same degree of upset all the way until the sound stops, and maybe even for some time after it ends. In fact, they may remain in a heightened brain and body state until they engage in specific coping strategies to encourage a return to their physiological baseline. They may also need to utilize specific coping strategies in order to encourage enough cognitive flexibility to resume their daily activities after the interruption.

How do NT and ND habituation differences relate to neurodiverse couple therapy?
Consider something as simple as the presence of an essential oil diffuser in a therapist's office. While most NT partners will have the biological ability to go "nose blind" by automatically habituating to this stimulus, some ND partners may not. If the scent is aversive to them, they may experience mental distraction or physiological restlessness that can easily be misinterpreted during couple therapy. This may persist all the way until the stimulus is removed, and even perhaps for sometime after. Some ND clients may also experience social anxiety from the need to advocate for the removal of this

object. Sensory insecurity and social anxiety, understandably, often go hand in hand. Acknowledging the reality of ND habituation differences can actually be a key factor in the effective support of Autistic clients who experience chronic anxiety.[31]

Partners in a neurodiverse relationship present to therapy with varying levels of education about sensory processing, with some having a wealth of knowledge and some having none. Similarly, some clients may have had past experiences with supportive therapies in this area (e.g., occupational therapy), while others have not. It's important to discuss whether or not any past therapies meant to improve sensory processing have been helpful or unhelpful, or maybe even traumatic. It's also important to provide clients with sufficient psychoeducation regarding sensory processing. Teaching neurodiverse couples that a NT partner and a ND partner both exist in different planes of Earth's sensory multiverse is a vital first step towards helping them identify their sensory similarities and differences. Only then can they learn how to validate each other. Formal tests or informal questionnaires may be used, if appropriate, to clarify each partner's sensory needs.

This chart lists a few common examples of the kinds of sensory-related issues those in neurodiverse relationships tend to report. While it obviously cannot list every single potential scenario, it does include examples of both hyper and hyposensitivity.

Table 6.2

NT Partner's Experience	ND Partner's Potential Underlying Sensory Challenge(s)
I never know when it's ok to touch them or not. They push me away a lot.	Hypersensitivity to touch.
I have to walk on eggshells around them since they find the sounds I make annoying. Yet, they can be super loud themselves.	Sensitivity to sound. (When one is in control of the sounds in their environment this may be more easily managed.)
We fight about the thermostat in our house way too much. My partner is always too cold or too hot.	Thermal interoception differences; ND persons can have marked difficulty modulating body temperature.

(Continued)

Table 6.2 (Continued)

NT Partner's Experience	ND Partner's Potential Underlying Sensory Challenge(s)
I'm tired of seeing them wear the same old things all the time.	Tactile defensiveness may lead to the need for the predictability of "safe" clothing.
My personal hygiene is a huge problem for them, but I don't understand why. I'm very clean!	Smell sensitivity to body odor, visual sensitivity to the appearance of sweat, tactile sensitivity to the texture of sweat, etc.
My partner doesn't ever seem to notice the smell of overflowing garbage or the cat's litterbox.	Hyposensitivity to smell.
My partner won't try new things that involve being active, like dancing, with me.	Proprioceptive differences.

As you can imagine, sensory differences are not only extremely relevant to clients' everyday life together, but also their sex life. Sexual interaction is biologically designed to have a sky-high sensory component! This may be experienced <u>more</u> or <u>less</u> intensely by a ND partner, and can vary from day to day. An example of this occurs when a ND person who is generally hypersensitive to touch partners with a NT person. The NT partner in this scenario not only tends to have difficulty understanding their partner's reactivity to everyday stimuli, but also can feel unattractive and rejected should their ND partner occasionally recoil from their touch. Alternatively, a NT person may partner with a ND person who is hyposensitive to touch. They may also take certain reactions personally, noting "Nothing I do seems enough to turn my partner on sexually. Do they just not find me sexy?"

Issue #7: Sexual Challenges

Numerous factors come into play when partners of any neurotype interact together sexually. Each partner's personal trauma history, toolbox of interpersonal skills, executive functioning skills, sensory processing issues, physical health concerns, gender expectations, spiritual beliefs, and much more all represent important considerations.

Neurodiverse couples often present to therapy with a wide variety of concerns about sex. Some partners struggle with touch and/or emotional intimacy to the degree they require practice with intentional coping strategies to allow them to enjoy non-sexual interactions, let alone sexual interactions. For them, sexual activity represents an extreme challenge. Other couples, however, may enjoy a satisfying sex life overall but seek clarification or improvement upon specific issues. Still others may want to use the therapy room to explore questions of sexual orientation.

Talking holistically about sex is always important, but perhaps especially so with neurodiverse couples. This is because there's often a greater degree of complexity to consider. For instance, the sensory component of sex <u>must</u> be top of mind when discussing the sexual experiences of neurodiverse couples. To understand why, consider the following two schemas.

Both schemas portray an outline for the exact same kind of consensual sexual interaction between two partners who are in a committed relationship. These schemas are vastly oversimplified, but nonetheless appropriate for comparison purposes.

NT-NT Sexual Schema.

1. Confirm mutual interest in sexual activity.
2. Remove clothing.
3. Begin lovemaking.
4. End lovemaking.
5. Return to baseline.

Apart from circumstances that involve recovery from trauma, sexual compulsivity, or other specialized concerns, NT couples' sexual problems tend to focus on deviations from the above script. Clients' stated goals for therapy often center around resolving sexual desire discrepancies, improving the quality of their sex life, learning how to cope with physical or mental challenges that interfere with their intimacy, or learning how to increase the frequency of their sexual interactions.

ND-NT Sexual Schema

1. Interpret one's own degree of sexual desire (*Interoception*).
2. Convey interest in sexual activity to your partner (*Communication*).
3. Confirm mutual interest in sexual activity (*Communication*).
4. Assess the sensory security afforded by the chosen environment for lovemaking (*Visual, Olfactory, Auditory Processing; Thermal Interoception*).
5. Make accommodations to the environment, as necessary, for sensory security (*Interoception, Cognitive Flexibility, Communication*).
6. Remove clothing (*Thermal Interoception, Tactile Processing*).
7. Begin lovemaking (*Communication, Sensory Processing – Hyper or Hyposensitivity will be a factor in arousal*).
8. End lovemaking (*Self-Monitoring, Communication*).
9. Return to individual emotional and physiological baseline (*Emotion Regulation, Interoception*).
10. Return to relationship baseline (*Self-Regulation, Communication*).

Note that NT-NT couples actually do experience the same brain-processing complexities and skill requirements during lovemaking that are clearly outlined in the ND-NT schema. However, they usually go unnoticed because NT persons generally consider them automatic. ND-NT couples, on the other hand, may become hung-up by any or all of these brain processes. These struggles will be piled on top of the basic concerns previously mentioned, i.e., resolving sexual desire discrepancies, improving the quality of their sex life, learning how to cope with physical or mental challenges that interfere with their intimacy, or learning how to increase the frequency of their sexual interactions.

Upon starting therapy, neurodiverse couples almost <u>never</u> attribute their sexual problems to any brain-based concerns. A client is far more likely to lament, for example, "My wife doesn't like to touch me" than to say "My wife appears to have difficulty, on a sensory level, with physical touch." Clients are also far more likely to state something like, "My husband requires an extremely high level of sexual stimulation for pleasure to even register for him, which makes me afraid he's some kind of pervert" versus "I find my husband's hyposensitivity to sexual touch troubling." Psychoeducation can help neurodiverse couples better conceptualize their sexual issues, put them into perspective, and decide how to address them. Therapists can guide rich discussions about how each partner's brain-based sensory hypersensitivity or hyposensitivity may play a role. Each partner's level of sexual desire, arousal preferences, and personal boundaries can be addressed.

A final point on this topic is the suggestion for neurodiverse couple therapists to stay current on research regarding ND sexual diversity, gender fluidity, and the need to expand this type of research. Because of the high incidence of neurodivergence within the LGBTQIA+ community, it's reasonable to expect that neurodiverse couples will bring concerns about sexual identity to therapy more often than NT couples.

One specific example of this can occur if a heterosexual male (NT) marries an Autistic female who was unaware of her asexual orientation when they first became partners, but who discovers this sometime later. If the husband is highly committed to the marriage for personal and/or religious reasons, he tends to feel unfairly forced into celibacy in this scenario. Meanwhile, the wife tends to feel distressed, guilty, and unsupported. Both partners may be confused about the direction they'd like their relationship to take. They wonder, "Can our relationship go on now that we have different sexual orientations from each other?" A therapist can join with this couple in support of their relationship discernment process, perhaps sharing the fact that research indicates Autistic females tend to self-identify as ace (asexual) more often than NT females.[32]

When significant differences regarding certain dimensions of sexual identity exist between two partners, clients may choose to use neurodiverse couple therapy in a few ways. Sometimes they wish to explore each partner's sexual identity, boundaries, and arousal preferences in detail with a goal to determine whether or not it's possible to create a mutually respectful sex life together. Or, they may request that the therapist help them transition to an entirely sexless relationship that still maintains non-sexual affection and emotional intimacy. Usually, though, these clients wish to use therapy to help end their relationship and focus on becoming healthy co-parents instead.

Depending on clients' stated therapy goals, neurodiverse couple therapists may wish to consider some or all of the following points:

The value each client places on their own sexuality within their overall identity framework differs from person to person.
Does a client view their sexuality as a fixed, immovable part of who they are as a person? If so, it's cruel of a partner (and unethical for a therapist) to suggest that this innate component can or should change. On the other

hand, does a client believe their sexuality represents a fluid component of their overall personhood?

Partners in a neurodiverse couple may answer these questions similarly or differently from one another. One or both partners may also express strong accompanying spiritual or secular values.

The value each client places on nonsexual and sexual touch in a relationship differs from person to person.
Some clients view either nonsexual touch, sexual touch, or both as crucial in a relationship. Others do not. Neurodiverse couples may benefit from first categorizing the various kinds of touch they share together (e.g., romantic, erotic, playful, nonsexual, etc.) and then assigning each kind a value according to personal preference. This simple exercise is potentially quite enlightening. It can even reveal vital nuance. Asexual persons are not necessarily always aromantic, for instance. They can be open to romantic behaviors (e.g., laying next to each other in the nude), yet draw the line at touching with the intention to promote erotic stimulation.

Neurodiverse couples have much to teach the field of relationship therapy regarding their lived experiences with sex. The current lack of data on this topic probably, at least in part, relates to the popular misconception that ND persons lack the interpersonal skills needed to maintain successful sexual relationships – especially when paired with NT partners. Yet, sexually satisfying neurodiverse relationships can and do exist!

Therapists should keep in mind the potential for bias as they review available scholarly information regarding sex and neurodivergence. For instance, subjective terms like *healthy sexual functioning* are not always thoughtfully defined. Far too much research focuses on what are presumed to be ND sexual deficits, and important contextual factors are sometimes not considered. Nonetheless, it must be stated that the available information regarding ND sexual habits indicates that neurodiverse couples are more likely to experience sexual concerns together than NT couples. A 2020 review of 11 studies found that ADHDers reported more sexual dysfunction, more frequent masturbation and less sexual satisfaction than NT persons.[33] This research agrees with a 2018 Dutch study that found sexual dysfunction in 39% of male ADHDers and 43% of female ADHDers (regardless of their use of psychostimulant medications), versus 17% for males and 20% for females in the general population.[34] They also found male ADHDers had more orgasmic problems, premature ejaculation, and sexual aversion than the general population, while female ADHDers had more orgasmic problems, sexual excitement problems, and sexual aversion. For Autistics, other research highlights increased sexual victimization histories, prevalent PTSD, increased risk of STIs, and reduced sexual interest.[35,36,37]

Issue #8: Parenting Stress

Any couple can struggle to work together as a loving, unified parenting team. But, some neurodiverse couples with biological children, who tend to be ND, can have a much harder time. Studies agree that couples with ND children are more likely to carry a higher stress level than NT parents with NT children.[38]

Neurodiverse parents tend to experience both mental and physical fatigue as they stretch themselves thin trying to balance parenting responsibilities with employment, self-care, marital connection, personal goals, and other life demands. Sadly, this may be amplified by low levels of support from family members and friends, financial burdens, and a lack of parenting resources relevant to their unique needs. Social shaming by those who cannot relate to their lives, or who are ignorant regarding neurodiversity, varies by geographical location and other contextual factors. Add to this the constant barrage of complicated decision-making tasks involved with raising children who differ from NT expectations and one can easily understand how neurodiverse parents of one or more ND children often report feeling isolated and overwhelmed.

Neurodiverse couples often present to therapy with elevated relationship distress, caregiver fatigue, and physical complaints as a result of their child-rearing challenges. This makes perfect sense because their ND children's emotional reactivity and challenging behaviors usually represent a clear increase in *frequency*, *intensity*, and *duration* when compared to NT children. For example, it's typical for children of any neurotype to struggle with separation anxiety from time to time. ND children, though, tend to experience more frequent bouts of high anxiety and/or panic that require skilled attention to effectively support. ND children may also have more frequent sleep struggles that persist for long periods of time or experience extensive challenges with feeding, communicating, toileting, etc.

Unless therapeutically appropriate, therapists should resist normalizing the stories neurodiverse parents tell about their home life. Deep invalidation can result from hearing such minimizing phrases as "all kids do that" or "that's a phase that will end soon." Chances are good that clients have already heard such hurtful words from well-meaning friends, family, teachers, doctors, and helping professionals. Effective therapists will learn how to correctly validate the fact that raising ND children is more stressful than raising NT children without going to the extreme of either demonizing or glorifying neurodivergence itself.

Therapists should recognize that ND children usually require much more involvement from their parents in order to meet their basic needs, and that parents can often disagree on the best methods to do so. Often, partners must learn totally new ways to parent via such focused support efforts as practicing co-regulation and creating different sensory diets unique to each child's needs. And, this challenge cannot be understated . . . the ND partner must do all of this while struggling with their own self-regulation!

Discussion thus far has presumed parents already have some level of awareness and acceptance regarding neurodivergence within their family. This is not always the case, of course. While some couples come to therapy in the midst of an intentional effort to understand the neurological make-up of each family member, others do not. Similarly, some couples may be in the process of deciding whether a formal diagnosis of neurodivergence for a child is wise, wanted, and needed. They may be weighing out the consequences of obtaining or not obtaining a diagnosis, while others may be in denial that brain differences in their family actually exist! Finally, those who do acknowledge their children's neurological differences may wonder who exactly needs to know about them.

Consider this chart that highlights some of the dilemmas regarding diagnosis and disclosure for a child. Partners may have opposing views, which can cause relationship tension.

Parents' Decisions Regarding Diagnosis and Disclosure of a Child's Neurotype

Table 6.3

Diagnose & Disclose	Don't Diagnose, But Disclose
"An evaluation revealed that our child is ND. This is good information to have and sometimes share. We'll choose what others need to know about our child's brain and disclose on an as-needed basis."	"Why seek a label? Diagnosis is expensive, inaccessible, intrusive, etc. We'll choose what others need to know about our child's brain and disclose on an as-needed basis."

Diagnose, But Don't Disclose	Don't Diagnose & Don't Disclose
"An evaluation revealed that our child is ND. This is good, private information to have. We won't disclose anything about our child's brain because this is undesirable, unsafe, a breach of their privacy, unwise, etc."	"Why seek a label? Diagnosis is expensive, inaccessible, intrusive, etc. We won't disclose anything about our child's brain because this is undesirable, unsafe, a breach of their privacy, unwise, etc."

There are far too many issues for parents to debate amongst themselves regarding their child's neurodivergence to list here. As just one example, the pros and cons of telling a child about their own diagnosis can be a sore subject – despite the fact that clear anecdotal and scientific evidence shows speaking openly with a child early on about their neurodivergence tends to bring about positive outcomes.[39] Parents may also debate what supportive treatment modalities to pursue (if any), how to afford them, and practical concerns such as driving to and from multiple sessions and implementing therapy homework at home. Having different opinions about how to handle a child's uncomfortable, or even potentially dangerous, behaviors at home or in public can also spark conflict.

Therapists should help neurodiverse couples attribute the root of their parenting tensions to underlying issues such as reduced self-care and couple-care practices, as well as manifestations of each partner's attachment wounds. Just as they would with a NT couple raising NT children, therapists should help each partner calmly discuss their own parenting preferences, expectations, and boundaries regarding child-rearing – as well as their origins. Socioeconomic considerations, gender expectations, and cultural factors should never be left out of these discussions. Each partner should be given the chance to process any hurts that surface from their own childhood, as well as any hurts they may have caused one another.

It can be helpful to talk about some common stereotypes of American parents of ND children en route to guiding clients toward healthy parenting roles and practices.

- *The Warrior Parent* tends to passionately fight to "rescue" their ND child via a cure for their neurodivergence. This parent is usually fueled by a sincere desire to make their child's life better, yet gauges success only by NT standards.

- *The Worrier Parent* tends to structure their life around protecting their ND child from actual (or perceived) concerns. This parent is fueled by anxiety regarding their child's safety and wellbeing.
- *The Wish it Away Parent* tends to outright deny their child's ND qualities. This parent may be fueled by apathy, ignorance, misinformation, fear, or perhaps even shame.
- *The Wounding Parent* tends to make their ND child a scapegoat, neglect them, invalidate them, or violate their personal boundaries. This parent may be fueled by unresolved trauma, insecurity, anger, repetition compulsion, mental illness, etc.
- *The Woeful Victim Parent* tends to make the "tragedy" and "burden" of their child's neurodivergence all about them. This parent is fueled by the attention that martyrdom provides.
- *The Healthy Parent** tends to be an emotionally differentiated person who strives for self-regulation. This allows them to attempt to support their ND child from a place of calm connection. This parent is fueled by accurate information regarding neurodiversity topics, social support, access to supportive resources, and copious amounts of self-care. They may also prioritize listening to ND voices and encourage their child towards healthy ND identity formation.

*This person is a living unicorn. If you see one in the wild, befriend them immediately

Therapists should also help clients who struggle with parenting stress to understand that their particular coping strategies can, logically, affect their intimacy. A sad but common example of this occurs when one parent copes via denial while the other partner copes with hypervigilance. This sets up a toxic neurodiverse couple dynamic in which the denying partner (generally NT) may insist on promoting NT parenting techniques, while the hypervigilant partner (generally ND) strongly opposes this. Naturally, this provokes interpersonal conflict. If the denying partner goes on to wrongly blame their child's behavior on a lack of discipline or maturity, the parenting style of their partner, their partner's "hypochondriasis," etc. then this dynamic can become extremely unfavorable for any level of trust and closeness to flourish. The hypervigilant partner often takes on an increasingly defensive position in order to advocate what their ND child needs. Even in less extreme situations than this example, however, partners who generally agree on what their child's brain-based needs are and how to work together to support them are not immune to periods of relational disconnection or resentment. The lack of supportive resources for neurodiverse parents can leave them especially vulnerable to taking out their frustrations on one another or relieving tension in other unhealthy ways.

Besides neurodiverse couple therapy, where can parents of ND children turn to for support?
Sometimes, healthy online or in-person support groups exist. However, clients and professionals must use good judgment to determine whether or not a group is truly healthy. This is often quite obvious, unfortunately, as many groups display clear red flag behaviors such as ableism, misinformation, parent-shaming, and learned helplessness. Avoid any group flooded with parents who use the space to practice toxic venting about their ND children. Unacceptable posts that include footage of ND children in the midst of meltdowns, toileting accidents, safety concerns, or other struggles also represent an immediate signal to leave the group. These horrendous privacy violations should never happen, no matter how much they represent a parent's desperate cry for help.

Regarding free parenting blogs and podcasts, therapists should be aware that the vast majority are presented from a NT perspective . . . even though some interesting content from ND perspectives is starting to emerge. Most of these resources will further parents' feelings of overwhelm and isolation because they simply don't reflect their actual experience. The same goes for some of the most popular parenting books on the market. The scope of these resources tends to be limited to teaching parents about typical child development patterns and how to control misbehavior. In both subtle and overt ways, some particularly cruel texts even blame a ND child's emotional dysregulation and developmental differences on the parents! (Mothers often get the worst of it.)

Where are the strength-based resources that promote holistic understanding of each parent's own neurotype and that of their child? Where are the voices destigmatizing atypicality? Where are the books inclusive of neuroaffirming coping strategies for neurodiverse parents and their kids?

Neurodiverse couple therapists have the distinct privilege and duty to help parents reduce stress while learning how to work *with* the reality of neurodivergence in their home instead of *against* it. All neurodiverse couples with children can benefit from developing a realistic plan for self-care, couple-care, and parenting. Therapists must remember, though, just how difficult it can be for neurodiverse parents to acknowledge and implement these plans. For one, it can be difficult to accept the ways one's parenting journey differs from others. There can also be sadness due to unmet personal expectations, not to mention ongoing fatigue due to the effort required from day to day (e.g., going to the park or a dentist appointment can be a monumental event). Even engaging with the American public school system, something most NT families take for granted, can be complicated! Although the IEP process in American schools may not cost money, the potential emotional roller coaster involved can be a lot to mentally endure. There may even be lost wages from taking time off to attend IEP meetings. For those who pursue homeschooling, this decision comes with its own set of blessings and challenges. The weight of supporting each family member's distinct neurological needs, managing the family's nutrition and other physical needs such as sleep, and monitoring educational needs can be all-consuming.

Successful parenting takes a lot of learning and unlearning about yourself, your partner, and your child. Encouraging clients to look beyond the rigidity of NT standards invites them to connect with who their ND child actually *is*, instead of who they (or society) wants them to be. It also, perhaps, invites each partner towards greater personal authenticity and radical self-acceptance.

As neurodiverse couples begin to realize their challenging parenting situations are not usually their ND child's fault, nor are they usually the result of intentional malice by either partner, their approach to conflict may soften.

Some healing reframes to foster cognitive flexibility, empathy, and healthy problem-solving regarding parenting challenges can be:

- "What if no one is to blame?"
- "What if you, your partner, and your child are all doing the best you can with the brains and bodies you have?"

Last, but perhaps most importantly, therapists can remind clients that any ND child displaying challenging behavior is very likely responding *proportionately* and *appropriately* to their developmental capacity, immediate physiological experience, and coping skills. Furthermore, this behavior is communicating something which deserves care and attention. Once a supportive plan is made to address these concerns and stress levels reduce, perhaps neurodiverse partners can unite around a fundamental truth: Their ND child is offering them a unique invitation to experience the world the way they do. This can increase parental empathy. Additionally, parents who are willing to attempt joining their ND child on their sensory plane at times can experience some heartwarming bonding moments! This may or may not be easier for the ND parent to do than the NT parent. For instance, an ADHDer may find it much easier to spontaneously join their ADHD child rolling down a small, snow-covered hill with reckless abandon. An Autistic parent may delight in introducing their Autistic child to the feeling of fingerpainting on a table with shaving cream or tracing the veins on a leaf with a crayon. NT parents, too, can definitely learn to have greater empathy for their ND child's experiences and enjoy sharing everyday sensory pleasures together.

Glossary of Bolded Terms

Autistic Burnout   Results from chronic masking, poor boundaries, environmental toxicity, unrealistic expectations, unhealthy coping skills, and/or a lack of validation and social support. This is often experienced as a period of intense physical and emotional exhaustion. Incoming stimuli may not be well tolerated, and a person may have difficulty engaging with everyday tasks.

Autistic Meltdown   Also known as a neurological emergency. This brain-based response and associated behavior occurs as a defense mechanism when an Autistic person experiences distress that exceeds their ability to cope. It can result from a single aversive stimulus, the accumulation of aversive stimuli over time, interpersonal dynamics, or chronic sensory understimulation.

Couple Identity   Refers to the way partners in a neurodiverse relationship conceptualize their partnership. This may include or exclude each person's neurotype and associated brain-based features.

Double Empathy Problem   Milton coined this term in 2012 to suggest that both NT persons and ND persons struggle to understand one another at times. This is due to having fundamentally different ways of experiencing and interpreting incoming stimuli. Also, NT and ND persons tend to have different communication styles, mannerisms, and patterns of behaviors they find mutually confusing.

Gender Dysphoria   A pervasive sense of unrest that stems from a perceived misalignment between one's own biological sex and their gender self-identifications.

Gender Expression   How one outwardly presents their gender to the world via their behavior, style of dress, use of pronouns, their name, etc.

Gender Identity   One's personal conceptualization of their own gender, which may or may not correspond to the biological sex they were assigned at birth or traditional categories for gender.

Learned Helplessness   Introduced by Seligman and Maier in 1967 after studying animals, this concept applies to people who experience stressors that do not abate regardless of their attempts to make things better. Sadly, they eventually internalize an external locus of control and stop trying to make positive changes happen.

Sexual Expression   Refers to the way one chooses to behaviorally express their own sexual thoughts, feelings, behaviors, and orientation. This may or may not include actual sexual interactions with other people.

Sexual Identity   One's personal conceptualization of their own sexual orientation as well as their erotic, romantic, or aromatic preferences.

Notes

1 Smith, R., Netto, J., Gribble, N. C., & Falkmer, M. (2021). 'At the end of the day, it's love': An exploration of relationships in neurodiverse couples. *Journal of Autism and Developmental Disorders*, 51(9), 3311–3321.

2 Mitran, C. L. (2022). Experiences of licensed counselors and other licensed mental health providers working with neurodiverse adults: An instrumental case Study. *The Family Journal*.

3 Thomas, M. D., Jewell, N. P., & Allen, A. M. (2021). Black and unarmed: Statistical interaction between age, perceived mental illness, and geographic region among males fatally shot by police using case-only design. *Annals of Epidemiology*, 53, 42–49.

4 Heylens, G., Aspeslagh, L., Dierickx, J., Baetens, K., Van Hoorde, B., De Cuypere, G., & Elaut, E. (2018). The co-occurrence of gender dysphoria and autism spectrum disorder in adults: An analysis of cross-sectional and clinical chart data. *Journal of Autism and Developmental Disorders*, 48(6), 2217–2223.

5 Strang, J. F., Kenworthy, L., Dominska, A., Sokoloff, J., Kenealy, L. E., Berl, M., . . . & Wallace, G. L. (2014). Increased gender variance in autism spectrum disorders and attention deficit hyperactivity disorder. *Archives of Sexual Behavior*, 43(8), 1525–1533.

6 Warrier, V., Greenberg, D. M., Weir, E., Buckingham, C., Smith, P., Lai, M. C., . . . & Baron-Cohen, S. (2020). Elevated rates of autism, other neurodevelopmental and psychiatric diagnoses, and autistic traits in transgender and gender-diverse individuals. *Nature Communications*, 11(1), 1–12.

7 George, R., & Stokes, M. A. (2018). Gender identity and sexual orientation in autism spectrum disorder. *Autism*, 22(8), 970–982.

8 George, R., & Stokes, M. A. (2018). Sexual orientation in autism spectrum disorder. *Autism Research*, *11*(1), 133–141.

9 Pecora, L. A., Hooley, M., Sperry, L., Mesibov, G. B., & Stokes, M. A. (2020). Sexuality and gender issues in individuals with autism spectrum disorder. *Child and Adolescent Psychiatric Clinics*, *29*(3), 543–556.

10 Milton, D., Neumeier, S. M., Walshe, R., Jackson-Perry, D., Taylor, K., Brown, L., . . . & Pountney, O. (2021). *Working with autistic transgender and non-binary people: Research, practice and experience.* Jessica Kingsley Publishers.

11 Mendes, E. A., & Maroney, M. R. (2019). *Gender identity, sexuality and autism: Voices from across the spectrum.* Jessica Kingsley Publishers

12 Keating, C. T., & Cook, J. L. (2020). Facial expression production and recognition in autism spectrum disorders: A shifting landscape. *Child and Adolescent Psychiatric Clinics*, *29*(3), 557–571.

13 Edey, R., Cook, J., Brewer, R., Johnson, M. H., Bird, G., & Press, C. (2016). Interaction takes two: Typical adults exhibit mind-blindness towards those with autism spectrum disorder. *Journal of Abnormal Psychology*, *125*(7), 879.

14 Heasman, B., & Gillespie, A. (2018). Perspective-taking is two-sided: Misunderstandings between people with Asperger's syndrome and their family members. *Autism*, *22*(6), 740–750.

15 Milton, D. E. (2012). On the ontological status of autism: the 'double empathy problem'. *Disability & Society*, *27*(6), 883–887.

16 Steenfeldt-Kristensen, C., Jones, C. A., & Richards, C. (2020). The prevalence of self-injurious behaviour in autism: A meta-analytic study. *Journal of Autism and Developmental Disorders*, *50*(11), 3857–3873.

17 Swannell, S. V., Martin, G. E., Page, A., Hasking, P., & St John, N. J. (2014). Prevalence of nonsuicidal self-injury in nonclinical samples: Systematic review, meta-analysis and meta-regression. *Suicide and Life-Threatening Behavior*, *44*(3), 273–303.

18 Bemmouna, D., Coutelle, R., Weibel, S., & Weiner, L. (2022). Feasibility, acceptability and preliminary efficacy of dialectical behavior therapy for autistic adults without intellectual disability: A mixed methods study. *Journal of Autism and Developmental Disorders*, *52*(10), 4337–4354.

19 Wise, S. J. (2022). *The Neurodivergent Friendly Workbook of DBT Skills.*

20 Quadt, L., Garfinkel, S. N., Mulcahy, J. S., Larsson, D. E., Silva, M., Jones, A. M., . . . & Critchley, H. D. (2021). Interoceptive training to target anxiety in autistic adults (ADIE): A single-center, superiority randomized controlled trial. *EClinicalMedicine*, *39*, 101042.

21 Porges, S. W. (2018). Polyvagal theory: A primer. *Clinical applications of the polyvagal theory: The emergence of polyvagal-informed therapies*, *50*, 69.

22 Fülling, C., Dinan, T. G., & Cryan, J. F. (2019). Gut microbe to brain signaling: what happens in vagus . . . . *Neuron*, *101*(6), 998–1002.

23 Kleinhans, N. M., Johnson, L. C., Richards, T., Mahurin, R., Greenson, J., Dawson, G., & Aylward, E. (2009). Reduced neural habituation in the amygdala and social impairments in autism spectrum disorders. *American Journal of Psychiatry*, *166*(4), 467–475.

24 Berger, J. M., Singh, P., Khrimian, L., Morgan, D. A., Chowdhury, S., Arteaga-Solis, E., . . . & Karsenty, G. (2019). Mediation of the acute stress response by the skeleton. *Cell Metabolism*, *30*(5), 890–902.

25 Bedrossian, L. (2015). Understand autism meltdowns and share strategies to minimize, manage occurrences. *Disability Compliance for Higher Education*, *20*(7), 6–6.

26 St. John, T., Woods, S., Bode, T., Ritter, C., & Estes, A. (2022). A review of executive functioning challenges and strengths in autistic adults. *The Clinical Neuropsychologist, 36*(5), 1116–1147.

27 Schulz, S. E., Kelley, E., Anagnostou, E., Nicolson, R., Georgiades, S., Crosbie, J., . . . & Stevenson, R. A. (2022). Sensory processing patterns predict problem behaviours in autism spectrum disorder and attention-deficit/hyperactivity disorder. *Advances in Neurodevelopmental Disorders*, 1–13.

28 Kerley, L., Meredith, P., & Harnett, P. (2022). Do childhood adversity and sensory processing sensitivity interact to predict meaningful activity engagement in adulthood? *British Journal of Occupational Therapy*.

29 Allely, C. S. (2013). Pain sensitivity and observer perception of pain in individuals with autistic spectrum disorder. *The Scientific World Journal, 2013*.

30 Jamal, W., Cardinaux, A., Haskins, A. J., Kjelgaard, M., & Sinha, P. (2021). Reduced sensory habituation in autism and its correlation with behavioral measures. *Journal of Autism and Developmental Disorders, 51*(9), 3153–3164.

31 Verhulst, I., MacLennan, K., Haffey, A., & Tavassoli, T. (2022). The perceived causal relations between sensory reactivity differences and anxiety symptoms in autistic adults. *Autism in Adulthood, 4*(3).

32 Bush, H. H., Williams, L. W., & Mendes, E. (2021). Brief report: Asexuality and young women on the autism spectrum. *Journal of Autism and Developmental Disorders, 51*(2), 725–733.

33 Soldati, L., Bianchi-Demicheli, F., Schockaert, P., Köhl, J., Bolmont, M., Hasler, R., & Perroud, N. (2020). Sexual function, sexual dysfunctions, and ADHD: A systematic literature review. *The Journal of Sexual Medicine, 17*(9), 1653–1664.

34 Bijlenga, D., Vroege, J. A., Stammen, A. J. M., Breuk, M., Boonstra, A. M., Van der Rhee, K., & Kooij, J. J. S. (2018). Prevalence of sexual dysfunctions and other sexual disorders in adults with attention-deficit/hyperactivity disorder compared to the general population. *ADHD Attention Deficit and Hyperactivity Disorders, 10*(1), 87–96.

35 Reuben, K. E., Stanzione, C. M., & Singleton, J. L. (2021). Interpersonal trauma and posttraumatic stress in autistic adults. *Autism in Adulthood, 3*(3), 247–256.

36 Li, J. C., Tsai, S. J., Chen, T. J., & Chen, M. H. (2022). Sexually transmitted infection among adolescents and young adults with autism spectrum disorder: A nationwide longitudinal study. *Journal of Autism and Developmental Disorders*, 1–8.

37 Attanasio, M., Masedu, F., Quattrini, F., Pino, M. C., Vagnetti, R., Valenti, M., & Mazza, M. (2021). Are autism spectrum disorder and asexuality Connected? *Archives of Sexual Behavior*, 1–25.

38 Haytham, A. O., Khuan, L., Lim Poh, Y. I. N. G., & Hassouneh, O. (2022). Coping mechanism among parents of children with autism spectrum disorder: A review. *Iranian Journal of Child Neurology, 16*(1), 9.

39 Oredipe, T., Kofner, B., Riccio, A., Cage, E., Vincent, J., Kapp, S. K., . . . & Gillespie-Lynch, K. (2022). Does learning you are autistic at a younger age lead to better adult outcomes? A participatory exploration of the perspectives of autistic university students. *Autism*.

Section III
Clinical Application

Neurodiverse Couple Assessment

7

Comprehensive assessment of each partner as an individual, as well as their relationship itself, is an essential part of any couple therapy process. To support this effort, this chapter begins with a series of brief questionnaires and ends with a discussion of the types of neurodiverse couple presentations frequently observed in a private practice therapy setting.

The following questionnaires have been intentionally designed for brevity and ease of integration with clinicians' existing procedures. They're not intended to encompass *all* necessary aspects of assessment. Rather, they're meant to hone in on concerns that may be particularly relevant to treating neurodiverse couples.

Safety, Trauma, & Boundary Assessment

Do <u>you</u> feel safe at home? Circle one.

Yes   No

Do <u>you</u> feel safe in your partner's presence?

Yes   No

Are <u>you</u> currently self-harming?

Yes   No

Are <u>you</u> currently suicidal?

Yes   No

DOI: 10.4324/9781003351337-11

If you're comfortable doing so, please mark any areas of significant pain within your life history:

☐ Physical abuse

☐ Sexual abuse

☐ Mental abuse, ex: gaslighting

☐ Spiritual abuse

☐ Housing and/or food insecurity

☐ Neglect

☐ Racial trauma

☐ Other:

Please rate your boundaries in the following areas. For each statement, circle either *Excellent, Ok,* or *Problematic.*

My boundaries with my . . .

Partner are:	Excellent	Ok	Problematic
Parents are:	Excellent	Ok	Problematic
Friends are:	Excellent	Ok	Problematic
Coworkers are:	Excellent	Ok	Problematic
Children are:	Excellent	Ok	Problematic
Eating and sleeping are:	Excellent	Ok	Problematic
Use of medication(s) are:	Excellent	Ok	Problematic
Use of illegal substances are:	Excellent	Ok	Problematic
Use of alcohol are:	Excellent	Ok	Problematic

Strengths Assessment

As a person, I have the following strengths:

My neurodiverse relationship has the following strengths:

_____

Intimacy Assessment

How would <u>you</u> rate the quality of *emotional intimacy* with your partner? Circle one.

Satisfying

Unsatisfying

Unsure

How would <u>you</u> rate the quality of *physical intimacy* with your partner? Circle one.

Satisfying

Unsatisfying

Unsure or Not Applicable

How would <u>you</u> rate the quality of *spiritual intimacy* with your partner? Circle one.

Satisfying

Unsatisfying

Unsure or Not Applicable

How would <u>you</u> rate the quality of *intellectual intimacy* with your partner? Circle one.

Satisfying

Unsatisfying

Unsure or Not Applicable

Executive Functioning & Sensory Processing Assessment

Please rate <u>yourself</u> in the following areas. For each statement, circle either *Excellent, Ok,* or *Needs Improvement.*

Remembering things that I need to remember:	Excellent	Ok	Needs Improvement
Starting tasks that I need to do:	Excellent	Ok	Needs Improvement
Planning things out:	Excellent	Ok	Needs Improvement
Organizing information in my head:	Excellent	Ok	Needs Improvement
Organizing items in my home or office:	Excellent	Ok	Needs Improvement
Thinking in flexible ways:	Excellent	Ok	Needs Improvement
Recognizing when I'm on or off task:	Excellent	Ok	Needs Improvement
Making adjustments when I lose focus:	Excellent	Ok	Needs Improvement
Controlling my own impulses:	Excellent	Ok	Needs Improvement
Regulating my emotions:	Excellent	Ok	Needs Improvement

Please mark any area(s) where your sensory processing is challenging. Provide details if you'd like.

□ Vision _____

□ Hearing _____

□ Smell _____

□ Taste _____

□ Touch _____

□ Balance _____

□ Awareness of my own internal body sensations _____

Brain Assessment

A set of characteristics that describe a person's brain wiring is called a *neurotype*. This may or may not also be referred to as a person's diagnosis.

Do you know your neurotype(s)? (You may have more than one.)

□ Yes, my neurotype(s) is/are: _____

□ I'm unsure about my neurotype(s)

□ No, I don't know my neurotype(s)

If you know <u>your</u> neurotype(s), how did this come about? Check all that apply.

☐ Self-diagnosis

☐ Diagnosis from a professional*

☐ Other

*If <u>you've</u> received a diagnosis from a professional, when did this occur? What type of professional did you see? _____

Somatic Assessment

Do <u>you</u> experience any of the following?

☐ Autoimmune disease

☐ Chronic fatigue

☐ Traumatic Brain Injury (TBI)

☐ PTSD

☐ Diabetes

☐ STD/STI

☐ Thyroid condition

☐ Hormonal concern

☐ Physical disability

☐ Sleep challenges

☐ Nutrition challenges

☐ Mental health concerns

☐ Cancer history

☐ Heart disease

☐ High/low blood pressure

☐ Transplant related concerns

☐ Skin condition

☐ Digestion problem

☐ Intolerance to cold or heat

☐ Alopecia

☐ Other: _____

Common Neurodiverse Couple Presentations

Some of the interpersonal dynamics that neurodiverse partners experience together in their relationship tend to follow certain observable patterns. Learning how to appropriately recognize whether or not these patterns may be occurring can assist a clinician to conceptualize a healthy treatment plan more quickly.

Often visible upon Intake, the following neurodiverse couple presentations seem to emerge time and time again. Each example presents a fictional couple.

The Uninformed Couple

Sometimes partners in an otherwise healthy relationship suddenly feel flooded with brain-based concerns – but, they have not yet properly identified them as such. These partners tend to be highly committed to one another, but uninformed about what is going on at a neurological level. They usually either lack access to information about the brain or have been deeply misinformed about what constitutes various neurotypes. These couples benefit from psychoeducation and thoughtful discussion about whether or not undiagnosed (or misdiagnosed) brain challenges may play a role in their stated challenges. All of the following example clients are fictional.

Shana (undiagnosed ADHD and SPD):

"I'm totally overstimulated by life at the moment. Our toddlers are constantly touching me, making tons of noise, and leaving sloppy messes all around the house. I used to love to cook before having kids, but now I can't keep up with even the most basic meal planning schedules anymore. Plus, the kids don't ever eat what I make. I feel guilty about everything that's piling up all around me. There are days when the smell of dirty dishes in the sink or spilled applesauce on the floor makes me cry. The sound of my kids' whining makes me reach for earplugs. There are so many messes, all the time . . . plus, I feel like a mess inside. With so many things to be responsible for, I don't even know where to begin. My brain is all jammed up."

Carlos (NT):

"I understand Shana's reached her limit due to the twins. They're at a tough age, and they're into everything. But, I don't understand how to help any more than I'm already doing. When I suggested Shana quit her part time job to be able to focus more at home, she got super defensive. That's her one escape from home chaos, I guess. I try to jump in with practical help like doing housework and cooking, but it doesn't seem to offer lasting relief. I even suggested something unconventional, like for her to work outside the home more and for me to work less. She didn't like that solution. She's always stressed out to the max, which stresses me out. I'm at a loss. We're arguing a lot lately over simple things, and that's never been how we've treated each other before."

In this example, Shana's *Brain Assessment Questionnaire* indicated she does not know her neurotype. The therapist notes she's displaying some signs of postpartum depression and anxiety, and that her level of self-care is fairly decent given her busy life circumstances. Most notably, though, the therapist notes that Shana has many indicators of undiagnosed ADHD and SPD. It's extremely common for neurodivergence to be missed in women up until some point in their adult life when their situational demands exceed their neurological ability to cope. This may be exactly what's happening here. Sadly, it appears none of this has been on the couple's radar at all! How different could their lives be once all applicable brain-based challenges are appropriately identified and supported?

Uniformed Couples can greatly benefit from psychoeducation about neurotypes, co-occuring conditions, family life cycle stages (inclusive of the postpartum period), sensory processing, executive functioning, and more.

Although they generally appreciate the invitation to discuss whether or not seeking a formal diagnostic process would be the right choice for them, some *Uninformed Couples* choose not to pursue formal testing.

The Proactive Couple

There are times when forward-thinking partners want to intentionally explore their brain qualities and associated couple dynamics during therapy. These clients tend to be young, energetic, educated, and genuinely intrigued by psychological topics. They're often aware of their different neurotypes, or at least highly suspicious that they may be a neurodiverse couple. Their stated therapy goals tend to prioritize global relationship improvement and maintenance strategies.

Juno (NT):

"We're considering getting engaged. There are some things about our relationship that I'm excited about, and one or two things that make me a bit nervous. We've been together for two years with no major issues, but I just want to make sure we can keep going strong. I want us to understand our different brains and how they work. I also want us to prepare for what we may be up against in society as a neurodiverse, gay couple. My main goal is for us to build a toolbox of skills we can use whenever we need them."

Isa (Autistic):

"I'm Autistic, but she's not. We've always known this from the start. Thankfully, we understand each other most of the time. Things are really good between us overall because we love each other and have taken steps to read books about how to communicate better. I'm definitely open to learning more relationship strategies through couple therapy, though. I want to do anything and everything I can to help us succeed as a couple. I'm not really worried about what society thinks of us. As long as we have each other, I'm good!"

Joining this kind of *Proactive Couple* to assess their strengths and areas of needed growth can help determine what healthy interpersonal skills and coping strategies they already have in place, and what additional skills they may benefit from learning.

Note that other *Proactive Couples* may seek therapy to specifically address anxiety centering around a very specific fear, (e.g., a family life cycle transition, a career decision, boundaries with in-laws, etc.).

Lenny (Dyslexic):

"We're engaged to be married next fall. We wanted to go to counseling before then to learn more about who we are as people and as a couple. I've really been wondering lately about how the learning disabilities I've had since childhood may show up in our relationship over the years - especially when we have kids. Could I even, genetically, pass on Dyslexia to them?"

Rosalind (NT):

"We want to have kids right away since we're getting married a little older than most people. But, I'm concerned about how our combined genetics might affect any future biological kids we have. In addition to his family history of Dyslexia, my side of the family has a history of Autism. Could I really be a 'special needs mom'? I don't even know if I can handle that thought. It's terrifying. I've been considering whether or not adoption would be a better path for us."

Psychoeducation can help this type of *Proactive Couple* gain accurate information about their concerns and put their worries into perspective. Teaching coping skills to manage anxiety and providing a nonjudgmental space to discern how they'd like to proceed regarding their specific concern is key.

The Reconsidering Couple

Sometimes a partner's adult diagnosis of neurodivergence shakes them, and/ or their partner, to the core. These partners tend to have identity questions (on an individual and a couple level) as they experience a period of heavy reconsideration. Partners in a *Reconsidering Couple* seek to re-examine themselves and what makes up the foundation of their relationship, often to varying degrees.

Toni (NT):

"When we got married, Mike didn't have a diagnosis. Now he does, and he talks about it all the time! I think he's starting to even use ADHD as an excuse. It's just a lot for me to take in. I thought I knew him, but I guess not. Even though a lot of things in our past make more sense to me now, it almost feels like I've been tricked. To be honest, I'm not sure I would have signed up to be in a relationship with someone who has ADHD. Will he always struggle the way he says he does? How can I ever expect to be able to depend on him as we get older?"

Mike (newly diagnosed ADHDer):

"That's really hurtful to hear. Can't you see that I'm still the same person I've always been? Now I just have an explanation for things that have always confused me about myself, which I tried to hide from others. I know it's hard for you to hear that I've been masking my everyday struggles. Honestly, though, I never thought they could be due to ADHD. I thought I just lacked the willpower to be consistent. Getting my diagnosis was a lightbulb moment for me. Why is this making you question our relationship instead of lean into it more?"

It's common for the NT partner of a newly diagnosed ND person to question whether or not the new label is being used as an excuse to underperform. They may also notice an "increase" in their partner's neurodivergent behavior. This is because having a diagnosis puts an understandable, temporary spotlight on each person's brain differences and their associated behaviors. It also may be because the ND partner is experimenting with unmasking at home.

In this example, Toni never envisioned herself in a neurodiverse relationship. She's scared of what this may mean going forward and feels betrayed by Mike's past masking behavior. Meanwhile, Mike is energized by finally understanding himself better. He feels let down that Toni doesn't share his eagerness to incorporate an understanding of ADHD (and thus, himself as an ADHDer) into their relationship.

A neurodiverse couple therapist can help *Reconsidering Couples* discuss their relationship expectations. Importantly, they can help each partner explore their own identity dimensionality in response to new diagnostic information and consider how this relates to couple identity. Will Toni choose to integrate acceptance of Mike's ADHD within their couple identity, or will ADHD be seen as an unwanted enemy?

The Cheerleader & Victim Partnership

This dynamic occurs when a ND partner has a negative relationship with their own brain combined with some degree of learned helplessness, low self-esteem, anxiety, and/or depression. Their chronic struggle to regulate their emotions exhausts their NT partner, who spends a lot of their own energy working to build them up and/or promote stability.

Cathy (NT):

"I love him, but I'm not sure how many more times I can say, 'It's going to be ok. You can do this.' It's terribly upsetting to hear him get so down on himself all the time. He needs to learn how to see himself more positively without my constant reassurance. I don't want to feel like I'm the only one keeping him from drowning. Also, if he's always drowning, when is there time to hear my needs?"

Colton (Autistic):

"It's an awful, guilty feeling knowing that I need so much help all the time from Cathy. I want to improve my self-esteem on my own, but it's hard not to fixate on all the problems I have due to my disability. My brain seems to sabotage all my efforts to improve myself, so I can't get ahead. I hate having Autism! I wish my brain was different. I'm thankful to my partner for being able to see me for more than my limitations. I don't know why I can't see myself like she does."

These partnerships usually benefit from extra assessment regarding depression, anxiety, trauma, self-harm, and substance use. If necessary, the therapist should refer the *Victim* partner to individual therapy, either as a break from neurodiverse couple therapy or concurrent with it. Therapy modalities that incorporate *Cognitive Behavior Therapy (CBT)* and/or *Dialectical Behavioral Therapy (DBT)* may be especially helpful to address shame spirals, anxiety attacks, persistent guilt, self-harm, trauma responses, or other concerns. The *Cheerleader* partner may also benefit from individual thearpy in order to privately discuss healthy boundaries.

If neurodiverse couple therapy is wise for *Cheerleader & Victim*, teaching about the various *stances* and *sentiments* used to describe one's relationship with their own brain may yield rich discussion. Psychoeducation about neurotypes, executive processing, sensory processing, self-regulation and assorted coping skills, codependency, and how to maintain healthy boundaries is essential.

The Frustrated Couple

There are times when a NT partner expresses chronic frustration about their ND partner's known brain issues, even sometimes claiming that their neurotype "dominates" their relationship. They typically lament about a lack of reciprocation from their ND partner, which is either perceived or actual, and usually express a desire for validation regarding the amount of personal sacrifice they've made over the course of the relationship to keep things afloat. The ND partner, meanwhile, tends to express a mix of gratitude for their partner's endurance and resentment. Their frustration is usually centered on the fact their genuine attempts to improve themselves and connect to their partner never seem successful.

Leslie (NT):

"His brain issues control our lives. At this point, what else can I do besides stay frustrated? I don't understand why we haven't been able to establish a normal sex life by now. I've already modified my sexual expectations – they can't get any lower – and he still can't meet them. Is it because he doesn't want to? It feels like I may never be satisfied in this relationship, and that scares me because it's against my religious beliefs to get divorced. Am I doomed to a life of sexual disatisfaction?"

Marcus (2e; Autistic and Gifted):

"I'm thankful for all you've done to try to understand my issues with sex. I've been trying really hard to understand your needs. I definitely don't want to be a burden on our relationship, but that's what it seems like you keep saying. You know I love you. I'm doing my best to be a loving partner. You keep telling me it's not good enough, though. I just don't know what else to do to improve our sex life. I'm not as frustrated as you are by the lack of sex . . .but I am frustrated that you're frustrated and that you can't see the ways I've been trying to make this better."

Depending on the source of each *Frustrated Couple's* distress, validating each client's concerns and providing psychoeducation on such topics as NT and ND differences, the Double Empathy Problem, healthy coping skills, and more can be important. The therapist can then help clients articulate their specific frustrations and unmet expectations. Skills-training in the area of executive functioning, communication, flexible problem-solving, and boundary-setting can be helpful. The couple can be coached to break down their *changeable* frustrations into manageable chunks and appropriately grieve the *unchangeable* frustrations.

Note that chronic frustration for some couples stem from a ND partner's undiagnosed or misunderstood Alexithymic qualities. Although it comes naturally to most non-traumatized NT persons within most sociocultural contexts to identify, interpret, label, and discuss their various body sensations, this is very difficult for Alexithymic persons. For example, most NT persons will easily notice the sensation of their own stomach growling and automatically label this as hunger. An Alexithymic person, however, may not truly feel their own stomach growl until it reaches quite a high degree of somatic signaling.

Similarly, interpersonal interactions may not automatically induce a readily identifiable somatic and / or emotional response for Alexithymic people. They often report a sense of feeling "neutral" most of the time. Their emotions tend to be difficult to label, and it may be difficult from them to differentiate between them. "I don't know how I feel" is a common answer to their NT partner's questions. As a result, NT partners of Alexithymic persons tend to describe feeling unfairly married to a "robotic," "clueless," "invalidating," and / or "emotionally-disconnected" person.

Slowing down to help Alexithymic clients learn ways to connect with the full scope of their internal experiences (and communicate about them with their partner) involves a great deal of patience and coaching in therapy.

Mindfulness techniques can help, but they should definitely not be used in a traditional way! Asking an Alexithymic client, for instance, to quiet their body and mind in order to tune into their internal sensations and emotions is typically unproductive. It's usually far more effective to encourage them to look for patterns in the way their heart, mind, and body respond within highly specific scenarios. Doing this work in vivo during sessions, in front of the NT partner, is important.

Connecting the dots between one's body sensations, thoughts, and feelings can be a slow but worthwhile process for Alexithymic persons that requires a lot of practice – and grace from their NT partner. Therapy that incorporates process comments, psychoeducation, scaffolding, and repetition is essential.

Therapist:	"I noticed you started rubbing the back of your neck as your conversation with your wife Cynthia got a bit heated just now. Can you describe how your neck feels at this moment?"
Alexithymic Client (AC):	"I don't know. I guess it feels tense?"
Therapist:	"Neck tension is a common indicator of stress. Are there other times in your life when your neck feels tense?"
AC:	"When I'm under pressure from my boss at work my neck can hurt enough to eventually motivate me to make a chiropractor appointment. Also, if Cynthia and I have been arguing a lot my neck will tense up."
Therapist:	"It seems like your neck gets tense in response to challenging interpersonal situations. This is probably a good indicator that you're feeling not only neck pain, but also some strong emotions. Connecting the dots between your neck tension and your emotions in those moments can help you navigate the interaction that's taking place.

Do any of the following emotion labels seem like they're the right fit? Could your neck tension during an argument with Cynthia be a signal you're feeling *nervous, frustrated, embarrassed, angry, sad,* or *overwhelmed?*" |
| AC: | "It probably means I'm feeling overwhelmed. I mean, really, when we're in an argument I just |

	want the conversation to be over as quickly as possible; I just want everything to be calm and good."
Therapist:	"Ok, so we've learned that your neck tension can equal the emotion of *overwhelm* – and this can be so intense that it makes you want to end a conversation. What can you do with this information? When you notice neck tension during a conversation, could you try asking for a break, agreeing on a time to come back to the issue later?"
AC:	"Sure. I mean, that sounds better than what usually happens. Usually, I walk away to organize my thoughts and stretch. Cynthia follows me around asking questions until I end up saying something hurtful or mean to get her to back off. She gets more upset, understandably."
Therapist:	"Can I suggest that learning how to tell your wife about your body sensations and feelings, as you start to notice them, may be quite meaningful? If you're consistent with practicing this, she's likely to start to trust that you'll share your thoughts and feelings on your own . . .without her having to chase after you.

Here's what this skill could look like . . .

1. Notice your neck tension.
2. Remember that your neck tension can indicate feeling *overwhelmed*.
3. Say out loud or write to Cynthia, 'I'm feeling too overwhelmed to talk right now. Can we stop now and try again after dinner?'

Does this seem reasonable?"

AC:	"Yes, I can try that."

Couples with Pursuer-Distancer and/or Parent-Child Dynamics

Just like NT partnerships, neurodiverse relationships can display well-known patterns previously described by counseling experts. In particular,

John Gottman's **Pursuer-Distancer pattern** and aspects of Eric Berne's **Transactional Analysis** contain helpful concepts to keep in mind during neurodiverse couple assessment.[1,2,3]

When a NT partner pursues their ND partner, who distances.
This dynamic frequently, but not always, involves a NT female who makes persistent attempts to connect to their ND male partner. As the ND partner withdraws, the NT partner feels highly rejected, abandoned, and confused – especially because the ND partner tends to poorly communicate their reason for distancing.

Identifying and discussing this couple dynamic often reveals that the ND partner's withdrawal tends to stem from physiological overload. Their withdrawal is an attempt to self-regulate – not reject their partner. Sometimes, but not always, it's also an attempt to avoid facing a hard truth (e.g., wanting to end the relationship but not wanting to hurt their partner's feelings, needing to admit a personal failure but feeling too ashamed to do so). Meanwhile, the NT partner's pursuing behavior tends to stem from their need for validation and understanding about what is really going on in the relationship. They may also fear abandonment.

When a ND partner pursues their NT partner, who distances.
This can occur if a ND partner emotionally smothers their NT partner due to general lack of awareness about healthy interpersonal boundaries, or perhaps because the NT partner and/or the relationship itself has become a hyperfixation. There is rarely any level of malicious intent involved in this type of pursuit. It's usually quite innocent, and may be addressed through psychoeducation about healthy relationship dynamics and coaching aimed at increasing <u>both</u> partners' interpersonal skills. Note that the NT partner in this situation generally withdraws in an attempt to set healthy boundaries. However, sometimes they actually do wish to end the relationship and are unsure how to do so without crushing the ND partner's feelings – which they perceive as fragile, intense, and/or underdeveloped.

Therapists unfamiliar with working with neurodiverse couples may be disillusioned to find that the traditional interventions used to address *Pursuer-Distancer* dynamics are frequently ineffective with this population. For example, unlike with most NT couples, simply encouraging a *Pursuing* partner to reduce interpersonal demand on their *Distancing* partner is not generally sufficient for the *Distancing* partner to feel safe enough to engage. A *Distancing* partner who is ND usually needs quite a bit of extra support and skill-building in the area of self-regulation in order to feel comfortable initiating interpersonal connection, if desired. A *Distancing* partner who is NT usually needs support sorting through their personal boundaries, needs, and expectations. Similarly, *Pursuing* partners of any neurotype in a neurodiverse relationship tend to need extra support to modify their interpersonal habits. Modeling by the therapist, providing opportunities for in vivo role-play regarding healthy versus unhealthy dynamics, and collaboratively analyzing enactments as they happen in session is vital.

When a NT partner parents their ND partner, who embodies a childlike role.
Sometimes NT partners in neurodiverse relationships express things like, "I want to be a wife, not a boss" or "my partner feels like another one of our kids." In these scenarios, the NT partner usually feels exhausted, unsupported, and resentful from having to bear the weight of their family's important tasks and decisions. They can also feel burdened by having to carry the bulk of the so-called emotional labor of their relationship.

By the time a couple with this dynamic enters therapy, interpersonal tension is typically high because of ongoing mutual frustration. The NT partner has often already expressed a critical need for their ND partner to improve their task initiation and follow through skills, and expressed anger and hurt that lasting change has not yet taken place in these areas. They also may have a habit of nagging, criticizing, or enabling. Meanwhile, the ND partner tends to feel micromanaged, undervalued, and helpless. They may also feel depressed. The combination of their own low self-esteem plus high interpersonal demand from their partner results in such "childlike" coping strategies as outright rebellion, self-sabotage, procrastination, deception, denial, projection, or avoidance.

Ironically, the very actions the NT partner craves from their ND partner may be the hardest for them to do. For example, challenges with task initiation and follow through are frequently hallmark characteristics of ADHD. Learning to acknowledge characteristics of each partner's neurotype can lead to a more grace-filled perspective on how *Parent-Child* dynamics emerge, what tends to trigger this, and how this may be resolved.

Fictional client Sita (NT) reports the following during an initial couple session with her husband Pavan (undiagnosed ADHD):

"Like clockwork, every few years Pavan is either let go from a job or he quits to go after something new. Even though he's starting to acknowledge how changing jobs so frequently is negatively impacting my feelings for him (not to mention our finances), he still can't seem to settle into one job for very long. I keep telling Pavan that this is unfair and unsustainable. I'd like to get an advanced degree to progress in my industry, but that just isn't possible when we keep having to drain our savings account to pay for living expenses while Pavan is unemployed. I don't want to keep paying for his next, best career experiment! I'm always nagging him to address this, but he keeps begging me to be more patient. My extended family doesn't understand why we're still married. They're extremely critical. It's to the point that it's uncomfortable to be around them lately. They expect Pavan, as a man, to do better. They keep reminding me that he's my husband, not my child. I'm starting to agree."

Pavan's response:

"Sita is the best wife I could ask for, and I love her very much. I'm driven to make her happy, but I just can't seem to do so regarding our finances. I've gotten excited about lots of career opportunities that could have panned out really well for us, but nothing has been successful so far. She expects good things to happen for us right away . . .just like both sets of our parents. The need for financial security and career achievement is ingrained in our culture, especially for men. There are definitely times I hide details related to our finances from Sita and the rest of the family because I don't want to admit I've taken another risk that didn't turn out well. Sometimes it just seems better to avoid talking about finances all together than to hear, again, that I'm a screw-up."

Here, Sita does not wish to be a parental figure in an intimate relationship where she bears the burden of maintaining financial security at the expense of her own professional goals. Although she does not want to micromanage her husband, she's unsure how else to proceed. His financial inconsistency is a valid threat. Pavan appears to feel trapped in a cycle of hoping for something great to happen in his career while denying the pattern of what is actually happening. He does not wish to embody a childlike role, yet cannot stop repeating impulsive and conflict-avoidant behavior.

If a neurodiverse couple therapist views this couple from a brain-based perspective, they may discover that Pavan has marked challenges with both self-regulation and executive functioning skills. As a result, he often faces negative interpersonal consequences. He uses defensive strategies to cope until impulsivity once again propels him towards risk-taking.

Pavan may be an ADHDer. It may help to discuss the characteristics of ADHD, the pros and cons of seeking a formal diagnosis (and whether or not to disclose this information to family members if so), and how to improve specific executive functioning skills. This couple could also benefit from discussing identity dimensionality, gender and cultural expectations, the difference between healthy and unhealthy coping skills, and how to set personal and interpersonal boundaries to promote an *Adult-Adult* dynamic.

When a ND partner parents their NT partner, who embodies a childlike role.
This usually occurs when a ND partner displays cognitive inflexibility, religious scrupulosity, micromanagement, or other characteristics the NT partner finds excessively logical and/or controlling. Sadly, it can also involve a ND partner's use of manipulative tactics to assert their own intellectual or spiritual superiority within the relationship. The NT partner tends to submit until they reach a point of extreme dissatisfaction, wherein they may start to rebel in passive-aggressive or "childlike" ways. While some NT partners in this scenario stay in the relationship and demand they work together toward a healthier interpersonal pattern, others may choose to leave the relationship altogether.

Consider the fictional couple below.

Brad (Autistic):

"I don't understand why managing finances has to be so difficult. I've made a spreadsheet and we meet once a week to talk about the numbers. Yet, Julia's spending still gets us off track each month. I hate nagging her about this so much, but I don't know what else to do. Does she really not understand the basics of cutting costs?"

Julia (NT):

"I resent so much of what Brad is saying right now. I'm a smart person who knows how to follow a budget. I'm not stupid. I don't overspend on purpose. The budget he created just isn't realistic! It's aspirational, not practical. I'm tired of feeling like a dumb teenager who is constantly being scolded for mismanaging her allowance. I've asked repeatedly for us to work on the budget itself together to improve it, and he refuses."

This couple is having difficulty connecting in an *Adult-to-Adult* manner to collaborate on sustainable, shared financial stewardship. The ND husband displays cognitive inflexibility that interferes with his ability to see the bigger picture. The NT wife's mounting resentment to this makes it unlikely for her to continue requesting change much longer. In time she may either give up on voicing her opinion, rebel in clear or passive-aggressive ways, or leave the relationship altogether.

A neurodiverse couple therapist can offer this couple psychoeducation regarding tendencies that may be associated with each partner's neurotype, as well to compare and contrast the qualities of an *Adult-Adult* dynamic versus a *Parent-Child* dynamic. Cognitive flexibility, mutual empathy and validation, and creative problem-solving skills can be modeled, coached, and practiced during couple sessions.

The Traumatized Partnership

Last, a specific type of intimate partnership dynamic deserves careful consideration. This interpersonal pattern fuels what has been termed the **Cassandra Phenomenon, Cassandra Affective Deprivation Disorder (CADD), Ongoing Traumatic Relationship Syndrome (OTRS),** or **Affective Deprivation Disorder (AfDD).**[4] Formerly called *Mirror Syndrome* and later renamed after a Greek myth in which a woman named Cassandra was given a gift no one believed, none of these named conditions has ever appeared in the *DSM*. Rather, they were designated by various professionals to give voice to certain NT females observed to suffer great distress when partnered with certain Autistic males.[5] Naming these conditions has been an attempt to summarize the psychological and somatic experiences these females attribute to chronic invalidation and insufficient emotional reciprocity within their relationship.[6] Criteria for these conditions varies, but does exist.[7]

Therapists should not presume that it's normative for every NT partner of a ND person to experience a *Traumatized Partnership*. However, they should know how to recognize the way this dynamic may present in some neurodiverse relationships. Therapists should also not assume that clients will recognize any of the above conditions by name because the American public is generally unfamiliar with such esoteric language. Note, though, that some self-advocates are familiar with these terms. They tend to dislike them and discourage their use, suggesting it's too risky to name these conditions due to the potential for therapists to overuse the labels and/or unfairly blame any ND partners who may be unknowingly perpetuating this dynamic.[8] While it is absolutely necessary to validate a NT partner's pain and identify relationship dysfunction, this cannot come at the price of their ND partner's miscategorization.

How can a BIC therapist appropriately assess this Traumatized Partnership?
If this dynamic is present, the NT partner tends to express that their relationship has become detrimental to their physical and mental health. They may report physical manifestations of emotional distress (e.g., headaches or other medical

problems) or negative changes to their eating and sleeping habits. Their symptoms may be more intense if they have a trauma history separate from the relationship and/or if their relationship recreates dysfunctional dynamics from childhood. A common theme is to describe feeling deeply neglected by their ND partner and dissatisfied in every aspect of their relationship's intimacy (e.g., spiritual, sexual, emotional, etc.). Meanwhile, the ND partner in this scenario usually reports a lack of insight about how to change the situation and no intentional malice regarding how it came about – that is, unless they have concurrent Narcissism.

A therapist should validate the NT partner's hurt while suggesting healthy self-care and boundary options, especially if they're experiencing clinical depression. Any codependent tendencies should be addressed. Importantly, and without minimizing the NT partner's experience, they should also assess the ND partner's underlying intentions and ability to use effective interpersonal skills. This is because it's critically important for the therapist to discern whether or not the NT partner's needs are being *knowingly* and/or *deliberately* dismissed. Keep in mind that it is quite tempting to presume a ND partner is aware of the relationship's dysfunction and either refusing to change or choosing to victimize their NT partner: It's easy for sympathy (and bias) to readily flow towards the NT partner given their level of distress. However, most ND partners in neurodiverse relationships do <u>not</u> mean harm. They don't wish to bring emotional dysregulation, cognitive inflexibility, social misunderstandings, executive functioning challenges, or other struggles into their relationship any more than NT partners wish to be barraged by these challenges!

Some ND partners who find themselves stuck in this dynamic can feel every bit as hopeless and helpless as their NT partner, yet there are no named syndromes for their feelings of chronic shame and inadequacy. Almost all ND partners crave emotional reciprocity and mutual respect within their relationship. Despite their longing for connection, though, they may have significant difficulty using the kinds of communication skills and self-regulation strategies required to foster it. They may struggle to demonstrate physical affection despite their high level of sexual attraction to their NT partner.

Because sometimes the ND partner in a *Traumatized Partnership* wants their toxic relationship patterns to change just as much as their NT partner does, both partners may report previous (unsuccessful) attempts to make changes. There may not be any malice behind either partner's actions and reactions to each other, but rather a great degree of misunderstanding back and forth that has gone on for a very long time.

Consider the nuances in the assessment process involved with properly conceptualizing the following two fictional stories that both have the same basic premise, with one important key difference: Narcissism.

A Traumatized Partnership <u>without</u> Narcissism

This is Sandra and Val's third attempt at marriage counseling, but their first time seeing a neurodiverse couple therapist. "What will be different this time?" they wonder.

Sandra (NT) reports years of emotional and sexual dissatisfaction in her marriage to Val (suspected ND). She feels her most intimate needs remain unmet despite attempts to scream her needs out loud, calmly discuss the changes she'd like to see, or even write things down. She says past relationship therapy hasn't mentioned Autism as a potential factor in their dynamic at all, but that she firmly believes her husband may be Autistic.

Sandra cries as she explains how unattractive and deeply rejected she feels. She laments that she's developed strong headaches and insomnia due to the degree of emotional and sexual disconnection she's suffered in their relationship over the years. At this point, she's made it clear to Val that she's considering divorce.

Val reports ongoing frustration, sadness, and shame regarding his marriage to Sandra. He says that no matter what he tries, his genuine efforts to connect (both sexually and nonsexually) end up failing. Val states he puts a lot of energy towards trying to understand and meet Sandra's needs by reading books about the differences between men and women, going to individual therapy, and even seeking out guidance about how to be a better husband from an older mentor at their church. He admits, though, that any positive behavior changes he makes as a result of these efforts tend to fizzle out after a while unless he has appropriate accountability. This makes him embarrassed and defensive. He also admits he shuts down emotionally and withdraws whenever he feels criticized by Sandra.

Val wonders if the kindest thing to do would be to get a divorce, despite the fact he really wants their marriage to work out. He says he's willing to explore whether or not he's Autistic if answering Sandra's lingering question could promote mutual understanding about their situation.

A Traumatized Partnership <u>with</u> Narcissism

This is Sandra and Val's third attempt at marriage counseling, but the first with a neurodiverse couple therapist. "What will be different this time?" they wonder.

Sandra (NT) reports years of emotional and sexual dissatisfaction in her marriage to Val (suspected ND with co-occurring Narcissism). She feels her most intimate needs remain unmet despite attempts to scream her needs out loud, calmly discuss the changes she'd like to see, or even write things down. She firmly believes her husband may be Autistic, but states that he refuses to consider this possibility. She says past couple therapy hasn't mentioned Autism or anything else as a potential factor in their relationship dynamics. "My individual therapist thinks Val may be a Narcissist just like my mother," she says.

Sandra notes on her Intake Form, "Val only cares about doing what serves Val. He's chronically self-centered and cannot handle my feedback. My needs just don't matter to him, not even my medical issues. He never listens and never changes. Because of this relationship, I've developed strong headaches and insomnia that I'm left to deal with all on my own. Past therapy hasn't made a lasting difference because Val performs for the therapist by temporarily love-bombing me before returning to his baseline behaviors when therapy ends."

Sandra cries as she explains how unattractive and deeply rejected she feels. She makes it clear to Val that she is considering a divorce. Meanwhile, Val reports anger and contempt regarding their situation. He states he's a good person who's given them both a good life together, and that he doesn't understand why she expects so much from him all the time. Val accuses Sandra of having unrealistic standards for marriage that neither he, nor anyone else, could ever possibly meet. Additionally, he says he finds her presumption that he may be Autistic an insult, pointing out his many major life achievements to justify that he's NT. "I'm not a Narcissist, either, Sandra. Maybe you're the one who's mentally ill," he tells her.

Val asserts he deserves happiness. He wonders if the most efficient thing for them to do is to give up on the marriage so they can stop wasting each other's time going around in circles.

Sandra experiences some form of *Cassandra Phenomenon*, *CADD*, *OTRS*, or *AfDD* in both scenarios. Although there's no specific named condition for this yet, the first Val experiences a unique form of mild depression that may be a potential counterpart to this. He has a behavioral history of sincere attempts towards personal and relationship growth, while the other Val does not. Remember, though, that both versions of these characters deserve the therapist's validation regarding their expressed feelings: The therapist should join every client and promote individual safety and wellbeing without displaying favoritism.

In any *Traumatized Partnership*, clients should be invited to prioritize their own self-care and healthy boundaries. Toxic behaviors that fuel the unhealthy dynamic (e.g., gaslighting, enabling) should be immediately addressed.

Clients alone decide how to engage with the therapy process, and each other. For either version of Val, this will include deciding whether or not to pursue a formal Autism evaluation. The therapist should discuss the pros and cons of this. Psychoeducation may help discourage any incorrect conflation of Autism with low achievement or mental illness. Similarly, the therapist must carefully assess whether or not Narcissism, which is distinct from Autism, is present.

Glossary of Bolded Terms

Cassandra Phenomenon, Cassandra Affective Deprivation Disorder (CADD), Ongoing Traumatic Relationship Syndrome (OTRS), or Affective Deprivation Disorder (AfDD)   These conditions describe the negative emotional and somatic experience of certain NT persons intimately paired with certain Autistic persons.

Pursuer-Distancer Pattern   A relationship pattern involving one partner who craves closeness while the other simultaneously craves space. It was first discussed by Thomas F. Fogarty in the late 1970s and has since been widely adapted by various therapy modalities.

Transactional Analysis   A psychoanalytic theory and therapy technique developed by Eric Berne during the 1950s that defines the social interactions between two people according to whether each party operates from their own *Child*, *Parent*, or *Adult* ego state.

Notes

1 Gottman, J. M. (1999). *The marriage clinic: A scientifically-based marital therapy*. WW Norton & Company.
2 Berne, E. (1996). Principles of transactional analysis. *Indian Journal of Psychiatry*, *38*(3), 154.
3 Harris, T. A. (2012). *I'm OK, you're OK*. Random House.
4 Aston, M. (2009). *The Asperger couple's workbook: Practical advice and activities for couples and counsellors*. London: Jessica Kingsley.
5 Arad, P., Shechtman, Z., & Attwood, T. (2021). Physical and mental well-being of women in neurodiverse relationships: A comparative study. *Journal of Psychology & Psychotherapy*, *12*(1).
6 Bostock-Ling, J. (2016). *Life Satisfaction of Neurotypical Women in Intimate Relationship with a Partner Who Has Asperger's Syndrome: An Exploratory Study* (Doctoral dissertation).
7 Simons, H. F., & Thompson, J. R. (2009). Affective deprivation disorder: Does it constitute a relational disorder. *Affective Deprivation Disorder*.
8 Yergeau, M. (2020). Cassandra isn't doing the robot: On risky rhetorics and contagious autism. *Rhetoric Society Quarterly*, *50*(3), 212–221.

Therapy Interventions for 8
Neurodiverse Couples

It's unfortunate that much of the information currently in circulation regarding neurodiverse couples seems to focus on quantifying their problems rather than proposing solutions. When solutions are proposed, only certain couple presentations tend to be highlighted (e.g., NT females partnered with Autistic males). Clients who like to dive into scholarly research may even come across the research-based suggestion that ND persons may be most satisfied in relationships with other ND persons.[1] This can be discouraging, as there are simply too few studies highlighting aspects of healthy neurodiverse relationships and too few relationship books written from an inclusive perspective for clients to arrive at therapy with a clear picture of what success could look like. There's also, of course, too little positive neurodiverse couple representation in the media.

For these reasons, it's important that neurodiverse couple therapists cast vision for their clients whenever safe and realistic to do so. Therapists have the opportunity to convey what society does not – it's entirely possible for neurologically diverse partners to learn how to flourish in a relationship together. Chronic relationship disappointment doesn't have to be an inevitability for partners of different neurotypes! Without providing false hope or unethical guarantees, therapists should seek to convey the same level of hope to neurodiverse couples as they would NT couples. Relationship satisfaction may be possible if both partners commit to an ongoing process of personal introspection and accountability, healthy boundary-setting, assertive communication, flexible problem-solving, and mutual respect throughout the therapy process and beyond.

DOI: 10.4324/9781003351337-12

This chapter introduces customizable relationship tools that encourage personal growth and skill-building from both partners, not just the ND partner. Some interventions are original to the author, while others build upon existing practices within the field of Marriage & Family Therapy to increase their inclusivity. Note that most empirically validated therapy methods in use today have been created from a NT perspective and also studied using NT participants. There's an urgent need to research how these interventions impact neurodiverse couples. Within existing data on this topic, sample sizes are often comically small. For example, a 2021 study found that 12 sessions of *Solution-Focused Brief Therapy* resulted in increased communication and emotional awareness for the <u>one</u> neurodiverse couple it studied.[2]

What distinguishes the types of couple therapy interventions a BIC practitioner uses from those of a traditional therapist?
This distinction actually sometimes has very little to do with the type of intervention in and of itself. Rather, what matters most is the environment of care in which the intervention takes place and the perspective through which the intervention is applied. For instance, consider one of the most basic forms of therapeutic intervention, the act of asking thought-provoking questions.

A traditional couple therapist may use phrases like:

- "How does that make you feel, emotionally?"
- "What thoughts just flashed through your mind when that happened?"
- "How would you describe the problems that brought you to therapy?"

A BIC therapist, by contrast, may have a distinctive twist to similar questions. This twist leaves more room for interoceptive processing differences and communication preferences.

- "Are you aware of any emotional reaction you may be having right now?"
- "When that just happened, did you notice your brain or body responding in any particular way?"
- "On your own terms, how would you describe the problems that brought you to therapy?"*

*There should be no expectation for an ND client to communicate verbally or provide eye contact. A white board should be provided for any client who prefers to write down or draw out their thoughts.

Furthermore, BIC provides a lot more **scaffolding** than traditional therapy when teaching interpersonal skills each session to ensure the clients are well-equipped prior to ever being asked to practice at home. This is not because neurodiverse couples are more developmentally immature or any less capable, though. It's simply because BIC therapists are more attuned to the executive functioning challenges or other brain-based issues ND clients tend to experience, and understand the benefits of providing structured support. Thoughtful scaffolding opportunities empower clients, not enable or infantize them.

Fictional couple Jorge and Juana state they've been to several therapists over the past year to try to improve their relationship. However, they report they usually attend only a few sessions before getting frustrated and giving up.

Jorge (2e; Autistic and Gifted):

"We just can't find the right fit for a therapist. Either they expect us to do too much homework on our own between sessions, or they don't give us anything specific to work on at home."

Juana (NT):

"Jorge is being a bit too picky, but I do agree that we haven't found a therapist who understands how best to help us yet. One counselor even seemed confused by our relationship altogether. For example, we want to do therapy homework . . . but we can only handle so much on our own."

This couple's persistence toward relationship growth is commendable. They're continuing to try to find a therapist who understands and who recognizes the executive functioning and emotion regulation challenges involved in their dynamic.

A neurodiverse couple therapist can explore whether or not past therapy homework has involved too many steps, was too abstract, required too much cognitive flexibility or planning to implement, or perhaps involved topics too intense to address without a therapist present. It's also possible past homework relied on the clients to apply interpersonal skills they had not yet learned.

The clients' expectations also deserve attention. Do they view a therapist as an elite, inflexible teacher (and themselves as subordinate students) versus an active collaborator? If so, a BIC therapist can invite them to consider entering into a therapeutic alliance that welcomes feedback. Together, a "just-right" homework assignment can be determined on a session-to-session basis. Ideally, this will take into account each partner's current ability to regulate their emotions and access their executive functioning skills. Homework can be broken down into manageable chunks determined by the clients' reality, not the therapist's assumptions.

Another important distinction of the BIC approach is its clear establishment – from the very start of therapy – of the type of service set to unfold. Neurodiverse couples usually benefit from a very high level of specificity, so it's essential to converse with every new couple about what kind of therapy seems most appropriate to their needs. Of course, this can be re-evaluated at any time.

The vast majority of couple therapy falls into three categories:

1. Relationship-Building Therapy.
2. Relationship Clarity-Seeking Therapy.
3. Relationship-Closing Therapy.

Relationship-Building Therapy

Relationship-Building Therapy is appropriate for neurodiverse partnerships in which each client is committed to relationship improvement, at least to some degree. (Their degree of commitment can vary.) It explores each partner's brain-based strengths and growth areas, noting how they contribute to relationship satisfaction or dissatisfaction.

Here, the therapist's role is to help clients create a shared definition for relationship success and determine what may be required from each partner to achieve and maintain this vision. Are these requirements realistic and sustainable? Do they honor each partner's innate personhood, values, needs, and life goals?

The therapist provides psychoeducation, supports the processing of hurts and dilemmas, teaches healthy boundaries, nurtures individual and couple identity formation, and offers guided practice with a wide variety of both self-regulatory techniques and interpersonal skills.

The *Relationship Mission Statement* Exercise

Step 1: Draft an initial *Relationship Mission Statement*

This is a brief saying that a couple creates to quickly capture their primary relationship goals. It should be easy to remember. Although memorizing this saying is certainly not required, doing so may help couples maintain focus and motivation throughout their time in therapy and beyond.

"Our marriage will honor God and each other."

Step 2: Get more specific

Add the phrase as evidenced by to make the goals measurable.

"Our marriage will honor God and each other, as evidenced by attending church regularly and talking through our problems together using respectful language."

Relationship Clarity-Seeking Therapy

This version of neurodiverse couple therapy seeks to make complicated relationship situations easier for clients to comprehend. During *Relationship Clarity-Seeking Therapy*, the therapist's role is to promote each client's individual wellness while they explore the current state of their relationship in order to discern its direction.

Here, the therapist provides an unbiased space where partners can discuss their concerns and learn the specific interpersonal skills needed to keep these discussions mutually respectful and productive. The therapist tends to focus on each partner's self-care strategies, self-regulation skills, and communication skills. Psychoeducation about brain differences and other topics is provided throughout.

Relationship Clarity-Seeking Therapy may be desirable in the following situations, among others:

- When a couple is deciding whether or not to get engaged, live together, get married, break up, have a biological child, adopt, take a job overseas, etc.
- When a couple is trying to determine how to proceed together (or apart) after an affair or other betrayal.
- When a couple is navigating a significant sexual desire discrepancy, unresolved conflict, neurological differences, spiritual disagreements,

a family life cycle transition, sudden onset of Disability, parenting stress, etc.

- When both partners disagree on the direction they'd like their relationship to take.

The *Relationship Clarity Statement* Exercise

Step 1: Draft an initial *Relationship Clarity Statement*

This is a brief statement clients create together in order to identify what they'd like to clarify throughout the process of couple therapy. This can make nebulous, intense, and/or complex issues seem more manageable. Memorization is not required. It can be helpful, though, to refer back to this statement from time to time as therapy continues.

"We want to understand whether we're better off together or apart. This means deciding if certain facts about ourselves and dynamics between us are deal breakers."

Step 2: Get more specific

Add phrases like <u>we will do this by</u> and <u>such as</u>, along with necessary details.

"We want to understand whether or not we're better together or apart. <u>We will do this by</u> talking through both scenarios. <u>We will also do this by</u> discussing what may or may not be deal breakers, <u>such as</u>: Partner A's inconsistent recovery efforts from gambling addiction, Partner B's low sex drive and tendency to shut down emotionally, both partners' difficulty with financial management, and Partner A's brain-based challenges due to ADHD."

Relationship-Closing Therapy

Most often, *Relationship-Closing Therapy* supports clients as they transition away from being intimate partners and toward being respectful co-parents due to separation or divorce. It's also appropriate when a couple (with or without children) seeks professional support after deciding to dissolve their dating relationship or engagement.

Here, the therapist provides psychoeducation, teaches each partner healthy coping skills for grief and other strong feelings, and encourages new boundaries. They also teach the specific interpersonal skills needed to keep discussions mutually respectful, with a special emphasis on emotional self-regulation.

The *Relationship Closure Statement* Exercise

Step 1: Draft an initial *Relationship Closure Statement*

Clients create this brief statement in order to recognize the ending of their relationship as well as the beginning of their new, separate lives. It reminds them that their stated goal is to gain closure and learn ways to be healthy, independent individuals – not to build intimacy. Memorizing the *Relationship Closure Statement* is not required. It can be helpful, though, to refer back to this statement from time to time as therapy continues.

"We want to learn how to be healthy co-parents instead of husband and wife. We each, separately, commit to prioritize both our individual mental health and our children's needs."

Step 2: Get more specific

Add the phrase <u>as evidenced by</u> to make the goals measurable.

"We want to learn how to be healthy co-parents instead of husband and wife, <u>as evidenced by</u> solving future parenting disagreements in a calm, timely manner. We each, separately, commit to prioritize both our individual mental health and our children's needs <u>as evidenced by</u> learning better self-regulation and communication skills."

What specific interventions tend to benefit neurodiverse couples?
Providing psychoeducation, using key reframes, applying CBT, teaching self-regulation and interpersonal skills, and encouraging couple identity work all tend to be impactful for neurodiverse couples.

Psychoeducation

- Refer to charts in this book and other resources to teach clients about executive functioning, neurotypes, the eight sensory systems, and the differences between ND and NT brains.
- Explain the role of each partner's amygdala, hippocampus, and prefrontal cortex during their interpersonal interactions.

- Discuss the pros and cons of diagnosing neurodivergence, as well as the difference between diagnosis and disclosure.
- Explain the difference between *changeable* versus *unchangeable* factors, on both a personal and interpersonal level. Some of each partner's individual characteristics may be flexible, while others are permanent. Accordingly, some couple dynamics may be flexible whereas others are not. Each person can only control that which is actually *changeable* within themselves – and only to the degree they desire change and have the capacity to move toward it.

There are three distinct concepts involved with this teaching:

1. Neurological permanence.
2. Desire for change.
3. Capacity for change.

First, whether or not certain changes are possible depends, at least in part, on each partner's areas of *neurological permanence*. It's important that each partner's permanent characteristics are identified and accepted (e.g., an Autistic person will never <u>not</u> be Autistic) in order to develop realistic expectations. This is frequently a process that involves identity work and sometimes even grief work.

Second, partners must recognize that they each might have a different level of *desire for change*. Everyone has the right to choose whether or not they'd like to try to improve upon that which may be flexible about themselves or their relationship. Change should never be pressured by a therapist, coerced by one's partner, or otherwise dictated.

Finally, each partner's *capacity for change* is a crucial consideration that cannot be overlooked. It's entirely possible, and quite common, for someone to *desire* to improve something *changeable* about themselves yet lack the physical energy and/or emotional capacity to move toward growth.

Consider the following fictional example.

Lexie (ADHD):

"I swear, my time management skills are going to change for the better. I'm going to hire a therapist to help me stay organized and follow through with things. I'm tired of struggling at work, and I'm tired of arguing with you at home. I really want to grow this part of myself and I know I need help to make that happen. I promise this time will be different."

Myles (NT):

"I'm thankful that you're taking this seriously. We'd argue less, for sure, if this improved, and I can see how it would help you at work. I've wanted this to change for years."

Presuming Lexie's existing time management skills aren't neurologically permanent (e.g., brain damage or inborn challenges), it's likely she'll respond well to executive functioning coaching during therapy because of her expressed *desire* for change . . . but only if she has the physical energy and/or emotional *capacity* for therapy. Too often, capacity isn't properly considered – not only do ND persons tend to have difficulty assessing and/or communicating about their own fluctuating energy level, NT persons tend to presume ND persons have (or should have) more energy at any given time than what they actually do! This is a frequently misunderstood topic amongst neurodiverse partners.

It's important to clarify *capacity* so that clients do not disappoint themselves and each other unecessarily, which often perpetuates dysfunctional relationship patterns. For persons of any neurotype, one's *capacity* to learn decreases in response to overwhelming feelings, interpersonal demand, perfectionism, physical illness, fear of failure, mental or physical exhaustion, or any number of other reasons. In this example, Lexie will only be able to deliver on her promise to herself and Myles if she, together with her therapist, commits to a realistic, ongoing assessment of her energy level throughout the course of therapy.

Given her strong *desire* for change, if Lexie experiences reduced *capacity* for growth at any point during the course of therapy it will probably be a perfectly logical response to life events or physiological factors. The therapist could easily offer support, structuring learning opportunities accordingly to keep things moving forward at an appropriate pace. Sometimes a temporary pause for therapy is needed. If so, the therapist can help keep the situation in proper perspective. To lose perspective regarding *capacity* is a recipe for relational disaster! This is because negative assumptions between partners are common; people tend to assume the worst. If Lexie truly needs to take a break from therapy but neither the therapist nor Myles properly understands that it's actually her *capacity* that is low versus her *desire* for change, they may view this as yet another disappointing example of her chronic lack of follow-through. While it's ok to feel disappointed, it's unfair to say Lexie broke her promise.

Key Reframes

Over time, neurodiverse partners can have increased difficulty relating to one another and solving their relationship problems due to their different "ways of being." They are, after all, living in two very different sensory planes of Earth's multiverse – all the while expecting each other to be able to consistently acknowledge needs, feelings, experiences, and expectations.

Consider the following reframes to provide neurodiverse couples specialized support, <u>when appropriate</u> to their situation. These reframes do not apply to abusive or otherwise unsafe dynamics.

Reframe couple therapy as an opportunity to learn how each partner's neurology plays a role in both their relationship problems and solutions.
When it comes down to it, most relationship partners come to therapy expecting to detail their own pain, receive validation, learn how to cope, and decide how best to move forward in life . . . together or apart. These expectations are not necessarily selfish, nor are they inherently wrong. However, what if clients were invited to expand their scope to include learning about their own brain and that of their partner?

Reframe a neurodiverse couples' presenting problems as stemming from brain-based differences, unrealistic expectations for themselves and each other, and underdeveloped interpersonal skills.
This is often an essential reconceptualization. Highly stressed couples, in particular, may have many negative assumptions about themselves and each other that fuel their dysfunction. For instance, they may view their relationship problems as stemming from intentional malice or a profound defect of character in their partner.

Reframe ignorance of brain wiring complexity prior to this point as understandable, and perhaps even protective.
Learning about neurological variability may have been too complex, too tiring, or too completely foreign of a journey to engage with until now.

Perhaps, too, there simply weren't resources available to do so. In some situations, denial may have been the only coping mechanism available to match one or both partner's overwhelm.

If a couple has had multiple failed therapy attempts in the past, offer the reframe that this indicates their keen determination to grow.
Some neurodiverse couples have had years of past therapy attempts and other unsuccessful efforts to understand themselves and their relationship. They tend to express grief and/or frustration regarding the time, energy, and money wasted prior to finally receiving effective support through BIC. It's important to acknowledge the cost that has accrued while also providing positive feedback about their persistence.

Reframe the problematic formulas for relationship success that almost all couples have subconsciously internalized.
Healthy relationships don't involve each partner giving an equal 50% toward relationship success. Nor do they involve each partner giving 100% of themselves all the time. Rather, healthy neurodiverse relationships acknowledge that it's normal for the "percentage" each partner has to give of themselves toward relationship success to fluctuate on a daily basis. (Remember the notion of *capacity?*)

How much a person has to give at any point directly relates to two things:

1. What's going on in their *internal climate*.
2. What's going on in their *external climate*.

Table 8.1

Internal Climate	External Climate
Level of hunger or thirst.	External sensory stimuli.
Physical energy level.	The U.S. economy.
Degree of physical pain or discomfort, inclusive of chronic or episodic conditions.	Office politics.
Thought processes (e.g., rumination, toxic positivity, etc.)	Immediate and/or extended family dynamics
Emotional intensity or numbness.	The weather.

(*Continued*)

Table 8.1 (Continued)

Internal Climate	External Climate
Stress level and corresponding somatic experiences.	Rules and regulations (e.g., work requirements, taxes, etc.).
Quality of sleep	Holidays and anniversaries.
Personal motivations.	How a favorite sport team is performing.
Brain-based concerns (e.g., ability to focus, sensory security).	Local and global news.
Low self-esteem or other personal hangups.	Interpersonal demands from one's partner.
Spiritual concerns.	Daily scheduling issues.

All clients can benefit from learning how to better identify and articulate what is going on in their own *internal* and *external* climate. Some of this will be within their control, whereas some will be totally outside their control. Some of this will relate to their partner and/or the relationship . . . and some will have nothing to do with it! Sharing this data back and forth (nullifying the tendency toward negative assumptions and mind-reading) can help partners feel more connected, and perhaps even more willing to collaborate.

The Same Situation, Two Ways

Partner A: "You've been acting really distant today. Do you even want to go on this date night tonight with me? I feel like it's not important to you at all."

Partner B: "Why do you always question my intentions? I said I would go out tonight, so I'm going. Can't you understand that work was just really stressful today? It's tax season."

In this situation, partners do not practice the skill of identifying and communicating about their *internal* and *external* climate. What would happen if they did?

Partner B: "Just a heads up that I'm operating at 40% capacity right now because work was super stressful today. Tax season has hit me really hard. I've had a headache today, too. I can try my best to give you all of the 40% I have to offer

> tonight on our date . . . but please understand why I may seem a bit off."
>
> Partner A: "Thanks for letting me know. It was starting to feel like going out with me tonight wasn't important to you. Actually, I've felt like you've been acting really cold and distant this week in general and I haven't been sure why. To me, it would be disappointing to have to reschedule tonight's date completely. I had a great day at work and I'm at 100%, so I can be flexible about what we do on the date, if that helps."
>
> Partner B: "I'm sorry for being distant without any explanation. I'll try to tell you sooner next time about what's going on. Thanks for understanding and offering to be flexible. Can we stay home and watch a movie for our date night instead of going out? You can pick the movie."
>
> Communicating about *capacity* and climate increases the likelihood of being understood, as well as finding creative ways to connect within each other's expressed limits

Reframe the path to personal growth.
Persons of any neurotype, but perhaps especially NT persons, often believe that "getting out of your comfort zone" is the one and only path to personal growth. However, this could not be farther from the truth for many ND people.

Brain-based research plus anecdotal evidence indicates that ND persons tend to grow best when allowed to safely experiment with change from a secure base. This base is distinct to each individual's needs, but is usually rooted in sensory security. Getting too far away from one's physiological comfort zone can lead to psychological and physiological distress (and corresponding defensiveness) versus positive change.

Every client deserves appropriate support to take incremental, and often non-linear, steps toward the changes they want.

Reframe what it means to "just do" a task.
From the perspective of most NT minds, the completion of any task follows the same simple formula: Action results from one's choice to match their behavior to an internal value (e.g., being on time is important to me, so I will get to work on time). One's neurologically-based ability to do the task without support, as well as sufficient emotional and physical *capacity*, is presumed!

Mathematically, this formula would be:

Behavior = Value

By this logic, when a person <u>doesn't</u> do a task, it means they must not value the task itself or some related factor (e.g., "My ND partner can't seem to show up on time to work, so that means she must not value her job or my opinion about her lateness.").

If Behavior = 0, then Value = 0

Sadly, this completely disregards an important truth. There are many reasons why it can be difficult to make it to work on time, particularly for a ND person, that have nothing to do with how much someone values their job . . . or their partner's opinion!

The ableist Behavior = Value formula is highly problematic. For one, the neurological ability to start a task and see it through to completion involves complex biological considerations and contextual factors. (Remember, task initiation is a key executive functioning skill of the prefrontal cortex.) One's strengths and challenges in executive functioning, degree of cognitive flexibility, level of resilience, access to resources, and connection to social support are all essential components of "just doing" a task. Most NT perspectives take for granted or invalidate these components.

It's unfair to focus on whether or not the entirety of a task is done or not without understanding this complexity. It's especially unfair to go on to make negative judgments and spiral into extrapolation about what this may mean about a person's character.

NT partner:

"My ND spouse can't seem to show up on time to work consistently, so that means she must not value her job. I've talked to her so many times about how this affects me negatively. Nothing changes, so she must not value my opinion either."

What if we used the following mathematical formula instead?

Behavior = Neurology x Capacity x Support

Here, the presence of favorable internal values is assumed! This allows broader consideration for the way one's neurology, *capacity*, and access to support can either enable or prevent task completion.

If Behavior = 0, then either Neurology, Support, or Context = 0

If a person <u>doesn't</u> complete a task this does not necessarily mean they don't value the task itself, what the task represents, or a partner's opinion. Sometimes, of course, it does, but not always! It's better for a therapist to offer clients the benefit of the doubt, modeling grace, as they keep discussions complex.

Many ND persons are actually trying very hard to demonstrate their values behaviorally, honor their partner's opinions, and meet their own personal goals for the betterment of themselves and their relationship.
ND partner:

"I value my job and I understand that lateness bothers my spouse. I try my best to get to work on time, but this is very hard for me. Even though I've learned to set two different alarms so I can wake up early and I also take a shower at night to save time in the morning, sometimes it's still difficult to get myself moving first thing in the morning. This is especially hard when my arthritis flares. Usually, though, what happens is that I get distracted. This makes it take longer to do all the steps involved with getting out the door. It's so much easier when my husband and I's schedules match up and we're able to leave for work around the same time together – getting ready side-by-side keeps me focused."

Moving away from the problematic Behavior = Value equation toward the Behavior = Neurology x Capacity x Support equation can reduce ableism and resentment in a neurodiverse relationship. It may even promote grace and creative problem-solving.

Reframe relationship health as a mix of proactive coping plus post-conflict recovery.
Measuring the health of a relationship by merely the presence or absence of conflict is not realistic. Some degree of conflict between partners (within acceptable limits) is inevitable and actually healthy!

Neurodiverse couples who learn ways to anticipate some of their most predictable challenges together, and also how to navigate unexpected ones, tend to report a sense of pride in their resilience. Therapy can teach each partner how to proactively identify their own triggers for dysregulation. They can then plan ways to cope and set boundaries. This helps a couple grow through their challenges and promotes faster and faster recovery when conflicts occur.

When clients' learned skills for proactive coping and post-conflict recovery understandably go out the window from time to time, especially during the beginning of therapy, the therapist can help them process their experience. If there were no deal-breaking boundary crossings, partners can learn what it takes to refocus on their self-regulation and relationship recovery efforts. These events can be incredible teachable moments.

Reframe relational teamwork.
Modern American social norms tend to condition couples to envision themselves as equal teammates engaged in a tug-of-war match against

an opposing team. Their shared goal is to win, of course, by both pulling together on the same side of the rope. What happens, though, when they don't pull at the same time or with the same force? Although the so-called stronger partner in this metaphor generally tolerates pulling more than their fair share from time to time, this kind of burden is not sustainable for too long or too often. Enter traditional relationship advice, which tends to help couples set boundaries regarding the equal distribution of effort, encouraging the so-called weaker partner to pull their own weight and the stronger partner to set boundaries so as not to pull too much weight. But, is this model helpful for neurodiverse couples?

The answer is usually no! For many, actually, the above conceptualization and its corresponding relationship advice is doomed to fail. While there's nothing wrong with encouraging healthy boundaries, fixating on the idea of fairness can be problematic. Instead, it's usually more important for neurodiverse couples to learn how to sustain flexibility regarding anything short of an uncrossable boundary. This is because partners tend to have very different skill sets, very different areas of neurological permanence, very different emotional and physical *capacities*, and very different support needs. "Pulling one's own weight" in a relationship can look quite different for each partner and vary from time to time. Sometimes this may even deviate significantly from dominant social norms or typical relationship expectations, while still being healthy.

All couples, but especially neurodiverse couples, can benefit from reenvisioning teamwork according to their individual characteristics, fluctuating abilities, energy levels, and variable needs. Instead of picturing each other sharing the same side of the rope(and pulling with equal strength) during a game of tug-of-war, it's better to envision each partner embodying one of any number the following positions.

- One partner securely hugging the other from behind to help anchor their feet to the ground, assisting them to pull the rope without falling.
- One partner pulling on the rope alone while the other cheers from the sidelines.
- Both partners pulling on the rope with different degrees of strength.

A second, entirely different visualization presents two neurodiverse teammates engaged in a track and field relay race. If the NT partner excels in task initiation, for example, while this represents a tough challenge for their ND partner, perhaps they can voluntarily get certain tasks started before passing the baton to their ND partner to complete. (This is not enabling or infantizing. It's teamwork!) This may be as simple as a NT partner printing out the right contact information the ND partner needs to schedule a home repair, which can eliminate some executive functioning fatigue. The ND partner can then take this baton and run with it to complete the task. If both persons can see themselves as respectful teammates in this example without becoming either parental or childlike, they can win the race (i.e., the task will get done, their relationship can thrive).

Whether or not this strategy is effective depends on the clients' various role and relationship expectations and if past hurts have been appropriately expressed and explored. Many neurodiverse couples do enjoy the relay race versus tug-of-war conceptualization of teamwork, though, provided that both partners agree to pass and carry the baton respectfully.

Naturally, a NT partner may crave a break from taking the lead regarding executive functioning considerations (e.g., task initiation, planning, organization) at times. If they can effectively communicate this need, perhaps their ND partner can find a way to tap into their energy reserves and/or obtain outside support to temporarily switch roles to provide relief. Flexible teammates know that occasionally switching positions is necessary, loving, and smart.

Reframe some ND traits traditionally considered to be deficits without resorting to toxic positivity or other forms of invalidation.
Asking the NT partner questions like, "Are there any ways your partner's ND hyperfocus benefits you as a person, or the relationship itself?" can be thought-provoking. This should not minimize a NT's concerns, of course. Rather, it should offer an expanded perspective. Potential ND traits to reframe may be:

- Literal thinking.
- Impulsivity/spontaneity.
- Heightened sense of justice.
- Distaste for social norms (or lack of awareness of them).
- Exactness.
- Sensory hyper or hyposensitivity.
- Emotional intensity.
- Non-traditional communication.

Cognitive Behavioral Therapy (CBT)

NT partners in a neurodiverse relationship tend to enter counseling with certain core myths about their ND partner as well as romantic love itself.

The underpinnings of these myths, and their accuracy, can be determined using *CBT* techniques. Consider two common myths below. Do not apply these techniques in situations where safety is an issue or abusive dynamics are present.

Using CBT to Address Common Myth #1

"If my ND partner truly loved me they would work harder and faster to change behavior I find challenging."
  What beliefs underlie this myth?

- Love should be "enough" to motivate change; A partner's love should equate to rapid personal improvement.
- Personal improvement should be demonstrable in ways that are quickly and easily recognizable to others.
- Existing perspectives about growth should not be challenged.

Without minimizing the NT client's concerns, what are some key discussion points?

- Discuss where these expectations may have come from, paying special attention to trauma.
- Discuss whether or not personal growth is always linear, quantifiable, and observable to others.

What are some Truth Statements to challenge this myth?

- Whether or not someone changes, and how quickly they do so, is not always just a matter of their heart. There are many other factors involved besides love.
- Neurology plays an important role in what type of personal growth is possible and at what rate it occurs.
- Like a competitive athlete needs a coach, ND persons often need specialized support from a trained professional to help make and maintain certain behavior changes.
- Some ND behaviors and/or tendencies may be *unchangeable* due to neurological permanency. Demanding that these change is both pointless and cruel.

Using CBT to Address Common Myth #2

"My ND partner's inconsistent behavior always equals disinterest and disrespect toward me and our relationship."
What beliefs underlie this myth?

- Consistency always equals interest and respect.
- Inconsistency always equals disinterest and disrespect.

Without minimizing the client's concerns, what are some key discussion points?

- Discuss where these expectations may have come from, paying special attention to trauma.
- Discuss whether or not a valid explanation for the ND partner's inconsistency exists, such as due to brain-based factors. Is their inconsistency within reasonable boundaries?
- Provide psychoeducation about any of the ND partner's specific brain-based factors that may contribute to (reasonable) inconsistency.
- Discuss whether or not it's possible for neurodiverse partners to convey interest and respect back and forth in ways other than just behavioral consistency.
- Discuss whether or not inconsistency can be tolerated in a relationship, and to what degree. Are there some behaviors that must be consistent no matter what?

What are some Truth Statements to challenge this myth?

- No human of any neurotype is ever perfectly consistent. A reasonable degree of inconsistency must be accepted in oneself and others in order to coexist. At the same time, healthy boundaries must be established.
- Regardless of neurotype, inconsistent behavior can be perfectly normal at times (e.g., when someone is learning a new skill or is under stress) and not at all indicative of disinterest or disrespect.

- Inconsistent behavior (within boundaries) can be a hallmark characteristic of certain kinds of neurodivergence. It's possible for someone's best efforts to still result in inconsistency.
- It's ok to feel upset by inconsistency and to express this. It's also perfectly ok to set boundaries regarding how much inconsistency is tolerable.

Self-Regulation Skills

The ND partner in a neurodiverse relationship is likely to struggle the most with self-regulation – but this isn't always the case. All clients can benefit from learning how to improve their interoceptive awareness, to identify triggers for dysregulation and associated coping habits, and to practice effective self-regulation strategies.

Neurodiverse relationship dynamics with regard to each partner's self-regulation challenges are often predictable. First, just like NT couples, struggles tend to occur in cycles maintained by interpersonal triggers. Second, once triggered, each partner usually requires an opposite pathway back to their emotional and physiological baseline! (This can be frustrating if misinterpreted.) Finally, a general lack of insight combined with low self-regulation skills usually exacerbate their problems.

Consider the following fictional situation.

Cindy (NT):

"You always shut down when things between us get hard and I want to talk it out. Do you have any idea how upsetting it is for me to have to get to the point of yelling before you finally decide to communicate?"
Johan (ND):

"Yelling isn't what makes me communicate any faster. You're right, I do go numb and hide when things get hard. This isn't because I don't care! I need that time alone to regroup and gear myself up to face the issue in a conversation."
Here, Johan admits to shutting down in response to relationship stress whereas Cindy reports agitation and the need to quickly connect.

These are opposite emotional and physiological responses. Accordingly, these partners will have opposite pathways back to baseline once triggered. Cindy needs to practice **physiological self-soothing**, while Johan needs to practice **physiological self-activation**. These brain-based differences must be acknowledged and mutually respected prior to learning how to break their *Pursue-Withdraw* cycle

Neurodiverse couples need many guided opportunities to practice identifying and expressing their thoughts, feelings, and body sensations in each other's presence. Hopefully, these efforts result in not only greater self-awareness, but also empathy for their partner's experience. Each partner will have a different learning curve with new skills: Patience with oneself and one's partner is essential. The following self-regulation exercises should be taught to couples together versus individually but may need to be reinforced via concurrent individual therapy (with a separate provider).

The Physiological Awareness Scale

Using the following *Physiological Awareness Scale* can emphasize each partner's interoceptive insights and encourage communication back and forth about them. Adapted for clients' daily use, it relies on a simplification of Dan J. Siegel's concept of the "window of tolerance."[3]

How do you use the Physiological Awareness Scale?

First, ask each client to draw a numeric scale from 0 to 10. This scale will be used to talk about <u>their own</u> brain responses, emotions, and physical sensations. Partners are never responsible for each other's self-awareness or self-regulation efforts, or lack thereof.

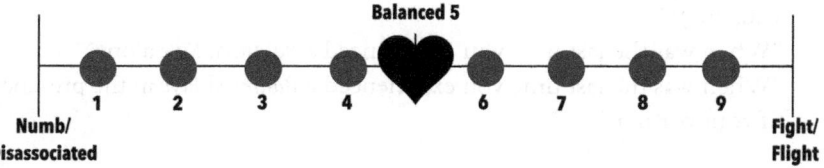

Balanced 5

1   2   3   4   6   7   8   9

Numb/
Disassociated

Fight/
Flight

Figure 8.1 The *Physiological Awareness Scale*

Next, the *Physiological Awareness Scale* is best explained by starting with the extremes. A zero is a state of emotional and physiological numbness or disassociation. This usually either involves shutting down (i.e., the brain's *Freeze* response) or going on autopilot (i.e., the brain's *Fawn* response). A ten is explained as a state of emotional and physiological hyperarousal (i.e., the brain's *Fight* or *Flight* response). This usually involves agitation or aggression. These extremes are automatic, defensive states in which healthy interpersonal growth is impossible.

Unlike the extreme ends of the scale, a *Balanced Five* is explained as a state of emotional and physiological regulation. This is characterized by feeling calm, present, cognitively flexible, and able to access one's own feelings, thoughts, and body sensations. Couple growth is most possible when both partners are at a *Balanced Five*, or at least close to it, because this state facilitates creative problem-solving. Positive feelings like joy, relaxation, and relationship satisfaction are most possible during a *Balanced Five* state.

Each partner is then asked to consider what they themselves experience at each numeric location of the scale. Clients with alexithymia will need extra support. Noncritical feedback between partners should be encouraged, with the therapist modeling how to do so (e.g., "I've noticed your cheeks flush when a subject becomes particularly heated. Are you aware this occurs?") The following questions can help:

- "What are your own behaviors at a 0, 1, 2, 3 . . . etc.?"
- "What physical sensations do you feel at a 0, 1, 2, 3 . . . etc.?"
- "What emotions do you feel at a 0, 1, 2, 3 . . . etc.?"
- "What do you think is happening in your mind/brain at a 0, 1, 2, 3 . . . etc.?"

Special attention should be paid to helping each partner describe themselves at a *Balanced Five*. Good questions to ask about this are:

- "How do you know when you're at a *Balanced Five* (i.e., what are you feeling in your body, what thoughts are you having, what behaviors are you doing, what emotions are you feeling, how are others responding to you, etc.)?"
- "When was the last time you experienced a *Balanced Five* alone?"
- "When was the last time you experienced a *Balanced Five* in the presence of your partner?"

Clients should be encouraged to get very specific, noting not only their internal experience but the exact environmental and interpersonal contexts in which they've most recently felt healthiest. It can be life-changing for partners to hear their similarities and differences about this. Frequently, this is the first time they're learning this about themselves and each other! For example, one partner may describe feeling best regulated when riding a horse. Their partner, on the other hand, may say reading a book alone at home feels best. Recognizing the neurological underpinnings here is crucial. Riding a horse (i.e., moving, receiving pressure on joints, being outdoors amongst variable stimuli, interacting with living creatures, etc.) and reading alone at home (i.e., being still, being solitary, being in a controlled environment with limited sensory stimuli, utilizing imagination and/or intellect, etc.) represent extremely different self-regulation preferences . . . which, of course, each stem from having a different neurological home base.

Last, but certainly not least, each partner is asked to consider how exactly they fluctuate up and down the scale. The following questions may guide discussion:

- "What events, thoughts, sensations, etc. are most likely to trigger your leaving a *Balanced Five*?"
- "When triggered, are you more likely to go <u>up</u> on the scale toward a ten or <u>down</u> on the scale toward a zero?"
- "How do you know you've left a *Balanced Five* (i.e., what are you feeling in your body, what thoughts are you having, what behaviors are you doing, what emotions are you feeling, how are others responding to you, etc.)?"
- "How can you bring yourself <u>down</u> toward a *Balanced Five* when needed?"
- "How can you bring yourself <u>up</u> toward a *Balanced Five* when needed?"

Again, it can be extremely eye-opening for partners to note similarities and differences in the neurological underpinnings of their respective dysregulation and self-regulation tendencies. Sometimes clients are knowledgeable about the self-regulation strategies that work for them and just need practice with identifying triggers and responding to them well. Other times, partners need help to learn fundamental skills.

Clients can be asked to place a blank *Physiological Awareness Scale* somewhere clearly visible at home in a spot they each regularly visit (e.g., the bathroom, the refrigerator). Each partner should check in with themselves whenever they find themselves naturally in proximity of the scale, using it as a visual cue to stop and examine their current state and to assign themselves a number. They should practice communicating together about their numbers at home only after being given the opportunity to practice healthy ways to do so during therapy.

The Brain/Body Break

Sharing life with an intimate partner requires learning how and when to both engage and disengage with each other. This dance may be especially challenging for some ND persons, who usually benefit from role-playing relationship scenarios during sessions – especially those that involve emotional intensity or conflict. Simultaneously, the therapist can highlight the role each partner's interoceptive skills can play in their relationship success. Any couple therapist who focuses solely on improving a ND partner's so-called "emotional intelligence" via traditional social skill training will only get so far. They've missed the point!

Healthy neurodiverse couple dynamics depend on each partner's ability to practice self-awareness and self-regulation strategies. Both partners need to understand how to identify and maintain their own mental, emotional, and physiological baselines in order to promote healthy interactions together. It's especially crucial that each partner learns how to recognize their own mounting overwhelm and take a *Brain/Body Break* before an extreme state. (Remember, partners are not responsibile for each other's extreme states – only their own.) Recall that it's normal for people of any neurotype to experience times of dysregulation, yet some ND persons may experience more frequent and/or more intense times like this. A therapist should normalize clients' expressions of dysregulation (within reasonable boundaries) in order to reduce stigma and offer appropriate support. For some clients, not all, dysregulation may even take the form of Autistic meltdowns – which look and feel different for each Autistic person. One person may hide under a blanket while rocking their body back and forth to disassociate from a triggering conversation with their partner, while another may beat on their own ears to physically block out the sensation of their partner's voice.* Some may repeat the same words over and over in a loop, while others find themselves unable to speak at all. Ideally, these clients can learn how to take a *Brain/Body Break* as a preventative measure prior to the occurrence of an actual meltdown. Sometimes, though, no matter how hard one tries a meldown is inevitable . . . and this is no one's fault.

*Self-harm in this scenario represents an attempt to focus on a sensation within one's control versus the external stimulus outside their control.

What's a Brain/Body Break?

This is a simple, easy to recall skill to reach for whenever personal distress begins to mount. It's designed to be used whenever someone recognizes that they themselves, not their partner, is becoming overloaded. This overload may occur on either a mental, physical, physiological, or emotional level.

Because it relies on interoceptive ability, the *Brain/Body Break* skill is best taught after a skill like *The Physiological Awareness Scale* has helped clients quantify their brain and body states. It should be taught in manageable chunks, with the therapist actively looking for ways to model its use during sessions whenever clients reenact problematic dynamics. Clients should be given opportunities to practice together during sessions prior to ever being asked to do this alone at home. Note, too, that when first assigned for homework, the *Brain/Body Break* should only be practiced while both parties are calm. This is to build muscle memory for the skill and promote recall when it actually becomes needed in a tense situation.

How to Take a *Brain/Body Break*

1. Recognize the somatic, mental, and emotional signals in yourself – not your partner – that mean you're leaving a *Balanced Five* on *The Physiological Awareness Scale*. This indicates you're headed in the direction of either a ten or zero. Both are extremes! Try to catch this in yourself early.
2. Clearly convey to your partner, "I need a break." You may speak this out loud, write this phrase down, text it, or use an agreed-upon hand gesture.
3. Clearly convey exactly where you're going and when you'll return. (If you don't know for sure, don't skip this step. Just provide a good estimate.) For example, "I think I need about 30 minutes to take a walk somewhere, and then I'll come back."
4. Use the break wisely. This may involve sensory-based strategies, *CBT* or *DBT* skills, spiritual practices such as prayer, or any number of self-regulation techniques your therapist is happy to teach.
5. Return exactly when you said you would, even if you're not back to a *Balanced Five* yet. If needed, it's ok to request a time extension to continue your self-regulation efforts.

How to Respond to a Partner's Request for a *Brain/Body Break*

1. All *Brain/Body Break* requests <u>must</u> be immediately honored. There's no use pushing your partner past their limits, as this will not result in the connection you crave!
2. Use the break wisely. This may involve sensory-based strategies, *CBT* or *DBT* skills, spiritual practices such as prayer, or any number of self-regulation techniques your therapist is happy to teach.
3. Return at the time requested, and no sooner. Again, it's not productive to rush the partner who called the *Brain/Body Break*. It may be helpful to remind yourself that your partner's recognition of their personal limits is a good thing. If you're not yet calm yourself, request an extension and continue your self-regulation efforts.

The Energy Audit

The *Energy Audit* exercise uses terms and concepts from Christine Miserandino's popular **Spoon Theory**. It allows each partner in a neurodiverse relationship to quantify their own energy levels at any given time. Units of mental, physical, and emotional energy are referred to as spoons. Each person's total number of spoons available to them per day differs, and this number fluctuates throughout the day. This is because some activities and conditions add spoons, while others deplete them. What determines this is unique to each person because it relies on brain wiring, coping skills, stressors, physical needs, preferences, etc.

A popular NT misconception is the assumption that everyone, regardless of neurotype or Disability status, starts each day with the same number of spoons (i.e., mental, physical, and emotional energy level). NT perspectives also tend to assume each person's number of spoons fully replenishes at the start of each day, and that everyone processes incoming stimuli throughout the day similarly. This could not be any further from the truth!

Some NT partners find themselves disappointed by what they perceive as their ND partner's oversensitivity and/or laziness. Their ND partner, who is often doing the best they can each day, can respond to this miscategorization with hurt and resentment.

Consider the following fictional couples.

Carol (ADHDer with Ulcerative Colitis):

"Sometimes the basics of life are hard for me. Even showering can be exhausting. There are times I desperately need to lessen my workload, but I'm not always able to do so. It's not like I can call in sick to work each and every time my ADHD challenges make me feel like a failure and chronic illness flare ups demand I'm near a bathroom."

Kris (NT):

"If you just woke up earlier and took a shower before work, I bet you'd feel more energized for the day. That always works for me. And, we talk a lot about you making diet changes to help your digestion . . . but they never happen. It doesn't seem like you're motivated to feel better."

Of course, sometimes it can be the ND partner who displays profound misunderstanding.

Justin (NT):

"Some things that come easily for you are extremely complicated to me. It's taking me way more time and effort to do these tax forms than you realize. You never give me credit for how much effort I'm giving."

John (ND):

"Come on, it's just simple mathematics. You've been working on these forms for weeks."

To promote mutual respect and empathy, neurodiverse couples often benefit from a perspective shift regarding energy gain and loss. Helping each partner complete their own *Energy Audit* in front of each other during a couple therapy session can be helpful. Partners need the chance to realize, in concrete terms, just how much effort it takes each person to meet the daily demands of life, how these values differ from one another, and how things can fluctuate based on various circumstances. In particular, NT partners tend to not realize how much the constant pressure to meet majority expectations weighs on their ND partner's mind, heart, and body. ND persons (especially those with concurrent chronic illness) may also need to expend far more energy each day to complete the same basic tasks NT persons do with little conscious effort. Some Autistic persons are far more easily depleted by social interactions than others, for instance, and Dyslexic persons expend far more energy on language-based tasks than others.

A therapist can help clients challenge their assumptions and unrealistic expectations for themselves and each other while providing psychoeducation. For example, most ND persons are usually energetically replenished via engaging with their own intense interests. This may or may not involve social interaction, even for those who are highly extroverted.

What are the Steps to an Energy Audit?

1. Ask each partner to list the personal behaviors, somatic conditions, interpersonal interactions, and environmental contexts that <u>add</u> spoons.
2. Ask each partner to list the personal behaviors, somatic conditions, interpersonal reactions, and environmental contexts that <u>take away</u> spoons.
3. Compare lists. In general, what tends to trigger energy fluctuation for each person? Furthermore, what factors tend to determine the pace of each person's energy recovery? For example, energy depletion can occur more often during stressful times and have a slower rate of recovery.

Sample *Energy Audit*

What <u>Adds Spoons</u> for Justin (NT):

- Being given a compliment or receiving recognition at work.
- Bowling with friends.
- Getting a good night's sleep.
- Playing guitar.
- Listening to worship music.

What <u>Takes Away</u> Spoons for Justin (NT):

- Occasional insomnia.
- Feeling misunderstood by my partner.
- Clothes not fitting right.
- Anxiety about finances.
- Traffic.

What <u>Adds Spoons</u> for John (ND):

- Watching a documentary.
- Keeping up my routines.
- Stimming.
- Working through a problem at work or at home.
- Knowing my partner is proud of me.
- Taking a nap.

What <u>Takes Away Spoons</u> for John (ND):

- Missing a meal or forgetting to take my medicine.
- Failing to meet my partner's expectations.
- Getting out of routine.
- Not having time to sit quietly with my own thoughts.
- Not expressing myself as clearly as I want to with my partner or boss.
- Not being able to move my body the way I need to (i.e., stim). while at work.

Interpersonal Skills

Brain-Informed Active Listening

Neurodiverse partners often long to be seen and heard by one another as they communicate, yet giving and receiving validation can be extremely difficult without targeted support. Remember, though, that these partners aren't any more guaranteed to fail due to their brain differences than NT partners are guaranteed success due to their brain similarities!

Teaching clients active listening usually takes high priority within most traditional couple therapy modalities. Unfortunately, applications of this skill tend to rely heavily on NT standards for "whole body listening" (e.g., maintaining a still body, making eye contact). These behaviors may bless most NT clients, but they can also completely invalidate ND clients' communication needs. Insisting upon these standards can have unfortunate outcomes. For one, it may distract and frustrate certain ND persons to the point their ability to focus, access their own thoughts and feelings, interpret their partner's expressions, and emotionally connect to their partner is greatly reduced. Simple accommodations are necessary to increase the inclusivity and effectiveness of any therapy intervention used with neurodiverse couples that involves active listening.

What makes Brain-Informed Active Listening different?

- *Brain-Informed Active Listening* does not prioritize spoken words. It can also involve helping partners type expressions back and forth or use any other form of communication.
- Some people connect to their own thoughts and the expressions of others best while fidgeting or pacing. Each partner is allowed, and even encouraged, to move their body as needed during *Brain-informed Active Listening*.
- The distance each partner is situated from each other is an important discussion point within *Brain-informed Active Listening*. A comfortable proximity for both should be established, along with a boundary regarding touch and eye contact. Neurodiverse couples should <u>never</u> be forced to sit close together, maintain eye contact, and/or hold hands during active listening.
- The therapist should provide intentional scaffolding for each of the basic components of active listening by teaching in manageable chunks:

  - How to know when it's your turn to speak or not.
  - How to assess what you're feeling.
  - How to ascribe a feeling word to what you're feeling.
  - How to formulate an "I statement."
  - How to non-defensively reflect your partner's "I statement" back to them.
  - How to give and receive feedback.

- If needed, the therapist can invite clients to safely experience the foundational elements of the natural flow of reciprocal information-sharing and validation between partners on a somatic level. Wendy Maltz's exercises entitled *Body Drawing* and *Magic Pen* are well suited for this purpose.[4] These exercises invite partners to practice non-sexual somatic engagement back and forth through light touch and simple movements. Generalization to conversational skills can easily take place, which can enhance partners' communication efforts.

I Wish/Because

The *I Wish/Because* exercise invites each client to take turns filling in the blanks of the following prompt written on a large white board. If the entire statement is too much all at once, it can be broken into two parts.

"I wish our relationship was (adjective) because then I would feel (emotion word)."

The therapist should then look for the underlying values and needs behind each client's statement (e.g., is there a desire to be chosen, sexually desired, comforted, excited, safe, peaceful?). Scanning for significant similarities and differences in the clients' expressions, they should then attempt to emphasize common ground in the form of a summary statement.

Fictional clients Pablo and Beatrice:

Pablo (ND):

"I wish our relationship was easier, because then I would feel relieved and hopeful."

Beatrice (NT):

"I wish our relationship was fun, because then I would feel happier."

Therapist:

"It sounds like you both view your current relationship as heavy, and that you both want it to feel lighter."

Next, if both clients agree with this summary, the therapist can encourage personal accountability. They can also offer a new perspective that shifts attention toward what each partner is attempting to offer versus how they come up short. Helpful questions to guide this discussion can be:

- "How are each of you genuinely trying to help the relationship feel lighter?"
- "Are there ways your partner may be genuinely trying to help the relationship to feel lighter that you may be missing, or even rejecting?"
- "Are there things that each of you might be unintentionally doing that keep the relationship feeling heavy?"

Therapy goals can be collaboratively drafted at this point in order to objectively define what a "lighter" (i.e., easier and more fun) relationship could look like and how to get there.

What if no unifying sentiment can be found during the I Wish/Because exercise?
The therapist can help each client more clearly define their relationship expectations, as in the fictional scenario below.

LeShawn (ND):

"I wish our relationship was <u>less entangled</u>, because then I would feel <u>more independent</u>."

Gemma (NT):

"I wish our relationship was <u>more connected</u>, because then I would feel <u>secure</u>."

Therapist:

"It sounds like there's tension between your wants and needs. One of you wants to build a couple identity around closeness, while the other craves more individuality."

If the couple agrees with this summary, the therapist can pose helpful questions to guide discussion:

- "Is it reasonable to think your relationship can accommodate both these opposing needs at the same time?"
- "LeShawn, what would your relationship look like if it was <u>less entangled</u>? Gemma, would this be acceptable?"
- "Gemma, what would it look like for your relationship to be <u>more connected</u>? LeShawn, would this be acceptable?"
- "Is there a mutually satisfying middle ground here? If so, what changes would need to take place to create and maintain this? If not, what could this mean for your relationship?"

Blesses Me/Blesses Me Not

This exercise invites each client to take turns filling in the blanks of the following prompt written on a large white board. The therapist should provide a clear summary statement after each partner's expression.* Responses should be as specific as possible.

*Clients who are skilled at *Brain-Informed Active Listening* may be able to summarize and validate their partner's expressions instead of the therapist, and should be invited to do so.

"It <u>blesses me</u> when you say/do this: _____."
"It <u>blesses me not</u> when you say/do this: _____."

**Sample *Blesses Me/Blesses Me Not* Exercise
with Fictional Clients**

Pauline (NT):

"It <u>blesses me</u> when you clean the kitchen without my having to ask."
"It <u>blesses me not</u> when I come home and see dishes stacked high in the sink and several other unfinished projects strewn about."
Therapist:

"It sounds like you value a clean home environment that you don't have to maintain all on your own."
Micah (2e; Gifted, ADHD):

"It <u>blesses me</u> when you give me time to get things done at my own pace."
"It <u>blesses me not</u> when you constantly remind me of everything I haven't accomplished yet."
Therapist:

"It sounds like you value being able to do housework according to your own routines, without feeling rushed."

If the therapist in the example above has made accurate summary statements, they can then discuss how the clients' use of effective communication skills and self-regulation may reduce criticism and defensiveness back and forth on the topic in question. New perspectives can be offered, too. Is the NT partner here truly nagging, or are they simply stating a reasonable expectation for cleanliness? Are her ND partner's preferred methods of completing housework effective, or do tasks never truly get done? Psychoeducation regarding any brain-based characteristics that may directly relate to the clients' situation can help promote mutual understanding, flexible problem-solving, and boundary setting. Ultimately, the therapist can help each partner decide what they're willing and able to do to contribute to an improved dynamic.

Using Cheat Codes as Communication Shortcuts

Many American children of the 1980s still have the infamous *Konami Code* memorized to this day: Up, Up, Down, Down, Left, Right, Left, Right, B,

A, and Start. Entering this code granted coveted gaming privileges within numerous games. Why do we still remember it? Because it was just that valuable! Using similarly valuable interpersonal cheat codes may provide lasting relationship benefits to some neurodiverse couples.

The TMB Rule

TMB is shorthand for "I Tried My Best" or "I'm Trying My Best." *The TMB Rule* states either partner can use this term in a variety of ways. Mainly, though, it can be used to quickly convey one's own genuine attempts at using healthy skills. This is important because NT partners frequently express difficulty trusting that their ND partner's brain-based challenges exist to the degree they claim. They also tend to be skeptical that their ND partner is truly trying to improve themselves and fear neurodivergence is being used as an excuse to justify underperformance.

Anyone of any neurotype deserves to be taken seriously when they state they're putting forth real effort toward accomplishing something. They also deserve to be trusted when they state they've genuinely reached their limit. Too often, though, neurodiverse partners criticize and/or doubt each other's motivations or intentions. They tend to invalidate, and even belittle, each other's efforts. This phenomenon may disproportionately affect ND persons, as their efforts may go unseen if they don't align with NT standards or involve observable and/or expected behavior.

Under *The TMB Rule*, the partner who uses the code <u>cannot</u> do so disingenuously. This means they cannot use it with the intent to make an excuse for themselves or otherwise manipulate the situation. In return, the person who hears the code <u>must</u> demonstrate trust.

Example Without Using *The TMB Rule*

ND Partner:

"I tried, but I just couldn't get to that task today. I'll try again tomorrow."

NT Partner:

"Yet, you found time to do other stuff? I don't believe you! How could this possibly be your best effort? I guess what I asked you to do just wasn't important enough to get around to doing. You always make promises you can't keep, so why should tomorrow be any different?"

Example Using *The TMB Rule*

ND Partner:

"TMB . . . I just couldn't get to that task today. I will try again tomorrow."

NT Partner:

"Even though it's hard for me to accept that because I didn't directly see your efforts, I'm learning to trust you. I'm trying to believe you when you say you've genuinely tried. Thanks for recommitting to try again tomorrow. It's important to me that this gets done."

What are some other applications of the TMB Rule?

1. To check in with each other:
   "I'm TMB. Are you?"
2. To cultivate personal accountability:
   "If I'm being honest with myself, am I really TMB? If so, are my efforts sustainable? If I'm not TMB, is there a reason why? Do I want to improve? Am I stuck? Do I need to ask for help or seek specific support to improve?"
3. To talk about *changeable* versus *unchangeable* factors:
   "I've been TMB for months on this. Actually, it seems like I've been working on this all my life! This particular thing just doesn't seem *changeable* about me. I'm not sure my brain will ever be able to do exactly what you're asking it to do. Can you accept that?"
   "We've each been TMB for months, and although this particular interpersonal pattern between us has definitely gotten better . . . it doesn't seem like it will ever fully go away. Can we accept that it might always be part of our relationship that shows up from time to time? If so, can we learn how to recognize it early and cope when it happens?"

Heart Card

There are moments when the kinds of loving verbal expressions and/ or behavioral gestures a NT partner expects their ND partner to provide are incredibly difficult or impossible. This usually occurs in an awkward, pressured, or socially complex scenario.

NT partners need to understand that increasing demand on their ND partner in these moments is not going to be productive. Meanwhile, ND partners need to understand that there's a much better option than freezing up in silence, masking, or retreating. The answer is the *Heart Card*.

A *Heart Card* is simply an index card or similar with a hand drawn heart on the front. Or, if the actual card is unavailable at the time, one can just draw a small heart somewhere clearly visible. This conveys "I love you, yet I'm unable to say or do anything else but produce this card at the moment." It's really that easy.

ND partners are encouraged to produce a *Heart Card* when their NT partner is urgently looking to them for connection, but they temporarily lack the ability to provide words or behaviors that reciprocate this.

Both parties benefit from the use of the *Heart Card*, as it can break unhealthy patterns of disconnection. The ND partner gets an easy-to-use, emergency tool for their interpersonal skill toolbox. Their needs for silence, space to process, reduced interpersonal demand, physiological soothing, etc. when too overwhelmed to speak or act are validated. The gesture is simple to remember and takes little energy to implement – even when physiologically overwhelmed. It's a valid way to convey love, compassion, and support and represents a healthy alternative to staying silent, masking, or retreating. Meanwhile, the NT partner gains at least some form of connection to their ND partner without resorting to demands or other unhealthy behaviors.

Consider the fictional couple below.

Sample Uses for the *Heart Card*

Justine (NT):

"Do you even care that my mom is in the hospital, Issac? I'm crying my eyes out over here, yet you can't even hug me and tell me it's all going to be ok? Why can't you just be there for me without me having to spell things out?"

Because Justine's partner Issac (Autistic) is currently at a loss for words but doesn't have the actual *Heart Card* they made in therapy available, he draws a small heart on the edge of a napkin and slides it over to her. Justine takes a deep breath and smiles.

Another Application of the *Heart Card*

Either partner can gently produce the *Heart Card* after conflict at the point when they're ready to re-engage. Here, the connotation of the card is similar to an olive branch. It's code for, "I love you and I want to try again to connect."

The Power of the Preface

Learning to use preface phrases can help clients who have difficulty expressing their thoughts due to anxiety, or maybe have a tendency to speak more bluntly than their partner can handle. The following phrases – when used sincerely – can provide a helpful jumpstart to get one's own words flowing in the right direction. This is usually far better than saying nothing at all or saying things without a filter!

- "I'm not sure if this is the best time to say this, but . . ."
- "I really don't want this to come across the wrong way, but . . ."
- "I'm not totally sure about how I feel about this yet, but . . ."
- "If I'm reading the situation right, I think what's happening is . . ."
- "I'm worried that you might not understand this about me, but . . ."
- "At the risk of sounding bad, I wanted to say . . ."
- "I'm not trying to get stuck on this, but I keep coming back to . . ."
- "I'm nervous to say this out loud, but . . ."

These are just a few examples. Therapists can brainstorm specific phrases that may be appropriate to each client's needs and invite couples to practice using "the power of the preface" with each other in session. The end result can be increased assertiveness and reduced defensiveness.

The Old Versus New Chart & Victory Journal

Neurodiverse couples can benefit from making a list of unwanted (i.e., "Old") relationship behaviors versus wanted (i.e., "New") relationship behaviors. The beauty of this exercise is in its simplicity. Rather than belaboring the past, it can quickly validate the clients' pain points while casting vision for improved individual and/or relationship health.

Making an *Old Versus New Chart* at the beginning of therapy can powerfully align clients together toward realistic goals while building up the therapeutic alliance. It should go without saying that this intervention should only take place in an atmosphere of nonjudgmental collaboration. The "Old" column should contain personal behaviors and/or interpersonal interactions that maintain distress, while the "New" column should contain healthy alternatives. Reducing the "Old" and encouraging the "New" is a prime focus of couple therapy. However, any item on the list that is actually *unchangeable*, or requires outside referral to support, should be addressed accordingly.

The *Old Versus New Chart* is also an accountability tool. A therapist can ask the following questions to guide discussion:

- "How are you intentionally choosing to behave in 'New' ways these days, both individually and as a couple?"
- "How have you been able to recover, both individually and as a couple, if something 'Old' happens?"

Sample *Old Versus New Chart*

Table 8.2

Old	New
Partner A uses blaming statements, e.g., "You always . . ." or "You never . . ."	Partner A uses "I statements"
Both partners become emotionally dysregulated during conversations to the point of emotionally shutting down (Partner B) and refusing to take a break (Partner A)	Both partners use self-regulation techniques and the *Brain/Body Break* to end their *Pursue-Withdraw* pattern
Partner B keeps their feelings to themselves without sharing, especially when stressed	Partner B uses sensory-based coping skills for stress, communicating their stress level and/or other feelings to Partner A using the *Physiological Awareness Scale*
There's no specific time set aside for fun and relaxation as a couple	Sacred times for fun and relaxation together are put on the calendar

The *Victory Journal* exercise goes hand in hand with clients' *Old Versus New Chart*. This is because all clients benefit from frequent, clear recognition of their personal victories – no matter how small. Therapists should actively look for <u>any</u> improvement in either partner's ability to self-regulate or utilize flexible, effective interpersonal skills during each session. They should then bring these to the clients' attention. Too often, clients miss out on giving themselves (and especially their partner) appropriate credit for growth. Modeling how to recognize positive change can improve a neurodiverse couple's awareness. After it has been explained and practiced in therapy, the *Victory Journal* exercise is given as homework so clients may record and celebrate their successes in between sessions. Asking about a couple's *Victory Journal* entries since the previous session is a wonderful ice breaker, especially if clients are able to tell each other their victories and their meaningfulness (versus simply report them to the therapist).

A *Victory Journal* is a simple chart with three columns: Partner A's Victories, Partner B's Victories, and Couple Victories.

Sample *Victory Journal*

Table 8.3

Partner A's Victories	Partner B's Victories	Couple Victories
Attempted an "I statement" during a conflict.	Suggested a fun activity to do together as a couple.	Talked together before a family outing to set reasonable expectations for how it may go.
Took a *Brain/Body Break* instead of pushing myself past my own limits.	Tried to take a calming walk outside in response to an argument with Partner A, but it was raining. Played video games instead. (This was an attempt to take a *Brain/Body Break*, but couldn't remember all the steps).	Had a satisfying sexual experience together.
Apologized for criticizing an aspect of Partner B's parenting.	Recognized that my stomach ache this week was in direct response to a tense incident at work.	Looked at the calendar to find time for relaxation as a couple. Realized we need a more consistent babysitter.

Personal & Interpersonal Maintenance Plan

Neurodiverse couples can benefit from collaborating with a therapist to make clear, specific plans toward success. The following *Personal & Interpersonal Maintenance Plan* provides an easy template. It's most beneficial to use after clients have at least been introduced to some of the skills presented in this chapter.

Sample *Personal & Interpersonal Maintenance Plan*

These are the specific triggers for dysregulation I commit to become more aware of from day to day:

Partner A:

_____

Partner B:

_____

These are the specific self-regulation skills I commit to practice:

Partner A:

_____

Partner B:

_____

These are the specific triggers for relationship conflict that we both commit to being more aware of from day to day:

_____

_____

These are the specific interpersonal skills we commit to use together in order to recover well from couple conflict:

_____

_____

Neurodiverse Couple Identity Work

Couple Circle Mapping

Just as each person gets to decide whether or not to integrate their own neurotype into their overall identity framework, each neurodiverse couple gets to decide whether or not to integrate acceptance of neurodivergence within their couple identity. *Couple Circle Mapping* provides a helpful framework for therapists to explore each partner's neurotype, identity dimensionality, strengths and challenges, and boundaries. Although it's intended to build upon *Individual Circle Mapping*, it can also stand alone.

What are the steps to Couple Circle Mapping?

1. Draw a large Venn Diagram on a white board. The two large outer circles represent each partner's individual identity. The space where the two circles touch represents their neurodiverse couple identity. Discuss the meaning behind the size of each circle (equal) and their location (slightly overlapping). This represents a healthy relationship characterized by both independence and interdependence.

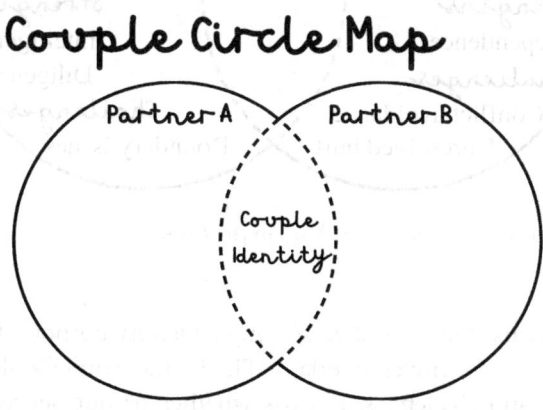

Figure 8.2 Blank *Couple Circle Map*

2. Next, ask if the couple agrees that this representation accurately characterizes their relationship dynamic. If not, give them each a turn to draw out what might be more accurate. For example, one partner may

draw two circles that don't touch at all, which is indicative of emotional distance. An invalidated partner may draw one very large circle to represent their partner and one very small circle to represent themselves, and a partner who feels smothered may draw the circles totally on top of each other.

3.   Return to a healthy, blank diagram. Fill in each partner's neurotype, with their guidance. (Remember, the placement of this – either inside or outside one's identity circle – can be meaningful. It can represent the choice to integrate one's neurotype within their overall identity framework, or not.) Also fill in each partner's prominent characteristics, values, strengths, and challenges. Remind each partner that they're only responsible for what's in their own circle, <u>not</u> their partner's circle.

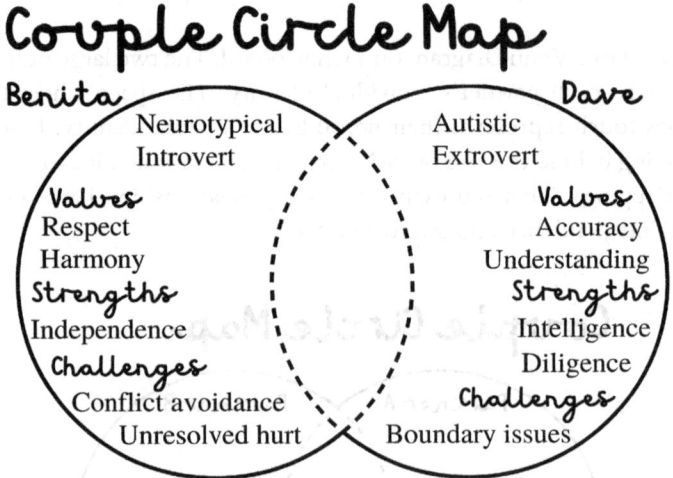

Figure 8.3 Sample *Couple Circle Map* in progress

4.   Finally, discuss the neurodiverse couple identity portion of the diagram (where the two circles overlap). Fill in the couple's shared values, strengths, and challenges. Discuss whether or not neurotypes impact couple identity (i.e., do they refer to themselves as a "neurodiverse couple?"). Why or why not? Do brain differences affect their shared values? Their relationship strengths and challenges?

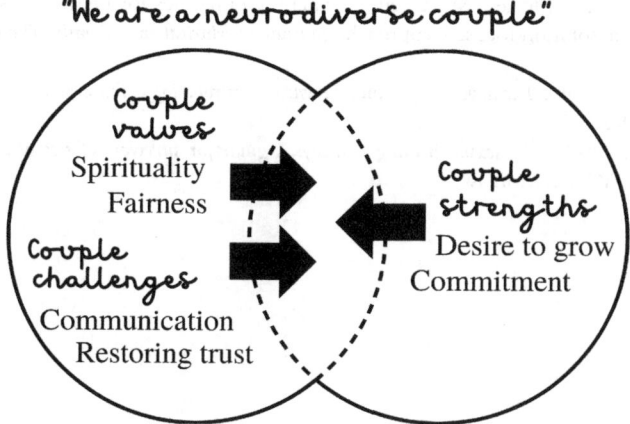

Figure 8.4 Sample section of a *Couple Circle Map*

Glossary of Bolded Terms

Scaffolding Inspired by Lev Vygotsky's concept of the *Zone of Proximal Development* for learning, *Scaffolding Theory* was further developed by Jerome Bruner in the 1950s. In the context of neurodiverse couple therapy, scaffolding refers to the therapist's efforts to actively coach partners in manageable chunks tailored to their unique needs. It also refers to the therapist's discernment regarding the type of homework that should be assigned at any given time.

Spoon Theory Christine Miserandino developed this in 2003 during a conversation with a friend in which she explained how lupus affects her everyday life. It represents a popular conceptualization of the ways each person's energy fluctuates based on their physical health, social dynamics, environmental context, and more.

Notes

1 Strunz, S., Schermuck, C., Ballerstein, S., Ahlers, C. J., Dziobek, I., & Roepke, S. (2017). Romantic relationships and relationship satisfaction among adults with Asperger syndrome and high-functioning autism. *Journal of Clinical Psychology*, *73*(1), 113–125.

2 Parker, M. L., & Mosley, M. A. (2021). Therapy outcomes for neurodiverse couples: Exploring a solution-focused approach. *Journal of Marital and Family Therapy, 47*(4), 962–981.

3 Siegel, D. J. (1999). *The developing mind: Toward a neurobiology of interpersonal experience.* Guilford Press.

4 Maltz, W. (2012). *The sexual healing journey: A guide for survivors of sexual abuse.* New York, NY: William Morrow.

What's Brain-Informed Neurodiverse Couple Therapy (BINCT)? 9

Brain-Informed Neurodiverse Couple Therapy (BINCT) is an original private practice therapy model inspired by two influential sources. The first is the *Myhill & Jekel Treatment Model for Neurodiverse Couples* introduced in 2015.[1] This provides a succinct framework for working with neurodiverse couples. The second, *Neurodivergence-Informed Therapy*, was introduced in 2022 by Chapman and Botha. This model promotes de-stigmatization of ND individuals by encouraging therapists to view clients' issues as primarily relational and to remove neuronormative bias.[2] BINCT respectfully acknowledges these and other groundbreaking works while seeking to expand upon them.

The Four Stages of *Brain-Informed Neurodiverse Couple Therapy*

Stage 1: Joining, Assessing, Teaching.
Stage 2: Practicing and Collecting Data.
Stage 3: Leaning into the New.
Stage 4: Maintaining Resilience.

First and foremost, *BINCT* upholds the six tenets of *Brain-Informed Care (BIC)*:

1. Commitment to non-ableist practices.
2. Sensory security.
3. Presumption of competence and strengths.

DOI: 10.4324/9781003351337-13

4. Acceptance of atypicality without manipulation or toxic positivity.
5. Listening to neurodivergent lived experience.
6. Authenticity of the therapist.

Furthermore, as discussed earlier in this text, a *BINCT* therapist:

• Invites each partner in a neurodiverse relationship to explore their own preferences and capacities regarding eye contact, as well as their physiological experience of it. Communicates permission for each client to direct their own eye gaze during therapy wherever they feel most comfortable at any given time: Eye contact is never mandatory, nor is it promoted as an essential life skill.

• Provides multiple seating options in the therapy room so that clients can dictate their own level of physical and emotional comfort, via proximity and other considerations, at any given time.

• Invites clients to stim freely during session, within boundaries, and validates this as a form of personal expression and/or self-regulation. Only attempts to redirect a client's stims in the event they're of a detrimental, hateful, or sexually inappropriate nature.

• Understands the historical context pertaining to the use of *Person-First Language (PFL)* or *Identity-First Language (IFL)*. Accepts a client's use of IFL, PFL, or a combination of both. Respectfully matches each client's chosen language, as this choice varies from person to person. Follows updated guidelines regarding the use of *IFL* or *PFL* when writing, speaking, or conducting research. Prioritizes any guidelines proposed by actual ND persons.

• Acknowledges society's longstanding history of atrocities against ND populations, which have often occurred under the guise of "curing defects." Recognizes ND populations are at a higher risk for psychological, physical, or sexual harm than NT persons. Also recognizes that past pathologization of a client's neurological differences may have resulted in physical harm and/or psychological damage– sometimes even at the hands of parents or caregivers, medical providers, teachers, or mental health professionals.

• Recognizes that sensory and executive functioning challenges vary significantly from person to person and fluctuates on a daily basis. Offers therapy accommodations accordingly.

• Does not act as an aloof expert during therapy, but rather an educated and collaboration-minded coach. Avoids the use of backhanded compliments and other forms of invalidating statements because of their potential for harm. Avoids any therapy modality that proposes to eliminate, conceal, or degrade valid aspects of a client's self-ascribed ND identity.

- Recognizes that each client's communication needs are fluid. Encourages clients to use whatever communication modality allows them to express themselves best at any given time (i.e., writing, utilizing *Augmented and Alternative Communication (AAC)*, speaking verbally, etc.).

- Respects that each client's own brain differences, chronic illnesses, and/or physical disabilities may or may not be important dimensions of how they self-identify. Recognizes that ND populations are not homogeneous regarding identity formation or any other topic.

- Recognizes the importance of each client's physiological stability to the process of therapy and collaborates with each client towards healthy self-regulation skills. Strives to learn more about human brain processes from both scientific research as well as ND persons themselves in order to promote effective clinical skills in this area and others.

- Validates clients' sensory experience during therapy, regularly initiating dialogue about this and encouraging them to share their sensory needs (to the degree they desire to do so). Challenges their own assumptions regarding clients' responses to environmental stimuli and validates ND lived experience. Invites clients to explore any aspects of their own neurology, or that of their partner, they experience as joyful or positive.

- Presumes each client's competence, mobilizing their individual strengths while properly assessing and supporting areas of struggle. Promotes individual and relational health in ways that honor each client's autonomy and innate personhood. Avoids perpetuating toxic positivity because of its potential for harm.

- Takes time to reflect upon the relationship they have with their own brain, their past and current interpersonal experiences within various kinds of neurodiverse relationships, and how their neurotype fits into the whole of their personal identity framework. Intentionally explores their own brain characteristics and self-identification as either NT or ND, acknowledging that every person (including themselves) should have the right to independently determine whether or not to disclose this personal information.

- Follows applicable ethical guidelines for the appropriate disclosure of their own brain characteristics to clients, if desired, within their marketing efforts and the everyday practice of therapy.

- Appropriately attends to their own sensory needs as they manifest in the therapy room, disclosing and discussing their own coping strategies (within boundaries) whenever clinically relevant to clients' goals.

Stage 1: Joining, Assessing, Teaching

The therapist's primary goal as *BINCT* begins is to join each relationship partner exactly where they are, without bias or judgment. Other foundational goals are:

- To display intentional respect for clients' unique racial, cultural, socioeconomic, spiritual, neurological, and Disabled characteristics.
- To offer equal empathy and support to each partner.

During Stage 1, demand from the therapist is very low. The therapist makes swift, reasonable accommodations to the therapy environment and/or the therapy process itself whenever necessary to support clients' sensory and/or executive functioning challenges. Should clients express interest in one or both partners or their child(ren) receiving an official brain-based label at this point, or at any other point in therapy, professional referrals are made. The therapist discusses the appropriate diagnosticians who may be of service, what the diagnostic process itself tends to involve, the pros and cons of diagnosis, as well as nuances of any potential personal disclosures the clients may be considering.

While hearing a couple's story, the therapist encourages realistic expectations for what *BINCT* may or may not provide. This includes clarifying the therapist's scope of practice. Together, the therapist and clients choose what type of treatment is to unfold (i.e., *Relationship-Building Therapy, Relationship Closure Therapy,* or *Relationship Clarity-Seeking Therapy.*) The therapist can use either the *Relationship Mission Statement, Relationship Closure Statement,* or *Relationship Clarity Statement* exercise accordingly. Obviously, treatment can be re-evaluated at any time per the clients' needs. The therapist should very loosely outline the four stages of *BINCT,* which are the same regardless of treatment type, using lay terms to give clients an accessible overview of the proposed process for change – without guaranteeing any particular outcome.

A skilled BINCT professional will integrate the brief assessment tools provided by this text during an Intake period that forms a strong therapeutic alliance. As needed, thoughtful discussions regarding any clinically significant level of anxiety, depression, or other co-occurring condition in either partner can take place. If needed, they can also help clients thoughtfully process any negative experiences they may have had with helping professionals in the past. The specific assessments provided by this text are: *Safety, Trauma, & Boundary Assessment*; *Strengths Assessment*; *Emotional & Physical Intimacy Assessment*; *Executive Functioning & Sensory Processing Assessment*; *Brain Assessment Questionnaire*; and *Somatic Assessment*.

Throughout Stage 1 and beyond, a *BINCT* therapist carefully considers the kinds of issues neurodiverse couples tend to face without prematurely jumping to conclusions or stereotyping. The therapist offers specific support for these concerns, which may relate to:

1.   Trauma or hardship.
2.   Identity dimensionality.
3.   Communication challenges.
4.   Emotion regulation differences.
5.   Executive functioning differences.
6.   Sensory processing differences.
7.   Sexual challenges.
8.   Parenting stress.

Note that some clients prefer to explore their personal and relationship history quite extensively during Stage 1. This often helps them feel they are providing the therapist detailed context to explain their current problems. For these clients, exercises like *Brain Branching*, *Writing a NeuroNarrative*, *Individual Identity Mapping*, and/or *Couple Identity Mapping* can be beneficial to experience early on in therapy. Other clients, particularly those who struggle with regulating their emotions and/or burnout, will want and/or need to focus on practical, here-and-now support instead of history. These clients will get more benefit from doing the above exercises at a slightly later stage of *BINCT* after enough psychoeducation and skill-building has taken place to encourage greater stability.

Once the therapist demonstrates sufficient understanding of a couple's dynamics, neurodiverse couples often appreciate collaborating to build a concrete visual representation of their situation in the form of an *Old Versus New Chart*. This exercise identifies the individual habits, interpersonal patterns, and unhealthy perspectives which maintain distress while contrasting them with those which may promote wellness. It organizes the huge and often nebulous frustrations clients bring to therapy, promotes stabilizing behaviors, and casts vision for a better future. It's key that the

"New" column contains specific, realistic, and measurable growth options. It's also key that the chart itself remains flexible enough to be updated at any time over the course of treatment. At the same time that this exercise is introduced, the therapist encourages clients to start logging any positive changes they notice in themselves and each other–no matter how small– in a *Victory Journal*. This journal will be maintained throughout the entire process of therapy, first only in session and then as homework in between sessions. At first, of course, it's normal for the therapist to take the lead in pointing out client growth. Partners are understandably too consumed by hurt and too caught up in "Old" dynamics to give and receive positive feedback back and forth. Just like any new skill, these interventions require an increased degree of awareness and self-regulation for clients to successfully implement them. Learning to produce and notice the "New" requires specific opportunities to practice.

BINCT's explicit shake-up of traditional couple therapy offers neurodiverse couples the chance to learn how each partner's brain wiring impacts their relationship. Providing accurate and accessible psychoeducation about neurotypes, human sensory systems, executive functioning characteristics, and ND-NT brain differences is a vital aspect of every stage of BINCT. It's perhaps most important, though, during Stage 1 in order to address myths and to fill in knowledge gaps. To this end, as presented in a previous chapter, the therapist uses *Cognitive Behavioral Therapy (CBT)*. Therapists who can provide this without morphing into a lecturing professor, always remembering that each client is the true expert of their own unique brain and body, are priceless.

Note that clients can either eagerly welcome psychoeducation or reject it; Teaching should never be forced. Each client has a right to react differently when learning about neurodiversity topics and the way they may apply to their life. BINCT therapists leave enough space for clients to share their beliefs, ask questions, and process their thoughts and feelings without invalidation.

If the therapist starts out by explaining such benign, but important, topics as the nonlinear nature of human growth, the concept of neuroplasticity, and the pivotal role that each partner's self-regulation plays within a healthy relationship . . . this is sometimes a better starting point than diving right into a discussion of each partner's specific neurotype. On the other hand, sometimes starting out with a detailed discussion of each partner's brain qualities is highly appropriate and effective. Psychoeducation can be supplemented via the therapist's use of reframes, discussion of *The Double Empathy Problem* and *Spoon Theory*, and exercises such as the *Energy Audit*.

Regarding teaching new skills, the most important interventions during Stage 1 of *BINCT* involve the *Physiological Awareness Scale* and the *Brain/Body Break*. This is because each subsequent stage relies on these skills and expands upon them. It may also be equally important, in some cases, to teach a quick version of *Brain-Informed Active Listening* using scaffolding (i.e., breaking the activity into small components and only discussing positive or neutral topics within the exercise). This is only appropriate, though, when each client has sufficient self-regulation skills and has a deep need for a taste of validation from their partner. The validation partners experience from each other via a successful experience with *Brain-Informed Active Listening* can be so powerful that it acts as a relationship defibrillator for certain couples! Most clients will benefit from placing this exercise at a later stage of therapy after they've stabilized. *Brain-Informed Active Listening* should <u>not</u> be assigned for homework yet.

Stage 1 ends when each client displays an appropriate understanding of the neurodiversity topics relevant to their lives as well as at least some movement towards their therapy goals – even if that means reaching a place of neutrality regarding a formerly negative habit, interpersonal pattern, or perspective. Movement to neutral can be a very good sign. Jumping straight from something negative to something positive is unrealistic and unsustainable: One must always pass through neutral first en route to lasting health. This not only applies to behavior, but also to emotions.

The Path to Positive

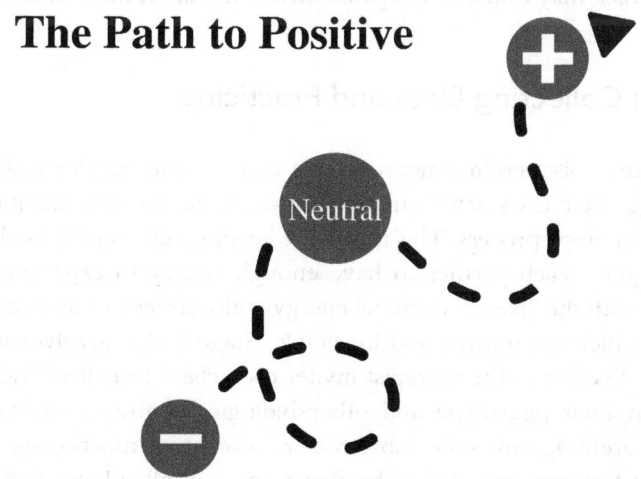

Figure 9.1 An illustration of the path to positive

Forcing oneself, or a partner, to move too quickly from negative feelings to positive feelings usually results in masking. It's better to move genuinely and incrementally from negative, to neutral, to positive . . . which may include a lot of twists and turns along the way. This allows time to more fully process one's own thoughts and feelings, and also promote lasting change.

An additional sign that clients are moving out of Stage 1 and into Stage 2 is their ability to use the *Physiological Awareness Scale* and *Body/Brain Break* in session. Clients will begin to at least attempt the use of these skills at home, with many blunders and misunderstandings amongst themselves, but also some delightful victories.

What can hinder a couple's transition from Stage 1 to Stage 2 in BINCT?
The effects of past trauma, low self-esteem, emotion regulation difficulties, contempt, or a lack of *desire* to grow are the most likely issues to hinder a couple's movement from Stage 1 to Stage 2. Sometimes *capacity* is an issue. It's possible, too, that either partner's choice of a *negative* stance and *sentiment* regarding their own brain (or that of their partner) means they're unlikely to want to progress with *BINCT*. The therapist must use discernment to thoughtfully address these circumstances. It may be necessary to suggest one or both partners attend individual therapy with a different practitioner in lieu of couple therapy, or concurrent with it. Some partners have the financial luxury, *capacity*, and *desire* to attend individual therapy as an adjunct and simultaneous treatment to couple therapy. Others may lack childcare, funds, or time, which may lead them to pause *BINCT* to pursue individual work.

Stage 2: Collecting Data and Practicing

A *BINCT* therapist reminds neurodiverse couples entering Stage 2 to keep prioritizing their own self-regulation, physical health, and mental health during the therapy process. This is because keeping relationship health going strong requires each partner to have enough energy to experiment more and more with the "New." Personal energy is also necessary to recover from setbacks, which are normal and inevitable. Stage 2 also involves increased personal reflection as the therapist invites each client to collect and analyze data about their neurotype and other biological features, environmental context, parenting stressors, job stressors, executive functioning, sensory processing features, etc. As in the first stage and all others, each client's experience of either sensory security or insecurity at any given time within the therapy environment continues to receive attention. Treatment always progresses at the clients' pace, with the therapist coaching practical self-care and couple-care strategies as needed.

The therapist frames Stage 2 to clients as an opportunity to objectively collect data about themselves, each other, and how their relationship looks and feels when they receive psychoeducation and experiment with suggested "New" dynamics. The therapist asks, "When you find yourself experimenting with the 'New,' how does this compare to how your relationship felt when it was 'Old'?" As therapy unfolds, clients become increasingly aware of their ability to <u>choose</u> whether or not to engage with healthy habits, interpersonal patterns, and perspectives through the use of their new therapy skills. They also become aware of their strong tendencies toward the "Old" and begin to understand why. The therapist encourages clients to initiate small experiments with personal and interpersonal change, both during couple sessions and at home, versus large leaps. Again, the *Victory Journal* serves as a vital data collection tool at this stage as the therapist seeks to balance the clinical tasks of helping clients process negative feelings and end dysfunctional habits while simultaneously acknowledging the emergence of healthy progress. It's normal for clients to default to many "Old" behaviors at this stage mixed in with blundering attempts at "New" behaviors. It's also normal and expected for clients to take healthy risks toward growth only to the degree their individual *capacity* and *desire* for change allows.

Each session, the therapist acts as an active interpreter of couple dynamics. They lead interactive discussions to analyze both clients' *in vivo* behaviors and their reported behaviors in between sessions. After repeated modeling of how to do this analysis themselves, clients can learn to identify that which represents "Old" versus "New." The therapist provides the necessary psychoeducation and scaffolding to coach clients toward discussing their data. The therapist may also incorporate role play during sessions to concretely reinforce differences between "Old" and "New" ways of thinking, feeling, and behaving. Coaching clients to practice identifying and communicating about their somatic experiences, thoughts, and emotions is important. Other helpful interventions to this end include the *I Wish/Because* exercise and the *Blesses Me/Blesses Me Not* exercise.

Note that clients will still miss out on recognizing a great many personal and interpersonal victories at this stage. This is expected! When this happens, the therapist doesn't miss out on the opportunity to gently point out their oversight and wonder aloud what this may be attributed to. They discuss how anxiety, defensiveness, contempt, resentment, trauma, criticism, fear, depression, or other factors can sometimes block one's ability to recognize positive change in themselves, their partner, or their relationship. The therapist gives special attention here to providing psychoeducation about amygdala-based responses, which may be quite active in one or both partners, and identifying triggers for dysregulation. These triggers can come from the immediate environment, internal body sensations, one's partner, or many other sources. Each client's reactivity, within reasonable boundaries, can be reframed as their brain's attempt to provide protection – which has likely served a very important role for them in the past. A big question at this stage becomes, "Do you need your brain to offer the degree of protection right now, in this specific circumstance, as it gave you in the past?"

The therapist teaches that one's defensiveness always involves a combination of their unique brain-wiring characteristics, automatic responses, and the influence of their past experiences. Often, but not always, it also can involve free will! Some reactions will always be automatic physiological responses due to *unchangeable* aspects of brain wiring. These reactions require either post-trigger coping or a bit of proactive support to attempt a reasonable degree of trigger prevention. Yet, many reactions only <u>feel</u> automatic . . . they're actually within one's control. That is, they're *changeable* due to the beauty of neuroplasticity. Regarding various scenarios the couple experiences together, the therapist poses the question, "Are your brain's attempts to defend yourself, to this degree and in these specific ways, actually needed right now with each other?" Another way to say this is, "Are your reactions proportionate to the actual interaction happening between you and your partner?"

As all this analysis occurs at the individual and systemic level, clients tend to express a mix of frustration, grief, and cautious optimism about change. To encourage realistic expectations and promote resilience, the therapist educates clients about the specific types of setbacks they're likely to face as therapy continues through the next stage, and normalizes them as they pop up. Certain predictable "failures" are a normal part of any growth process, after all. The first to look out for is that neurodiverse couples tend to get stuck trying to change *unchangeable* factors about themselves and each other. The therapist may need to provide grief support for any feelings that may emerge about that which the clients realize is neurologically permanent. Similar support should be provided as clients process what is *unchangeable* about their past, their environment, or perhaps some aspects of the future (e.g., the need for a Disabled child to live with them through adulthood versus launching on their own). Specifically, too, each couple tends to struggle with triggers for individual dysregulation. The therapist collaborates with each partner to brainstorm coping strategies – which may or may not involve sensory-based strategies – to use when triggering internal sensations, environmental conditions, or interpersonal interactions occur. These experiences can be positively reframed as valuable opportunities to collect data and practice new therapy skills. The therapist can gently challenge each partner, "Will you act 'Old' or 'New' when dysregulation occurs?"

Healthy interpersonal skills, self-regulation techniques, and neurodiversity concepts are all still very fresh during Stage 2 of *BINCT*. The frequent dysregulation that occurs as clients revert to the "Old" and experiment with the "New" provides rich experiences to analyze together. While doing so, the therapist models grace and empathy. Common discussion questions after clients experience dysregulation during session, or in between sessions, are:

- "What *internal climate* and *external climate* factors were involved in this situation? How many *spoons* did you have at the time?"
- "At what point did you feel yourself begin to leave a *Balanced Five*, and in what direction did you go on the *Psychological Awareness Scale*? What were you thinking and feeling as this happened? What were your body sensations? If you experienced an interoception challenge at the time, how can your mindfulness increase in the future?"
- "What behaviors resulted after you left your *Balanced Five* on the scale? How did this affect you? How did this affect your partner?"
- "What therapy skills could have been helpful to remember in this scenario? For example, how do you think that experience would have gone differently had you used the *Brain/Body Break*?"
- "Did you feel free to utilize stimming or any other type of brain-based coping, such as sensory-based techniques, if you wanted to do so? Why or why not? If you did use them, were there any social consequences?"
- "Did you need any specific brain-based support during that experience? Was this available? If so, were you able to request it? If your communication ability was limited, or if no help was available, what may be needed in the future to help quickly connect you to support?"
- "How long did it take you to return to your own personal physiological baseline? What helped promote this the most?"
- "How long did it take to return to your relationship baseline? What helped promote this the most?"

During analysis, the therapist praises any and all growth by either client. They expand the definition of success to encompass <u>any</u> attempt by either partner to use healthy skills, regardless of the outcome. At this stage, taking any healthy risk in an intentional effort to cope is what counts! As clients begin to experience slight to moderate increases in individual and interpersonal stability as a result of their growth attempts, interpersonal skills such *Using Cheat Codes as Communication* and *The Power of the Preface* can be taught. These represent even more specific ways to experiment with "New".

Stage 2 ends when clients show proficiency in distinguishing "Old" versus "New" on their own, actively participate in either therapist-led or client-led analysis, and more readily identify personal and interpersonal victories. Couples begin to do better self-care that may incorporate what they're learning about how to nurture their specific brain and body-based needs. They may also start doing better couple-care. From a big picture perspective, clients begin to move towards having an **internal locus** of control instead of an **external locus of control** as personal accountability increases in proportion to insight. If not previously requested, more complex topics such as intimacy and identity dimensionality may start to become the clients' requested focus of therapy going forward.

What can hinder a couple's transition from Stage 2 to Stage 3 in BINCT?
As before, the effects of past trauma, low self-esteem, emotion regulation difficulties, contempt, or a lack of *capacity* or *desire* to grow can hinder a couple's movement to the next stage of *BINCT*. At this point, too, some clients may also wish to pause relationship therapy in favor of exploring emerging individual identity narratives via individual therapy with a different practitioner, potentially resuming *BINCT* at a later date. If either partner embodies a *negative* stance and *sentiment* towards their own brain (or that of their partner), they are not likely to desire to progress with *BINCT*.

Stage 3: Leaning into the New

In Stage 3, each partner displays a notable increase in their own ability to self-regulate and regularly initiates healthier interactions during and outside of couple sessions. Clients express a greater depth of understanding and acceptance about many things at this stage: Their relationship with their own brain, their relationship with their partner's brain, aspects of individual identity and couple identity, the brain-based factors that impact their dynamic, and how both *internal* and *external climate* factors contribute. Endearingly, clients tend to use their favorite therapy terms fluently, such as *spoons* or *Cheat Codes*. Also, clients begin consistently taking the lead during sessions to analyze their personal and interpersonal data. They tell stories about how using specific therapy skills helped them to neutralize a previously tense conversational topic, resolve a conflict, promote sexual or emotional closeness, set or maintain a healthy boundary, handle parenting stress, etc. Each partner starts to more regularly give themselves, and each other, proper credit for the ways they're demonstrating such "New" traits as patience and resilience. They also, of course, still tell some stories of intense personal and interpersonal struggles. At this point, these usually can be linked to chronic triggers or *unchangeable* factors. Yet, clients tend to respond far better, faster, and with more insight. Now more aware of their vulnerabilities, strengths, and differences they each start to more consistently utilize better coping tailored to their neurotype. They demonstrate greater acceptance of their own limitations and those of their partner. Their couple interactions tend to indicate greater consideration of ND-NT differences. Each partner's *stance* and *sentiment* towards their own brain (and that of their partner) is usually becoming either neutral or positive at this point. The "New" is starting to take root.

Like all other stages, the therapist continues to coach self-regulation skills as a priority while encouraging the couple to lean into their emerging insights. *Brain-Informed Active Listening* becomes a central technique in order to help clients share their physiological experience, heal from interpersonal hurts, and explore increasingly complex topics. Note that alexithymic clients and some other clients may need extra support regarding the identification and discussion of their physiological or emotional states as this happens. The therapist should avoid NT bias when coaching communication skills. Remember, too, that some Autistic clients in particular may benefit from role playing some of the social principles behind reciprocal conversation via Wendy Maltz's *Magic Pen* and/or *Body Drawing* exercises.

As couples practice the foundational principles for healthy communication on their terms, and using strategies unique to their needs, they may begin to experience increasing relationship satisfaction. Although the specific topics to be discussed in *Brain-Informed Active Listening* vary according to each couples' goals, content from the *NeuroNarrative*, *Brain Branching*, *Individual Circle Mapping*, or *Couple Circle Mapping* exercises can provide excellent subject matter. (Of course, *Relationship-Closure Seeking* couples who intend to peacefully co-parent will only be using topics related to their children. Their focus is to solidify a foundation of mutual respect that promotes healthy boundaries and problem-solving going forward.) At first, all couples should practice *Brain-Informed Active Listening* during sessions only. This allows the therapist to provide appropriate scaffolding, which minimizes unnecessary obstacles to client success. To be able to use this skill alone at home is a highly advanced skill, yet many neurodiverse couples can learn to do so if they desire.

Increased self-regulation, improvements as a result of executive functioning coaching, and increased relational stability can not only be a sense of relief – sometimes it sets the stage for serious introspection and even social-justice analysis in some clients. If not previously explored, such in-depth exercises as the *Masking Exercise* and certain key reframes may be helpful to use with any clients who wish to explore how neurodivergence intersects with identity, society, spirituality, Disability, advocacy, justice/injustice, etc.

Couples begin to show marked personal and interpersonal resilience by the end of Stage 3, which officially takes place after they've navigated at least a few major personal and interpersonal triggers well on their own together (or with minimal coaching from the therapist). When "Old" relationship dynamics or personal dysregulation emerges, clients demonstrate an ability to use their strengths and resources to return to baseline.

What can hinder a couple's transition from Stage 3 to Stage 4 in BINCT?
Couples who are satisfied with their progress thus far in *BINCT* may decide to end therapy. This is a little disappointing because it eliminates an important component of maintaining gains, i.e., Stage 4, but is understandable. Rarely, around the end of Stage 3, a couple experiences an extreme setback. For example, sometimes a partner suddenly feels safe enough in the relationship to reveal hidden information. Their partner, naturally, finds the omission of this information distressing. They may feel like this disclosure negates all the efforts put forth in therapy thus far. This is especially true if it happens to violate a sincerely held value, sparks intense identity re-examination, or represents sexual or financial betrayal. Rarely, too, one or both partners become so dysregulated (often in an "Old" way) that they cross a firm relationship boundary – an occurrence that clients sometimes decide warrants discontinuing the relationship entirely. In short, one or both clients may choose not to proceed to the fourth stage of BINCT either due to feeling successful and ready to end therapy, or in response to some occurrence from which they deem their relationship cannot or should not recover.

Stage 4: Maintaining Resilience

For couples who proceed to Stage 4 of *BINCT*, each partner is encouraged to take appropriate accountability for their own efforts to move away from "Old" and toward "New." To do so requires an ability to quantify growth. Clients regularly use healthy self-regulation skills and interpersonal techniques at this point in therapy, demonstrating increased grace and flexibility. Importantly, the couple has learned to set healthy personal and interpersonal boundaries, recognize triggers for dysfunction, and to recover well in response to emotional dysregulation and/or other challenges neurodiverse couples face. Perfection in all of these areas, obviously, is certainly not the goal! Relationship satisfaction always looks like a combination of partners' combined efforts to:

1. Proactively recognize problems *before* they occur, and
2. Recover quickly <u>after</u> something goes awry.

Since interpersonal tension is reduced and clients' initial therapy goals are met by now, clients attend *BINCT* during Stage 4 on a reduced frequency, i.e., for maintenance purposes. The therapist's role becomes to provide ongoing encouragement, troubleshooting, and customized self-care and relationship strategies as client's needs fluctuate. In terms of specific interventions, the therapist does collaborate with the couple to intentionally safeguard and maintain their victories via the *Personal and Interpersonal Maintenance Plan* exercise. The therapist also incorporates aspects of *Narrative Therapy* by inviting partners to retell the story of their lives as individuals, the story of their relationship, and the story of their therapy process. This allows clients to articulate and reinforce any valuable lessons they've learned and/or meanings they have made from their experiences. It can also be powerful to invite clients to share their *Individual Circle Map* with one another, pretending as if they were meeting for the first time. The therapist can even ask the couple to read their *Couple Circle Map* out loud as if they were introducing themselves, as a couple, to the therapist for the first time. If appropriate, another form of the *Relationship Mission Statement* can be made. This can energize and unite a couple towards continuing their shared vision for health after therapy ends.

Stage 4 can be a precious time of renewal and bonding for *Relationship-Building* couples. Some, but not all, may even experience a paradigm shift that propels them towards advocacy. For *Relationship Closing* and *Relationship Clarity-Seeking* couples, this is usually a time to take action upon the decisions they have discerned regarding their relationship through the embodiment of their chosen roles, goals, and boundaries.

Glossary of Bolded Terms

Brain-Informed Neurodiverse Couple Therapy (BINCT) Based on the principles of *Brain-Informed Care (BIC)*, this therapy modality prioritizes understanding and utilizing each partner's unique brain features en route to personal and interpersonal health.

External Locus of Control When a person feels disempowered due to the belief that what happens to them in life is due to fate, luck, circumstance, or the actions of others. Because they believe their efforts have no identifiable impact, which may be the result of trauma, they can remain in a state of passivity and helplessness unless they receive appropriate support. Alternatively, this also may apply to someone with an overinflated ego and/or victim mentality who chronically avoids taking personal responsibility.

Internal Locus of Control When a person feels empowered due to the belief that what happens to them in life results from their own efforts. They believe they're responsible for their own actions, which have an identifiable impact.

Notes

1 Myhill, G., & Jekel, D. (2015). Neurology matters: Recognizing, understanding, and treating neurodiverse couples in therapy. *FOCUS*.
2 Chapman, R., & Botha, M. (2022). Neurodivergence-informed therapy. *Developmental Medicine & Child Neurology*.

Section IV
Case Studies

Wanda & Ben 　　　　　　　 **10**

Fictional client Wanda is a 32-year-old neurotypical (NT) female of Jamaican descent partnered with Ben, a 27-year-old Autistic transgender male of Caucasian descent. They begin *Brain-Informed Couple Therapy (BINCT)* in an online format from their home in upstate New York.

This case study highlights the following interventions over the course of Wanda and Ben's experience within 18 one-hour virtual sessions of *BINCT*:

- *Relationship Clarity Statement.*
- *Couple Circle Mapping.*
- *Writing a NeuroNarrative.*
- *Physiological Awareness Scale and Brain/Body Break.*
- *Brain-Informed Active Listening.*
- *Relationship Mission Statement.*
- *Personal & Interpersonal Maintenance Plan.*

BINCT Stage 1: Joining, Assessing, Teaching

The therapist provides a free, brief consultation to each partner separately prior to the couple's decision to begin *BINCT*. Neither requests any reasonable accommodation to complete their Intake paperwork, inclusive of simple brain-centric assessments. For optimal convenience and sensory security, the clients request therapy take place online. The therapist assesses this format as both safe and appropriate.

DOI: 10.4324/9781003351337-15

To begin, the therapist joins each client and hears their presenting concerns while reviewing their Intake paperwork together. She then loosely describes the four stages of BINCT and the types of neurodiverse couple therapy that could potentially unfold: *Relationship-Building Therapy*, *Relationship Clarity-Seeking Therapy*, or *Relationship-Closing Therapy*.

Wanda expresses strong commitment to the relationship and requests *Relationship-Building Therapy*. She explains the main reason for seeking couple therapy at this time, after five years of living well together in a loving relationship, is to understand the reason behind Ben's emotional withdrawal. She laments nothing seems to cheer him up anymore since he lost his job six months ago, and that she's been consumed by frustration and worry over him and the state of their relationship:

"I just don't understand. Ben's always been quiet, but never distant. I've been by his side ever since before he transitioned, and he knows I support him unconditionally. Why shut me out now? Nothing I say or do gets through to him, and his moodiness is only getting worse the longer he's unemployed. He won't let me in on whatever he's going through. Being rejected like this hurts so much. I want to fight for us to succeed. I'm losing sleep over the fact he's pulling away from me for no good reason."

Ben expresses a preference for *Relationship-Clarity Therapy*. He states his motivation for attending *BINCT* is to improve his low mood, help Wanda be less anxious, and make a decision about how to handle their relationship going forward:

"I thought I knew who I was and what I wanted from life before I lost my job. Corporate downsizing threw off my routine, my career goals, and even my sense of purpose. Since I'm big on the benefits of counseling because it's helped me a lot in the past, I decided to see a vocational counselor. She encouraged me to pursue a formal diagnosis of Autism and some other kinds of tests. This was supposed to help me get to know myself better so that I could start looking for a new job well-suited to my strengths. I agreed to pursue testing because I'd already self-diagnosed myself as Autistic long ago. What harm could there be in getting a formal diagnosis? I had no idea going through the testing process would kick-off intense self-doubt and overanalysis. That was not what I was expecting. I know I've been spiraling and pushing Wanda away, and I also know she wants us to get back to the way we were before . . . but I'm just too overwhelmed right now."

The therapist normalizes and explains the couple's current *Pursue* (Wanda) – *Withdraw* (Ben) dynamic. She also provides psychoeducation about such topics as identity dimensionality, family of origin dynamics, neurotypes, and contextual factors as related to relationship stress. She suggests the couple begin *Relationship-Clarity Therapy*, offering to help them re-evaluate their preferred treatment style or therapy goals at any time. She then guides the couple to create a *Relationship Clarity Statement* together:

Wanda and Ben's *Relationship Clarity Statement*

"We want to understand how we've arrived at this uncomfortable place in our relationship and consider what our path forward (either together or apart) will be. Specifically, we want to decide whether greater relational intimacy, as evidenced by reduced verbal conflict and increased emotional connection, is mutually desirable."

The therapist notes Ben may be experiencing mild depression without suicidal ideation or self-harm. After she shares this observation with him, he states:

"I've worked so hard over the course of my life to figure myself out and go after what I want. I think I'm just really, really tired. Just learning who I really am and how to be myself in the world can be exhausting. Wanda's been a great support, but I hate that I don't have the energy to be there for her the way she's been there for me. I don't want to disappoint Wanda after all we've been through together, yet I'm not sure I can offer much to our relationship right now. Maybe being single is better so I can sort all my feelings out."

As therapy continues, Ben indicates *capacity* and *desire* to learn healthy coping strategies to help reduce his depressive symptoms. He hopes this will help reduce emotional fatigue and even certain sensory processing concerns. Together, in front of Wanda, he and the therapist develop a self-care plan for him that consists of a few simple *Cognitive Behavior Therapy (CBT)* and *Dialectical Behavioral Therapy (DBT)* strategies. The therapist also coaches sensory soothing and/or sensory activation activities customized to Ben's specific needs. She suggests some of these techniques for Wanda, too, to support her anxiety reduction efforts. Together, in front of Ben, Wanda and the therapist make a self-care plan for her inclusive of increased social support and sleep hygiene strategies. The couple agrees to temporarily prioritize their individual self-care efforts over couple-care efforts at this time.

Ben states he's previously taken an antidepressant during a moderate bout of depression during his 20s and that he may be interested in taking this medication again since it had worked well during that time. The therapist provides a referral to a psychiatrist should he wish to discuss starting an antidepressant again while also encouraging him to discuss his emotional state with the doctor that prescribes his testosterone. Wanda expresses concern that Ben's current level of testosterone supplementation may be affecting his mood. Ben agrees to discuss his hormone levels with his prescribing doctor to understand if there may be a connection. He also volunteers to check in with the individual therapist with whom he had worked positively in the past regarding gender identity issues in order to secure one-on-one mental health support concurrent with *BINCT*.

The therapist continues to validate more of the clients' personal and relationship concerns as they talk about their personal and interpersonal history. She offers psychoeducation about each partner's neurological and physiological characteristics that may factor into the verbal conflicts they seek to reduce. For example, Ben's Autistic neurology may explain why he's more likely than Wanda to experience emotional, mental, and physiological shutdown in response to arguments. Wanda admits she rarely experiences shut down: She usually ramps up in response to arguments. Both clients report frustration regarding their recent communication and conflict resolution patterns:

"At the start of our relationship, I appreciated that Wanda never wanted to go to bed angry. She always knew how to get me talking. What I'm going through now mentally can't be so easily explained or resolved, though. The more she brings up sore subjects, the more I want her to stop."

"It never used to be this hard to communicate with Ben. I'm getting tired of being the one to initiate conversation. And, lately, conversations don't even go anywhere. It's like living with the ghost of the person I once knew. Trying to get him to understand how this makes me feel is painful."

The therapist teaches the *Physiological Awareness Scale,* helping each client identify and articulate their own mental, emotional, and physiological experience throughout everyday scenarios and also during couple conflicts. Because neither client is alexithymic, they are quickly able to acknowledge Ben's tendency to go <u>down</u> on the scale while Wanda tends to stay calm at first . . . until she eventually goes up the scale in an anxiety-fueled response to Ben's disengagement. This usually takes the form of criticism and tearfulness. The therapist teaches the *Brain/Body Break* as a "New"coping strategy to avoid overwhelm and promote more instances of being a *Balanced Five*. She coaches each partner to practice the individual components of this skill during their sessions.

Collaboratively, the therapist and clients make an *Old Versus New Chart.* She also introduces the *Victory Journal* as a way for the couple to chart both individual and couple progress.

Wanda and Ben's *Old Versus New Chart*

Table 10.1

Old	New
Inability to recognize the combined effects of personal, interpersonal, and environmental triggers on couple dynamics.	Ability to identify many kinds of triggers and their effects, using healthy coping strategies as needed.
Reduced interoceptive awareness.	Increased interoceptive awareness via the use of the *Physiological Awareness Scale*.
Poor anxiety management.	Use of *CBT* and *DBT* strategies, including sensory soothing or activation activities as needed.
Poor self-care.	Creation of individual self-care plans that include sensory strategies, social support, sleep hygiene, etc.
Pursue (Wanda) – *Withdraw* (Ben) behavior.	Use of the *Physiological Awareness Scale* and *Brain/Body Break* to promote healthy self-regulation and an *Adult-Adult* dynamic.

BINCT Stage 2: Practicing and Collecting Data

Ben participates in an abbreviated version of the *Writing a NeuroNarrative* exercise, which highlights how the accumulation of his own physiological experiences plus contextual factors have led to a bottleneck effect at the moment. The therapist provides psychoeducation about Autistic Burnout, which Ben says describes his current experience well:

"Some days even traffic sounds and the itch of my clothes are too much. Sometimes talking to Wanda is just too much."

He also talks about how losing his job activated an intense sense of injustice upon which he can't seem to stop ruminating. In a journal entry he drafts at home and brings into therapy, Ben reads out loud:

"My life hasn't been fair. Why are some of my family members unsupportive? Why did corporate downsizing derail my career goals? It's not just depression that I'm feeling, it's an existential dread. It's an intense burnout. I don't even know what I have to offer the world or Wanda anymore. My brain and body get all locked up when I think about finding a new job. It's easier just to disconnect. The confirmation that I'm Autistic explains why I feel things so strongly and why layered noises, some food textures, and certain stressors bother me so deeply. It's also why losing my job has been so hard on me, I guess. But, why do I have to be like this? I really don't like my brain sometimes. Why should Wanda have to put up with someone so complex for a partner?"

The therapist provides a safe space for Ben to process how he feels about various aspects of his identity, his family, and his relationship with Wanda. Via a modified version of *Couple Identity Mapping*, the therapist and clients discuss the potential *stances* and *sentiments* one can have regarding their own brain and how this can affect both one's overall view of themselves as well as their relationship. She discusses how various self-identifications may be integrated (or not) within couple identity. Ben asserts that he recognizes the value of returning to at least a *neutral* relationship with his brain because this is what he had prior to receiving his formal diagnosis. Meanwhile, Wanda states she's always accepted Ben inside and out. She says she sees their differences (including neurological and cultural differences) as part of what makes them strong as a couple.

Wanda expresses deep hurt that Ben has not let her in on the details of his recent internal struggle until now and sadness from his neglect of her emotions:

"I don't know what more I could do to prove that I'm here for you as a partner and that I accept you. I don't deserve to be shut out! I also deserve emotional support, too. I can't carry all the emotional labor of the relationship on my own. You can't just give up on yourself and us after we've come so far together."

In response, Ben states:

"I don't really want to give up. My *capacity* for being a relationship partner right now is just really low. I thought finally having a formal answer about my Autism would help me figure out my next career steps. I was even excited about that process, actually, just like I was excited to begin gender confirmation efforts years ago. Just like I've always known I'm a 'he,' I've always known I'm Autistic. But unmasking, this time, was so different. Instead of feeling more and more comfortable in my skin, the opposite happened. I got more and more self-conscious and insecure. Noticing more of my sensory challenges even made me get angry at my brain. I started asking myself questions like, 'Who would want to hire me?' and 'Who would want to be partnered with me?' I guess I haven't really been able to say all this clearly to you until now."

The clients practice lots with their "New," noting progress in their *Victory Journal*. They soon start responding quite well to each other's observable behavioral changes regarding self-care, both in session and in between sessions. When they miss a victory, the therapist gently points it out and provides the opportunity to process both the victory itself and the fact that it was missed. Additionally, the couple displays a good amount of empathy back and forth as they tell stories of key challenges they've weathered together (both over the entire course of their relationship and in between sessions). The therapist helps them analyze these interactions, providing psychoeducation about NT-ND differences as needed.

As the couple explores the roots of their relationship expectations, Wanda reports a history of significant rejection from certain influential schoolmates that led her to cling to her boisterous family for support. Raised by a vivacious single mother and grandmother, she describes these women as more like best friends, noting they were not at all surprised when she first came out as queer to them.

"I fell hard and fast for Ben when we first met. My family liked him, too. We've faced judgment from others, like his family, but I've always pushed for us to persevere together. I guess my 'Jamaican passion' can put pressure on him to match this energy . . . which isn't always fair. He's wired differently and had a totally different family life growing up. My family taught me to love fiercely and didn't mind that I fell in love with a woman who then transitioned into who he really is. I must have learned along the way that low energy equates to giving up on someone. Now, I'm learning that low energy can mean many other things, like depression or self-doubt."

Ben reports a family history marked by passive-aggression and aloofness:

"Let's just say there wasn't a lot of hugging going on in my childhood. I'm still in contact with my parents these days, but they always find a way to sneak in their negative opinion about my 'life choices.' I've learned to tune this out, but the feeling of being chronically misunderstood is rough. Weirdly, the feeling of being understood is also hard for me. I'm learning how to receive all that Wanda and her family selflessly give to me in terms of acceptance and love . . . without feeling smothered."

The therapist helps the couple navigate minor experiences of emotional dysregulation that occur during session, and to analyze that which they report occurs in between sessions. They soon see improvements in each partner's ability to self-regulate in response to triggers and a corresponding reduction in the interpersonal tension at home. Ben reports his new antidepressant may be making a positive difference, and that adjusting his testosterone level has also helped his mood.

Ben states, "I'm starting to be able to think more clearly, and I feel less burned out; I'm no longer at a level two or three on the *Physiological Awareness Scale* every day. I actually have brief moments of feeling like a *Balanced Five*."

Wanda states, "I really appreciate how Ben is starting to share his inner thoughts and sensory processing concerns with me. When he shares his numbers, I feel much more connected. It also helps me better understand how his brain and body works differently than mine. I'm trying, too, to listen to his thoughts about our relationship dynamic without getting defensive. It's hard to hear that what I consider a 'normal' level of connection is actually pretty intense for him sometimes. I feel bad that I didn't realize how draining it can be for him just to get through the day sometimes, let alone have enough energy to meet my needs. Sometimes I need to accept that he needs time and space to get back to a *Balanced Five* before he can connect. I'm allowed to have needs, but pushing him to meet them before he's ready doesn't work."

Through journaling at home and feeling increasingly comfortable sharing during session, Ben is able to articulate how his recent bout with situational depression caused him to overanalyze everything about himself - something he says his Autistic brain is prone to do. Coming out on the other side of depression and re-establishing a *neutral* relationship with his own brain in the process, he states he <u>doesn't</u> actually want to end the relationship with Wanda:

"I think my brain thought being single would somehow magically end my feelings of burnout. But really all I needed was the space to process my racing thoughts, learn sensory strategies, and practice with unmasking. Individual therapy and couple therapy is helping me feel okay with myself again and my potential new career steps. The medication is helping my depression. I want to learn how to give back to Wanda in loving ways. She deserves it. We deserve it, actually! We've come so far, and I want us to get back on the path to being healthy together."

Both partners decide they've met their initial therapy goals and request to switch to *Relationship-Building Therapy*. Their favorite interpersonal technique to use at home becomes writing brief emails to each other back and forth during those times when Ben finds engaging with a verbal conversation too taxing, but Wanda craves connection. They also utilize communication cheat codes such as the *TMB Rule* and the *Heart Card* and regularly review their *Victory Journal*.

BINCT Stage 3: Leaning into the New

The therapist guides the clients to complete the *I Wish/Because* exercise and the *Blesses Me/Blesses Me Not* exercise.

Ben begins to take accountability for emotionally shutting Wanda out before, to validate her feelings of abandonment, and apologize:

"It's not ok to totally shut you out, Wanda, when I'm overwhelmed. I'm learning how not to do that."

Wanda begins to reframe this experience in their couple story as the logical result of Ben's temporary Autistic Burnout versus malicious rejection. She also begins to take accountability for the times she's been critical or demanding of his attention:

"I'm realizing just how fast and often I can go up on the scale from a *Balanced Five*. There have been times when I've been harsh with you, Ben, and that's not how I want to react when I'm feeling rejected."

The clients continue to note successful behaviors associated with living in their "New" versus their "Old" using the *Victory Journal*. They participate in *Individual Circle Mapping*, and the therapist teaches *Brain-Informed Active Listening* to discuss their results together. The clients state that these efforts help them gain a renewed sense of personal identity, couple identity, and emotional closeness. Ben begins to apply for jobs again. They continue to practice *CBT* skills, *DBT* skills, sensory-based activities, the *Physiological Awareness Scale* and the *Brain/Body Break* as needed through the ups and downs of his job search.

BINCT Stage 4: Maintaining Resilience

The clients elect to end therapy upon Ben's acceptance of a new job in an adjoining state where the therapist is not licensed to practice. As *BINCT* comes to a close, the therapist guides the couple to create a *Personal & Interpersonal Maintenance Plan*. She provides a referral to a new therapist should they wish to continue couple therapy after they move, offering to coordinate care with this clinician to facilitate their transfer should both clients wish to sign the type of written authorization form allowing her to ethically do so.

Celia & Julio

11

Celia (fictional client) is a 47-year-old neurotypical (NT) female of Puerto Rican descent. Her extended family settled in the American South three generations ago, and she was born in the United States. Her husband, Julio, is 50 years old. He grew up in Colombia before moving to America as a teenager along with his parents. The couple has three biological children who range in age from 13 to 17 years old, and have also been raising Celia's five-year-old nephew since he was an infant. At Celia's insistence, they begin attending *Brain-Informed Couple Therapy (BINCT)* in-person at a therapist's office near their home in Florida.

This case study highlights the following interventions over the course of Celia and Julio's experience of twenty-five non-consecutive, in-person sessions of BINCT:

- *Blesses Me/Blesses Me Not.*
- *Relationship Mission Statement.*
- *Reframes.*
- *Physiological Awareness Scale and Brain/Body Break.*
- *Cognitive Behavioral Therapy (CBT).*
- *Brain Branching.*
- *Brain-Informed Active Listening.*
- *Personal & Interpersonal Maintenance Plan.*

DOI: 10.4324/9781003351337-16

BINCT Stage 1: Joining, Assessing, Teaching

The therapist provides a free, brief consultation to each partner separately prior to the couple's decision to begin *BINCT*. Notably, Julio asks detailed questions about what *BINCT* entails and what makes it different from other forms of couple therapy. Celia, on the other hand, demonstrates better than average knowledge about neurodivergence and a variety of topics related to neurodiversity. She asks if the therapist can provide a formal diagnosis of Autism to her husband – should her husband agree to this type of testing, that is. The therapist clarifies that her scope of practice does not allow this and provides an appropriate referral. Neither partner requests any reasonable accommodation to complete their Intake paperwork, which includes simple brain-centric assessments. Both clients state they prefer to attend in-person sessions versus virtual sessions.

As the therapist welcomes Celia and Julio into her office for their first visit, she clarifies what was previously discussed on the phone regarding her service offerings and limitations. She then offers various seating options and accommodations to promote sensory security, such as adjusting the room's temperature or lighting. The clients deny any need for sensory accommodations at this time, but do elect to take one of the seating options which allows more physical distance between partners. Julio also chooses to occasionally stand up to lean his back against the wall during the session. While explaining that he does this to ease lower back pain, Celia interjects:

"Julio is too stubborn to see a doctor. One of the reasons why we're here, actually, is his inflexibility."

The therapist joins each client and hears their presenting concerns while reviewing their Intake paperwork out loud together. The clients each describe how their respective cultural backgrounds and families of origin have influenced their expectations for marriage and parenting. While these expectations reflect similar values, their views on neurodiversity and health do not.

Julio remembers with fondness how he entered America with the hope of attending college, starting a career, meeting a wife, and having a family:

"I now have everything I've ever wanted. I have a great job, Celia is amazing, and our kids are amazing. The circumstances around adding her nephew to our family have been difficult, but it's nothing we can't handle.

What's there to be so anxious about? Where I grew up, no one had any diagnosis or took anxiety medication."

Tearfully, Celia responds:

"Being a wife and mom was always my dream, but lately marriage feels like a nightmare. My anxiety and our 17-year-old's Autism are real, organic, issues that Julio minimizes. He also won't consider that he may be Autistic himself. I've never held resentment for my husband before, but I'm starting to do so now. That scares me for our future as a couple. Things can't always be so positive and easily fixed the way you think they should, Julio. You need to be less set in your ways and take my feelings seriously."

The therapist loosely describes the four stages of BINCT and the types of couple therapy that could potentially unfold: *Relationship-Building Therapy*, *Relationship Clarity-Seeking Therapy*, or *Relationship-Closing Therapy*. Both clients express strong commitment to their relationship and decide to begin *Relationship-Building Therapy*.

Celia tells the therapist that the main reason for seeking couple therapy at this time is due to her long-standing frustration with Julio's inability to converse about her concerns, leaving her feeling invalidated. She explains:

"Yes, I'm an anxious person. That comes from my mom's side of the family. Even though they don't believe in taking medication or therapy, I do. I'm open-minded like that. Sometimes new solutions are needed, but Julio is just like them . . . too traditional to consider new options. I absolutely love his positive attitude, but not when it turns into denial and inflexibility. For example, even though he shows so much love to our son Felix, he glosses over his struggles and doesn't take the time to understand Autism. I've been doing a lot of research, and Julio seems like he might also be Autistic. If he acknowledged all this, maybe we could connect better."

Julio says he's attending therapy to make Celia happy because her happiness is important to him. Regarding Autism, he disagrees with her recent decision to have their 17-year-old son, Felix, diagnosed. He also explains why he's not interested in pursuing a similar diagnosis for himself:

"Just because I'm an engineer doesn't mean I'm Autistic. In Colombia there wasn't any Autism! In America there's a diagnosis for everything. Everybody takes medication. When I talk with my parents about Felix, we agree he's an extremely bright kid who just needs extra coaching when it comes to socializing. He also has quirks, yes. Why does Celia want to put a label on him that will stay with him forever? He's going to be fine in college, where his intellect will shine and he'll be able to reach his full potential in life. As for me, I already speak English with a heavy accent, so if I go and get some big diagnosis . . . that just gives society another reason to discriminate against me. Celia worries too much. Life is good! But when I try to get her to relax, she just gets mad. We hardly even have sex any more these days because she stresses out too much about the kids."

The therapist provides psychoeducation about male and female sexual desire differences, the brain mechanism involved with anxiety, Autism as a neurotype, common neurodiverse relationship dynamics, issues related to parenting a neurodivergent child, etc. She then guides the couple in a brief *Blesses Me/Blesses Me Not* and *I Wish/Because* exercise, offering scaffolding as needed, to observe how each partner speaks and listens to each other and provide gentle feedback. She notes that Julio frequently, yet unintentionally, interrupts and invalidates Celia. In response, Celia responds with tearful frustration. She explains, using concrete examples, the difference between validating and invalidating conversation. The therapist then helps the clients create a *Relationship Mission Statement* together.

Celia and Julio's *Relationship Mission Statement*

"We want a marriage where each partner's opinions and personal characteristics are valued, as evidenced by mutually validating communication. We also want to learn flexible problem-solving techniques to address hot topics, like parenting and sex, to increase our connection."

The therapist validates more of the clients' personal and relationship history as sessions continue, offering psychoeducation about each partner's neurological and physiological features as observed *in vivo* or within the stories they tell.

Along the way, the therapist offers key reframes and discussion points:

- *BINCT* is more than just an opportunity to make your partner happy. It's a chance to learn about each partner's unique neurology and how this may play a role in both relationship problems and solutions.
- Celia's frustration, anxiety, and reduced sex drive are all logical human responses to chronic invalidation and stress from parenting children with high support needs. These symptoms aren't something Julio's positivity can cure. Looking at the relationship factors that maintain her distress (e.g., brain-based processing differences, *The Double Empathy Problem*,

etc.), improving the couples' interpersonal skills, and learning anxiety management strategies may help.

- Julio's ignorance about brain wiring may be an understandable, automatic defensive reaction in response to both his cultural background and fear of discrimination. Learning more about brain wiring within the privacy *BINCT* offers may offer valuable insight, not to mention provide long-awaited validation for Celia.
- Validation is a two-way street. Like Julio must learn to stop invalidating Celia's anxiety, her appropriate use of anxiety medication, and their son Felix's Autistic challenges, Celia must choose to recognize that it's Julio's choice whether or not to pursue a formal diagnosis of Autism for himself.

The therapist teaches the *Physiological Awareness Scale*, helping each client identify and articulate their own mental, emotional, and physiological experience throughout everyday scenarios and couple interactions. This proves somewhat difficult for Julio at times, who benefits from increased support from the therapist as the couple practices using the scale in her office. The therapist teaches the *Brain/Body Break*, coaching each partner to practice the individual components of this skill during their sessions.

Collaboratively, the therapist and clients make an *Old Versus New Chart*. The therapist introduces the *Victory Journal* as a way for the couple to chart both individual progress and progress as a couple.

Table 11.1

Old	New
Julio's (unintentional) use of invalidating statements with Celia.	Julio's intentional use of validating statements with Celia.
Celia's (unintentional) expectation for Julio to "just know" what she's feeling, physically or emotionally, and to expect him to "just know" how to respond accordingly.	Realistic expectation setting, by each partner, that takes into account *The Double Empathy Problem* in neurodiverse relationships. Each partner's use of clear communication regarding their own thoughts, emotions, body sensations, and needs.
Julio's cognitive inflexibility, particularly regarding the potential neurotypes within his marriage and family.	Julio's increased cognitive flexibility and recognition of the brain-based characteristics within his marriage and family.

Old	New
Celia's use of passive-aggressive behavior and critical statements towards Julio when upset.	Celia's use of the *Brain/Body Break* and self-regulation strategies as needed.
Julio's reduced interoceptive awareness.	Julio's use of the *Physiological Awareness Scale* plus sensory-based mindfulness skills.
Celia's occasionally heightened state of interoceptive awareness due to anxiety triggers, and overall high stress level.	Celia's identification of anxiety triggers and corresponding use of the *Physiological Awareness Scale* and *Brain/Body Break* plus physiological soothing or other healthy coping strategies (e.g., appropriate use of anxiety medication, *CBT* homework, self-care techniques, etc.)
Reduced physical intimacy.	Increased physical intimacy via awareness of medication side effects, human anatomy, male versus female sexual responses, etc. Increased couple-care strategies inclusive of improved communication and conflict resolution skills, mutual empathy, mutual respect, better non-sexual bonding, etc.

BINCT Stage 2: Practicing and Collecting Data

Both clients participate in *Brain Branching*, an exercise that highlights each partner's family history of possible neurodivergence as well as prevalent attitudes and beliefs. The couple realizes that Celia's sister may have had undiagnosed ADHD in addition to the complications from alcoholism that led to the unfortunate necessity to adopt and raise her son after her untimely death. They also each identify several extended family members with anxious traits, Autistic traits, and/or ADHD traits. As a result of this exercise, Julio begins to acknowledge some of his own brain-based qualities that may indicate an Autistic neurotype. The therapist discusses the pros and cons of formal diagnosis, the difference between diagnosis and public disclosure, and the concept of identity dimensionality. Julio decides to not pursue an Autism diagnosis for himself. Celia expresses grief over this decision, but also gratitude for his willingness to keep exploring their brain-based differences with her in neurodiverse couple therapy.

The therapist helps the couple navigate experiences of emotional dysregulation that occur during session and to analyze that which they report occurs in between sessions. Invalidation from Julio is the most common trigger for interpersonal tension, with Celia often responding with tearfulness and passive-aggressive statements. For instance, in his attempt to lessen Celia's anxiety about their son Felix's approaching transition to college, Julio often uses cliche statements. Celia finds this irritating and invalidating:

"We live in the land of opportunity. Some of Felix's quirks are considered superpowers in the engineering field – he's going to be fine. Stop worrying!"

"Optimism doesn't dry tears, Julio. Can't you see how much it upsets me when you hype Felix up about going away to college? He acts excited because he wants to please you, but he confides in me that he's really worried about going to college. You can't deny that he has a meltdown once a week right now whenever he gets too stressed about friend drama or his schoolwork. Who's going to help him manage that when he's living away from home? What good will all your optimism be when he has to quit school because he's gotten too overwhelmed? We need to discuss realistic options for his college experience."

The therapist coaches the clients toward improved validation, self-regulation, empathy, and creative problem-solving skills. In doing so, the therapist often finds herself returning to the concreteness of the *Blesses Me/Blesses Me Not* exercise:

"Julio, it <u>blesses</u> <u>me</u> when you let me talk to you about my worries and brainstorm ideas. It <u>blesses me not</u> when you become single-minded and try to comfort me using invalidating positivity. I do need encouragement sometimes, but lately I need a partner in flexible problem-solving more."

"Celia, it <u>blesses me</u> when you don't focus on the worst outcomes for situations with Felix and other things. It <u>blesses me not</u> when you become critical of my encouragement."

Role playing, with scaffolding by the therapist, becomes an important feature of therapy sessions going forward. The therapist guides each partner to actively demonstrate to each other the kind of communication they'd like to receive versus that which they find off-putting. She shares her observations of potential ND-NT differences regarding each clients' unique thought processes, physiological responses, communication style, and behaviors. For example, Julio displays some alexithymic traits, which may or may not be associated with an Autistic neurotype. Celia displays mostly NT features, yet reports a lifelong struggle to regulate her anxiety. The therapist provides psychoeducation about these qualities and actively models grace for each partner's developing skill areas (i.e., interoception, self-regulation, communication).

Celia expresses grief at times as she rates Julio's progress towards greater interoception, and what she calls "social awareness," as disappointingly slow:

"Julio and Felix are so similar. Like father, like son! Both are very upbeat, intelligent, and enjoy fixing things . . . including other people's sadness. They're always quick to offer love. But, they're also both very concrete thinkers and can get stuck on what <u>they</u> consider to be the one 'right' way to do something. Socially, that doesn't always work. It's too rigid. Julio seems clueless about how this makes me feel."

"I'm not clueless, Celia. I just don't know how else to respond. Truly, some things are just not worth the amount of worry you put into them. And, usually there's an efficient answer to our problems. I hate to see you upset, so I try to cheer you up the best I can. I suppose that hasn't been as helpful as I thought."

The therapist validates both clients while simultaneously normalizing their learning curve for the "New" they're starting to practice. She then discusses what kinds of *changeable* versus *unchangeable* factors may be embedded at the individual and relational level. She refocuses each partner on an internal locus of control for only that which is actually *changeable* in themselves and within their relationship.

Along the way, the therapist periodically uses *CBT* to explore certain myths that seem to underlie some of the couple's major conflicts. For example, she helps Julio critically examine the following notions he holds regarding neurodivergence:

Autism is an overdiagnosed, modern American phenomenon; There's no Autism in Colombia.
Without judgment, the therapist encourages Julio to share any life experiences or other data points associated with this belief. She then summarizes his thoughts for objective examination:

Autism always has the same visible look; I never saw anyone with Autism when I was growing up in Colombia.

Modern Americans are too quick to diagnose Autism. They should be more careful, because this label can lead to discrimination.
The therapist, next, offers a mix of psychoeducation and Truth Statements:

- Autistic people have always existed across the world and throughout history. There are valid reasons why they may not be visible to others.

First, research shows that Autism does not have one specific look. One's Autistic features are not always observable – especially when they utilize masking. Second, some cultures and/or social systems intentionally exclude, conceal, or even seek to eliminate neurodivergent people from mainstream view.

- There are many opinions about the current diagnostic criteria and assessments for Autism in the United States. Yet, research indicates Autism is influenced by genetics and may actually be <u>underdiagnosed</u> in certain populations around the world. Science continually proves that the Autistic neurotype is valid, as it's just one of many identified variations of human neurology. The increase in Autism diagnoses in recent years is likely due to changes to diagnostic criteria and increased awareness.
- Fear of discrimination may reflect past trauma, which deserves attention. It's important to consider, though, how these fears may be more rooted in the past than in the present reality. In geographical regions with active stigma against neurodivergence, for example, disclosure may indeed have very real negative consequences. Yet, in other regions, disclosure may have neutral or even positive consequences. Sadly, no one can ever predict exactly when or why any kind of injustice may occur regarding neurodivergence or anything else. Senseless acts of prejudice and discrimination do happen for any number or reasons: Injustice is totally outside of anyone's control regardless of diagnosis and/or disclosure.

The therapist also helps Julio examine another perspective that tends to invalidate Celia:

Celia should be able to manage her anxiety without medication.
Again, the therapist offers a mix of psychoeducation and Truth Statements:

- Anxiety is a valid mental health issue that can negatively affect physical wellness, sex drive, etc. Medication usually represents just one part of a comprehensive anxiety reduction plan.
- In some cases, medication is not vital to managing anxiety, whereas other times it's essential. Celia's diagnosis of *Generalized Anxiety Disorder* given by her primary care doctor appears to be accurate. Her use of medication as one component of a comprehensive self-care plan also seems appropriate.
- The ability to manage anxiety without medication isn't an accurate measure of a person's strength or courage. Managing anxiety with medication is not an indicator of a person's weakness or laziness.

- Some anxiety medication does have the potential side effect of reduced libido. (But, so does untreated anxiety!) It's ok to express concerns about your partner's use of medication. However, ultimately, it's Celia's decision whether or not to take anxiety medication just like it's your decision whether or not to pursue an Autism diagnosis.

In response to *CBT*, Julio states:

"It's been interesting to think about all this. I've been valuing my parents' assumptions and my own assumptions about Autism and anxiety over neuroscience, which just isn't logical. I also didn't realize how much my early experiences with discrimination when I first arrived in this country and my memories of growing up in Colombia affected my perspective. Even though I don't see my parents ever understanding any of this brain stuff, I'm starting to. I understand now why Celia pushed so hard for Felix to be diagnosed and supported by an IEP at school. I also see now how my brain has some Autistic tendencies that affect our relationship, just like how Celia's anxiety affects our relationship."

As the clients begin to experiment with "New" attitudes and behaviors during sessions and at home, they also begin to recognize the specific ways things get worse between them whenever the "Old" crops up. Working through those times with the therapist to find good coping strategies, they begin to experience personal and interpersonal victories. Celia begins to express feelings of greater validation and cite examples of Julio's improved cognitive flexibility. Julio expresses appreciation to Celia for her recognition of his efforts to put therapy skills into practice at home. He also notes she seems less anxious, less critical, and more open to his initiation of physical affection.

BINCT Stage 3: Leaning into the New

The clients continue to note successful behaviors associated with living in their "New" versus their "Old" using the *Victory Journal*. They find using the *Physiological Awareness Scale* and the *Brain/Body Break* helpful when discussing hot topics like parenting and sex. Julio sometimes needs support from the therapist to correctly identify examples of unintentional invalidation and inflexibility in his interactions with Celia, but demonstrates genuine efforts to make things right once they're brought to his attention. Learning how to use *Brain-Informed Active Listening* during couple therapy becomes extremely helpful.

Celia occasionally needs support to practice her self-care plan in order to reduce her overall stress level, but reports a vital part of anxiety management involves setting more realistic expectations. She states she's willing to do the work to reduce her stress and enjoy life more to break the anxious cycle passed down from previous generations in her family. She also recognizes that a tendency toward anxiety may be *unchangeable* about herself – what is changeable is her response to anxiety triggers. She expresses satisfaction with she and Julio's renewed emotional connection:

"Being on the same page with Julio about our son's Autism and the communication challenges we face as a couple makes me feel so much better. I'm much more attracted to him when I see his intentional efforts to face tough issues together and talk them through."

At the clients' request, the therapist provides sex therapy inclusive of psychoeducation about the sensory aspects of sex and potential ND-NT differences in the bedroom. She also provides parenting support inclusive of psychoeducation about common needs of Autistic teenagers who are preparing to launch to college. During this time, the couple demonstrates increased ability to communicate together. They successfully use "New" skills to create and implement key parenting decisions.

BINCT Stage 4: Maintaining Resilience

As *BINCT* comes to a close, the therapist guides the couple to create a *Personal & Interpersonal Maintenance Plan*. She uses an engineering example to remind them that an earthquake resistant structure depends on flexibility. A rigid structure collapses easily in an earthquake, but a flexible structure often survives. Lasting ND-NT relationship success is similar in that flexibility (within healthy boundaries) is often more important than rigid adherence to a plan. The couple requests to move to monthly visits to maintain their progress.

Walker & Lizbeth   **12**

Walker and Lizbeth are a fictional neurodiverse couple who attend *Brain-Informed Couple Therapy (BINCT)* mostly in-person at a therapist's office outside of Houston, Texas. However, they also utilize online therapy visits with this therapist as necessary due to childcare needs. Walker is a neurotypical (NT) 29-year-old Caucasian male, while Lizbeth is a Gifted (ND) 27-year-old Caucasian female. The couple have been married for three years and have an eight-month-old biological son. The child was delivered at full term without complications. He's currently meeting all developmental milestones, but does struggle with acid reflux.

This case study highlights the following interventions over the course of Walker and Lizbeth's experience of 18 non-consecutive, in-person sessions of BINCT and three sessions of virtual BINCT:

- *Relationship Mission Statement.*
- *Couple Circle Mapping.*
- *Physiological Awareness Scale* and *Brain/Body Break.*
- *Energy Audit.*
- *TMB Rule.*
- *Personal & Interpersonal Maintenance Plan.*

BINCT Stage 1: Joining, Assessing, Teaching

The therapist provides a free, brief consultation to each partner separately prior to the couple's decision to begin *BINCT*. Lizbeth mentions she vaguely

DOI: 10.4324/9781003351337-17

remembers being diagnosed with ADHD at some point in her early childhood, but indicates she hasn't thought much about this label since then. She does, though, vividly remember attending Gifted classes throughout Elementary and Middle School. She self-identifies as a *Highly Sensitive Person (HSP)* due to feeling strong emotions and having certain sensory issues. Neither partner requests any reasonable accommodation to complete their Intake paperwork, which includes simple brain-centric assessments. Both clients state they prefer to attend in-person sessions versus virtual visits, but are open to an online session should this be more convenient or necessary regarding their childcare needs. The therapist assesses that telehealth is an appropriate option for the couple to use as needed.

As the therapist welcomes Walker and Lizbeth into her office for their first visit, she offers various seating options and accommodations to promote sensory security. The clients choose to sit near each other on one couch, and Lizbeth requests that the shades directly behind them are closed to prevent the strong sunlight that day from heating up the back of her neck. The therapist notices that Lizbeth alternates between chewing on a fingernail and bouncing her leg throughout the visit. She briefly discusses the concept of stimming as a potential self-regulation and/or self-expression tool and encourages both clients to stim freely, should they desire to do so.

The therapist joins each client to hear their presenting concerns while reviewing their Intake paperwork out loud together. She provides psychoeducation related to Lizbeth's self-report of sensory processing concerns, emotional dysregulation, and executive functioning issues. This may all relate back to her childhood diagnosis of ADHD, not just her recent transition to motherhood! Lizbeth replies:

"Really? I remember my parents and doctor saying I'd grow out of ADHD. I figured what I'm going through right now might just be postpartum depression. I don't want to take medication, by the way, since I'm still nursing."

The therapist takes Lizbeth's concern about postpartum depression seriously, screening her for this. Lizbeth denies any hallmark symptoms other than feeling more tired than usual, being stressed out, and being irritable. Mostly, she reports being increasingly bothered by certain physical sensations (e.g., the feel of her clothing, the smell of certain foods) and frustrated with not being able to perform housework to the same high level she did prior to having a baby. She also reports clear signs of executive functioning strain. The therapist provides psychoeducation to compare and contrast ADHD, Giftedness, Sensory Processing Disorder, and postpartum depression – noting that it's certainly possible for all of these to co-occur.

The therapist explains that emotional dysregulation, executive functioning strain, and heightened sensory sensitivity can be a big part of the ADHD neurotype that's often misidentified and misunderstood. She clarifies that it's common to discover (or re-discover) these kinds of multiexceptional neurodivergent features in adulthood during a meaningful life transition like having a baby, after a series of stressful events, or even after something like a promotion at work. Having to adapt to new circumstances and new expectations or responsibilities can easily overwhelm an ADHDer's executive functioning and sensory systems. Things that may have come easily before, or have been easier to cope with, may suddenly take much more energy or even seem impossible. Add the lack of sleep from having a new baby and this is a recipe for feeling tired, stressed, and irritable!

As the couple tells the story of how they met ten years ago up until the present moment, the therapist jots down a quick relationship timeline on a whiteboard to list their milestone moments as individuals and a couple. She asks about moments where Lizbeth has noticed executive functioning challenges or sensory issues and includes them on the timeline. Lizbeth explains:

"Well, a few years ago I did choose to switch jobs. I have a pattern in my career where I expect a lot from myself and push myself to perform at a really high level. But, that kind of drivenness to succeed is only sustainable for so long. I end up taking on too many responsibilities and doing too many people-pleasing things. Eventually, I reach a breaking point where I'm forced to slow down. I've had to walk away from getting overinvested in some amazing projects over the years, which has been really painful for me. Walker's always trying to help me notice the slow boil effect toward mental and sensory overload. He's probably annoyed with me that I never listen. I've always had to learn things the hard way, I guess. I'm an all or nothing person. Thankfully, God has blessed me with tons of energy and lots of different interests and talents, so I always end up back on my feet again somehow after getting burned out – even if it means having to change roles or jobs. After having a baby, it's bothering me that I can't seem to rebound as quickly."

The therapist guides the couple towards a quick *Couple Circle Mapping* exercise in which Walker draws the circle that represents himself quite small relative to Lizbeth's circle. He states one reason for this size difference is the pattern Lizbeth mentioned above, in which he feels unheard:

"Lizbeth throws herself 100 mph at life and then gets mad at me whenever I ask her to slow down or choose just one main thing to focus on. It feels like I have no influence; If she's passionate about something, she's going to go in that direction no matter what. You should see our house right now. There are so many unfinished home improvement projects and art pieces that she's either lost interest in or run out of steam before completing. I don't want to feel like a critical parent all the time or a buzzkill, so sometimes I just don't say anything at all any more. But now she's talking about getting a puppy. How can I not put my foot down about something like that? What on earth makes Lizbeth think adding a puppy into our home right now is a good idea?"

Walker also explains how Lizbeth's sensory processing concerns have become more and more noticeable over the years:

"When we first met it was easy to show compassion and work around Lizbeth's occasional sensory aversions, such as handling raw meat. When we cooked together, I'd just prepare the meat while she prepared other parts of the meal. Now she can't even stand the sight or smell of raw meat. We're not vegetarians, so this requires me to do a lot of the cooking without her or for us to order prepared food. I also can't play my music any more . . . yet, somehow, she's ok when her music is playing. Don't even get me started about sex. Sometimes she's super interested in sex and initiates. Other times she can't even stand to hear me chewing food in the same room as her, so sex is totally out of the question. It's confusing."

The therapist wonders out loud about what having more equally sized identity circles in their *Couple Circle Mapping* exercise might represent, and what it may take to get there. She provides psychoeducation about the relationship between sexual desire and sensory security, as well as information about ADHD, Giftedness, sensory processing, executive functioning, neurodiverse relationship dynamics, the family life cycle, and a variety of other topics pertaining to the couple's concerns. She also guides the couple to recognize each partner's individual strengths, plus valuable aspects of their couple identity (i.e., the shaded part of the Venn diagram where the individual identity circles overlap). The clients indicate Christianity, love for their son, commitment to personal and interpersonal growth, and good financial stewardship represent dimensions of their couple identity. The therapist wonders out loud, "How does neurodivergence fit in?"

Lizbeth says she primarily agreed to attend couple therapy at this time to improve communication in her marriage so Walker can understand what she's going through – but also to find out more about herself. She explains:

"I've always felt 'too much' for other people. I feel too much, think too much, want too much, do too much. When I first learned the term *Highly Sensitive Person (HSP)* a few years ago, I was relieved. It made me feel so seen. I'm really doing my best to cope with all the new demands of a nursing baby while still trying to go after what makes me feel alive as a person. I want to have a good marriage, a healthy family, a social life, and eventually return to my job after this extended maternity leave. I'd love to get another dog. It's so frustrating that I haven't fully bounced back yet mentally and physically after having our baby. Part of my irritability is that I seem to have zero short-term memory any more. It's as if 'pregnancy brain' never left."

Walker states he's been confused and upset about their marriage dynamic lately and hopes therapy can help them get back on the path to being a healthy team:

"We've always had some level of conflict in our relationship, but we've always been able to work it out pretty easily. Not, though, Lizbeth calls childish outbursts directed at me 'venting,' but it doesn't feel like venting. I can't help but get defensive. What more can I do here? On top of my job, I've tried to lessen her mental load by taking on lots of our practical concerns like cooking, finances, and cleaning. But she <u>still</u> talks about how hard it is to get things done around the house. Why is there always time for random projects and playdates with the baby, but never tidying up afterwards? It gets tiring asking her to finish the latest project she's abandoned on the kitchen table so we can sit down there as a family to eat together. I don't want to nag, but I don't know what else to do."

The therapist loosely describes the four stages of *BINCT* and the types of couple therapy that could potentially unfold: *Relationship-Building Therapy*, *Relationship Clarity-Seeking Therapy*, or *Relationship-Closing Therapy*. Both clients agree they'd like to begin *Relationship-Building Therapy*. She then guides the couple to make a *Relationship Mission Statement* together.

Walker and Lizbeth's *Relationship Mission Statement*

"We want a marriage where we both feel like balanced, fulfilled Adults (versus *Parent-Child*) as evidenced by the way we practice self-regulation and teamwork."

The therapist validates more of the clients' personal and relationship history as sessions continue, offering psychoeducation about each partner's neurological and physiological features as observed in vivo or within the stories they tell about their interactions in between visits.

The therapist offers some of the following discussion points:

- For couples with any combination of neurotypes, the definition of "teamwork" in their marriage usually has to change a bit after they have a baby. Neurodiverse couples may need lots of additional flexibility with this definition because an ND partner's sensory and executive functioning needs can sometimes increase dramatically and require a new level of support. Similarly, their NT partner may also have new needs or develop unmet needs that deserve attention.

- It's normal for major life events to bring out a couples' best and worst features. As they navigate new territory together, partners often realize the need for new or updated coping skills. . . yet don't know where to start.
- ADHDers and/or Gifted individuals who stay home to raise an infant after having previously had an extremely on-the-go lifestyle may feel a unique mix of both overstimulation and under-stimulation. Figuring out new roles, routines, and ways to meet their brain-based needs can be difficult without specific support.
- Irritability is an understandable reaction to one's own sensory overwhelm and executive functioning strain, while defensiveness is a common reaction to a partner's irritability.
- Neurodiverse couples can easily fall into a *Parent-Child* dynamic with each other at times until they learn better self-regulation, communication, and conflict resolution skills.

The therapist teaches the *Physiological Awareness Scale* so each client can better identify and articulate their own mental, emotional, and physiological experiences. Neither client displays characteristics of alexithymia. Lizbeth benefits from learning sensory-based strategies (e.g., breathing exercises, smelling lavender, and other methods of physiological soothing) to counteract her brain's tendency to have rapid, emotional responses to Walker and other incoming stimuli (e.g., the sight of raw meat). The therapist normalizes this type of automatic reactivity as a fairly typical feature of some forms of neurodivergence – it doesn't mean Lizbeth has a lack of discipline, a personality defect, is being malicious, or is being "too much!" She suggests a customized self-care plan for Lizbeth inclusive of a sensory diet meant to reduce overall overwhelm. (She also helps Walker create a self-care plan.)

The therapist introduces the *Brain/Body Break* as a new coping strategy for both clients to use to avoid the personal extremes of overexcitability or shutdown, noting that this can also be a vital tool to correct their problematic *Parent-Child* couple dynamic.

Collaboratively, the therapist and clients make an *Old Versus New Chart*. The therapist introduces the *Victory Journal* as a way for the couple to chart individual and couple progress.

Table 12.1

Old	New
Lizbeth's reduced interoceptive awareness, leading to unsustainable energy output and eventual burnout.	Using an *Energy Audit* periodically; Using *Spoon Theory* to communicate; Lizbeth's use of the *Physiological Awareness Scale* plus sensory-based mindfulness skills and self-regulation skills; Lizbeth noting the signs in herself of impending burnout without Walker having to point them out.
Lizbeth's lack of a sensory diet to support sensory processing challenges.	Lizbeth's creation and maintenance of a balanced sensory diet as part of an overall self-care plan.
Parent (Walker) – *Child* (Lizbeth) couple dynamic.	*Adult-Adult* dynamic, as evidenced by each partner's self-regulation efforts and use of healthy communication and conflict resolution skills; Reduced nagging behavior from Walker and reduced verbal outbursts from Lizbeth.
Improved communication regarding NT-ND brain-based differences.	The couple's use of the *Physiological Awareness Scale* and *Brain/Body Break* as needed; Walker using assertive communication skills versus avoidance; Both partners reducing defensiveness in order to give and receive healthy feedback to each other.

BINCT Stage 2: Practicing and Collecting Data

The therapist guides the couple towards healthy *Adult-Adult* communication via the *I Wish/Because* exercise:

"Lizbeth, I wish our household responsibilities were <u>more equally distributed</u>, because then I would feel <u>more respected</u> by you."

"Walker, I wish our relationship had more <u>understanding</u>, because then I would feel <u>encouraged</u> as I'm figuring out ways to have better life balance."

Therapist:

"It sounds like you both view your current relationship as deflating. Walker feels trapped into having to shoulder more of the household burdens, which makes him feel disrespected. Lizbeth feels misunderstood and discouraged as she tries her best to self-regulate."

The therapist then poses some key questions:

1. "How can you both contribute to a marriage atmosphere of greater understanding?"
2. "Could greater understanding lead to more connection, a more creative definition of teamwork in this season of life, as well as mutual respect?"
3. "What do your different neurological characteristics make possible in your marriage?"

The couple participates in the *Energy Audit* exercise, which highlights their ND-NT differences. The therapists guides discussion about important topics such as how they each acquire dopamine, self-regulate, start tasks and follow through with them, manage their time, receive sensory input, process auditory information, respond sexually, etc. The therapist provides psychoeducation accordingly. She also teaches *Spoon Theory* as a "New"way for the clients to talk back and forth about what either <u>adds</u> to their life satisfaction and balance, or <u>depletes</u> it.

Lizbeth's experience of multiexceptionality and its effects on Walker also become a discussion topic. He states, in all seriousness:

"I'm both in awe of Lizbeth's ability to function as a human hummingbird and annoyed by it. She's in constant motion. I'm more like a bear. I do what I need to do every day, and then I rest."

Meanwhile, Lizbeth laments:

"I've spent my whole life trying to be more disciplined. Things just don't seem to work for me like they work for other people. I can't just take things step by step, A-B-C. For example, I need to have a 'just right' amount of stress going on at any given time to be able to function. Too much stress, and I'll collapse. Too little stress, and I'm not motivated to get started. Part of what Walker sees as 'constant motion' is me trying to figure out how to find a balance between stagnation and warp speed. Believe me, I really do try. I also like to rest, by the way, but being still isn't always what I want. I'd rather be doing something like listening to music (that is, when my brain doesn't decide sounds are too much to handle that day) while using my hands to work on a project. That's my definition of relaxation. I'm so glad there are people in the Bible like James and John who were so fierce in their loyalty to Jesus. I can understand how they acted. Not everyone is wired to sit still and be calm all the time."

The therapist helps the couple navigate emotional dysregulation that occurs during their sessions, paying special attention to times when Lizbeth verbally snaps at Walker and Walker snaps right back at her with defensiveness. As this occurs, she discusses potential *internal climate* and *external climate* factors that may have contributed to the clients' perception of each other at the time and their resulting reactions. She coaches use of the *Physiological Awareness Scale* and *Brain/Body Break* during their sessions.

The therapist validates both clients while simultaneously normalizing their learning curve for the "New" they're practicing. She discusses what *changeable* versus *unchangeable* factors may be embedded at the individual and relational level for them as a neurodiverse couple. As she refocuses each partner on an internal locus of control for only that which is actually *changeable*, it naturally promotes their emerging *Adult-Adult* dynamic.

The clients display an increased ability over time to identify "Old" versus "New," as well as incremental progress to personal and couple victories. Both partners struggle to understand each other's preferred forms of self-regulation at times, but regularly find common ground via couple-care, e.g., attending a weekly fellowship group at their church. They learn how to more respectfully negotiate parenting tasks and household responsibilities, showing increased awareness of each other's brain-based characteristics. Not surprisingly, their sex life improves in correlation to their nonsexual improvements. When a sensory-related issue emerges regarding sex, the therapist provides psychoeducation and nurtures validating dialogue between the partners.

The couple experiences a setback after Lizbeth forgets about a scheduled couple therapy appointment, triggering Walker's "Old" feelings of disrespect upon finding himself alone at the therapist's office. At their next couple session, Lizbeth displays defensiveness and hurt by verbally lashing out at Walker in response to his "scolding" of her for the mistake. As their couple dynamic briefly, and intensely, returns to *Parent-Child*, the therapist coaches self-regulation strategies. She encourages them to practice reacting to this situation in "New" ways, providing appropriate scaffolding. Each partner subsequently demonstrates an ability to analyze this incident with the therapist. The couple mutually decides to switch to virtual therapy for a few sessions after this due to its convenience, and also to avoid another scheduling mishap.

BINCT Stage 3: Leaning into the New

As the clients begin to more steadily add to their *Victory Journal*, the therapist keeps reminding them of any improvements she observes. The clients start to report increased satisfaction in certain areas of their marriage, and pride in their ability to recover from "Old" patterns as they emerge. Lizbeth becomes better at predicting times of impending self-dysregulation, and also starts to recognize how certain brain-based tendencies (e.g., hyperfocus) negatively affect Walker. Walker becomes more educated about and understanding of Lizbeth's neurodivergent qualities, displaying increased empathy. He learns to more assertively state his concerns about the household with Lizbeth and initiate creative problem-solving efforts versus resorting to nagging or scolding.

The partners increase their communication skills, learning how to speak from a *Balanced Five* position as much as possible and taking *Brain/Body Breaks* as needed. The therapist introduces the *TMB Rule*, which is an intervention the clients like very much. This language, plus language associated with *Spoon Theory*, becomes pivotal to improving their problematic communication patterns. Lizbeth's newfound self-acceptance and self-identification as multiexceptional, bolstered by Walker's acceptance of her, promotes the following tender moment during a couple session:

"Walker, it's nice to feel seen on a deeper level now. That's what I've always wanted. . . to understand myself and to be understood. We're definitely wired in opposite ways, but I believe God can use those differences to help us have a strong marriage. You have gifts that I don't have, and vice versa. Our baby is blessed by us both, as long as we keep working together in flexible, grace-filled ways. It means a lot to me that you trust I'm doing my best, and I'm learning to forgive you for misunderstanding me before. I won't apologize for being overwhelmed as a new mom, but I can apologize for the times I lashed out at you."

"Lizbeth, it feels great to be married to a passionate *Adult* instead of a messy *Child*. Sorry, I know that might sound harsh. But, that's what I used to think when times were rough between us. I never want you to feel like a *Child* with me ever again, and I never want to feel like I'm your *Parent*. It means a lot to me that we figured out the triggers for that cycle. I've forgiven you for how you treated me at times after the baby was born. That period in our marriage makes a lot more sense now, and I think in the future we may actually be thankful God allowed us to go through it. Please forgive me for all the times I was critical towards you. I'm so sorry I misunderstood what you were actually going through as a ND new mom."

BINCT Stage 4: Maintaining Resilience

The therapist guides the couple to create a *Personal & Interpersonal Maintenance Plan* to keep up the momentum of their "New." They make a plan to visit the therapist again in three months. In the interim, Lizbeth wonders whether or not individual therapy may be beneficial for her to continue learning about her identity dimensionality as a mother, ADHDer, wife, child of God, etc. She jokes that personal growth may be a newfound hyperfocus, while Walker playfully responds that he'd be fine with that if this were the case. The therapist affirms individual therapy as a great idea to support self-care and self-insight, provided it makes sense for the couple financially. At Lizbeth's request, she makes a referral to another *Brain-Informed* counselor who operates from a Christian worldview and has a heart for new mothers. Without taking on a *Parental* stance or otherwise infantilizing Lizbeth, the therapist gently suggests that she takes individual therapy at a sustainable pace. This is because personal growth can absolutely become a hyperfocus, and it is actually possible to experience burnout from intense self-reflection!

As *BINCT* comes to an end, the therapist introduces the notion of the various *stances* and *sentiments* one can have with one's brain at any given time, noting that it seems Lizbeth has developed a more positive relationship with her brain throughout therapy. (Walker, too, seems to have a better relationship with it!) As a final intervention, the therapist takes a *Narrative Therapy* approach in order to invite the partners to tell each other the story of their lives inclusive of their transition to parenting and their overall experience of *BINCT*.

Index

Page numbers in *italics* refer to figures. Page numbers in **bold** refer to tables.

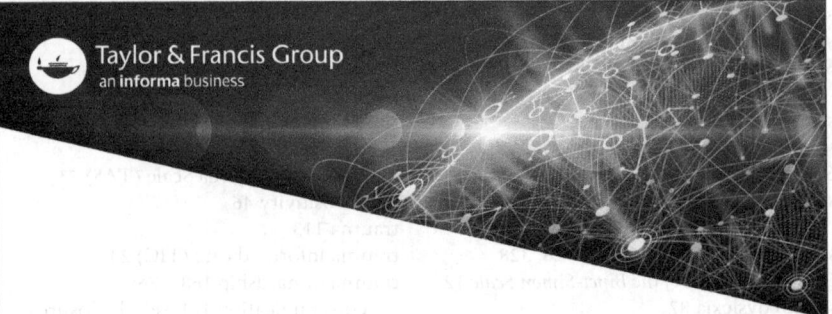
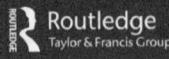
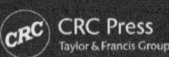